Endoscopic Approaches to the Skull Base

Progress in Neurological Surgery

Vol. 26

Series Editor

L. Dade Lunsford Pittsburgh, Pa.

Endoscopic Approaches to the Skull Base

Volume Editors

Amin B. Kassam Ottawa, Ont.

Paul A. Gardner Pittsburgh, Pa.

109 figures, 24 in color, and 13 tables, 2012

KARGER

Basel · Freiburg · Paris · London · New York · New Delhi · Bangkok · Beijing · Tokyo · Kuala Lumpur · Singapore · Sydney

Amin B. Kassam, MD
Chief, Division of Neurosurgery
The Ottawa Hospital – Civic Campus
1053 Carling Avenue, Box 615
Ottawa, ON K1Y 4E9 (Canada)

Paul A. Gardner, MD
Assistant Professor
Department of Neurological Surgery
University of Pittsburgh School of Medicine
Co-Director Center for Cranial Base Surgery
University of Pittsburgh Medical Center
200 Lothrop Street, PUH B-400
Pittsburgh, PA 15213 (USA)

Library of Congress Cataloging-in-Publication Data

Endoscopic approaches to the skull base / volume editors, Amin B. Kassam, Paul A. Gardner.
p. ; cm. -- (Progress in neurological surgery, ISSN 0079-6492 ; v. 26)
Includes bibliographical references and index.
ISBN 978-3-8055-9210-9 (alk. paper) -- ISBN 978-3-8055-9211-6 (e-ISBN)
I. Kassam, Amin B. II. Gardner, Paul A. (Paul Andrew), 1973- III. Series: Progress in neurological surgery ; v. 26. 0079-6492
[DNLM: 1. Skull Base--surgery. 2. Brain Diseases--surgery. 3. Neuroendoscopy--methods. 4. Sphenoid Sinus--surgery. W1 PR673 v.26 2012 / WE 705]
617.5'140597--dc23

2012001494

Bibliographic Indices. This publication is listed in bibliographic services, including Current Contents® and Index Medicus.

www.karger.com
Printed in Germany on acid-free and non-aging paper (ISO 9706) by Kraft Druck, Ettlingen
ISSN 0079–6492
e-ISSN 1662–3924
ISBN 978–3–8055–9210–9
e-ISBN 978–3–8055–9211–6

Contents

Editor's Note

Volume 26 of the continuing series of *Progress in Neurological Surgery* indeed reveals one of the most innovative and game-changing modern evolutions of skull base surgery. Transsphenoidal techniques were first envisioned more than 100 years ago, but were hampered by lack of visualization and illumination. While traditional transsphenoidal surgery using microsurgical techniques blossomed in the 1970s and 1980s, the introduction of the expanded endoscopic approach in the 21st century has been a very powerful addition to an array of neurosurgical technologies. The expanded endoscopic method was facilitated by the revolution in image guidance using computed tomography and magnetic resonance imaging, and the remarkable growth of endoscopic devices. This volume provides a broad overview of the expanding role of transsphenoidal approaches for a wide spectrum of skull base diseases. A number of centers across the world have been major innovators and adopters of endoscopic expanded techniques. These centers are well represented in the author list of this volume, which should serve as a potent reference for students and practitioners of neurosurgery. The endoscopic approach is firmly integrated within the modern multidisciplinary management of skull base tumors. I am grateful to the editors for their leadership in this volume, as well as to the many co-authors who have been willing to share their ever increasing experience with the readership of *Progress in Neurological Surgery.*

L. Dade Lunsford, MD
Pittsburgh, Pa.

Kassam AB, Gardner PA (eds): Endoscopic Approaches to the Skull Base.
Prog Neurol Surg. Basel, Karger, 2012, vol 26, pp 1–6

Historical Perspectives

Paolo Cappabianca · Felice Esposito · Oreste de Divitiis

Università degli Studi di Napoli Federico II, Division of Neurosurgery, Napoli, Italy

Abstract

Endoscopic surgery has grown slowly, but in parallel with the simultaneous developments of microsurgery and skull-base surgery. In this report, we describe the early innovations in skull-base endoscopic approaches as well as the pioneers who first popularized transsphenoidal surgical approaches. Endoscopy has been used by an increasing number of surgeons over the last 25 years and represents a major advance in the transsphenoidal and endonasal technique.

Endoscopic Surgery of the Skull Base

Modern neurosurgery, as all other surgical specialties, has passed through a chronological development. First, owing to the lack of proper diagnostic tools, inadequate illumination during surgery and the relatively huge size of pathologies which were usually discovered late in the disease course, neurosurgical approaches have always been relatively extensive and disfiguring. Later, with improvements in the previously mentioned factors and the introduction of the concept of microneurosurgery, the rationale relating to neurosurgical approaches has changed to more precise, smaller, and effective ones. Recently, with the advent of the conceptual thinking of reduction of mortality, morbidity, cosmetic disfigurement and financial burdens, the concept of 'minimally invasive' and 'keyhole' surgery has been adopted in a continuously increasing number of conditions. This concept in particular led to the interest in searching for new innovative trajectories together with surgical instruments and optical tools, amongst them, endoscopes [1, 2]. Smaller skin incisions, less bone removal during craniotomy or craniectomy, less brain retraction with better visualization and easier closure, decreased morbidity and mortality rates and improved results for pathology control, attaining patients, surgeons and third party satisfaction, constitute the rationale behind the concept of key hole surgery.

Therefore, during the last two decades, endoscopic applications in skull base surgery reflected the chronological development in neurosurgical approaches rather than reflecting two parallel, distinctive endoscopic methods of approaching the brain, i.e. endoscope-assisted skull base surgery and endoscope-controlled skull base surgery.

Although the term 'endoscopically assisted microneurosurgery' was used by Matula et al. [3] in 1995, Perneczky and Fries [4] were the first to popularize such technical advancement. Endoscope-assisted skull base surgery implies the application of different angled lens endoscopes in order to enhance the illumination within the target field, explore the complicated anatomy of certain skull base regions, identify any alteration in the anatomical landmarks by the effect of the current pathology dealt with, and view the hidden angles and blind spots that can't be properly visualized with the surgical microscope as the sole visualizing tool. Furthermore, it provides video documentation and last but not least, specific benefits to each approach for the lesion dealt with. The surgical microscope is still indispensable for these types of approaches whereas the endoscope should be considered as an additional surgical instrument with a different role than that of most surgical instruments currently in use [4]. There are many surgical routes for which endoscope-assisted skull base surgery have been explored, such as supraorbital, transglabellar, retrosigmoid and transsphenoidal.

The term endoscope-controlled skull base surgery implies performing the surgical procedure exclusively under endoscopic view. In other words, the endoscope is the sole visualization tool (video surgery). This concept developed over time and dates back to the first applications of the endoscope in the cerebral ventricles, which is known now as neuroendoscopy. Nevertheless, in its earlier applications, this technique provided very limited space in terms of surgical instrument maneuverability and was, therefore, not satisfactory for many neurosurgeons. Hence, the concept of endoscope-controlled surgery was developed, especially for the skull base, in which has been introduced the use of rigid endoscopes with rod lenses of different diameters, lengths and viewing angles and moreover without working channels. What is really interesting is that the first extraventricular neurosurgical endoscopic application was performed via the transsphenoidal approach [5], and the first purely endoscopic skull base application was performed via the transsphenoidal approach [6].

The history of transsphenoidal surgery might be traced back to the old Egyptian embalmers who were able to evacuate the brain during the process of mummification without disfiguring the face [7].

In the modern neurosurgical era, a similar route through the nose and the sphenoid bone has been developed in the last century as a surgical procedure for the treatment of tumors of the sellar region and more recently of the skull base. This contributed to a significant decrease of the overall morbidity and mortality rates which has been the basis of the great popularity of minimally invasive surgery for both patients and surgeons alike. At the end of the 19th century [8], Davide Giordano, chief surgeon of the Hospital of Venice, was the first to perform an anatomical study that after a transfacial exposure provided an approach to the sella turcica through an extracranial transsphenoidal route. As a matter of fact, renewed interest was born in such a technique and at the beginning of the 20th century, a series of European and American innovators, first

Schloffer, followed by Kocher, Hirsch, Halstead and Cushing [9–12], rendered transsphenoidal surgery, either with a sublabial or directly transnasal approach, a surgical reality for patients. Nevertheless, one of the pioneers, Harvey Cushing, after popularizing this new approach via a sublabial procedure with the surgeon standing rostral to the patient's head in the supine position, abandoned it in favor of the transcranial route. This choice once again caused a rapid decline of the transsphenoidal approach. Only the Scottish neurosurgeon Norman Dott, one of Cushing's fellows, continued to use this surgical technique. It was the second half of the 1950s when the French neurosurgeon Gerard Guiot, who learned the technique from Dott, implemented the standard procedure by introducing the use of intraoperative fluoroscopy thus restoring importance and centrality to the transsphenoidal approach, and moreover attempting to extend it even to supra- and parasellar pathologies. Jules Hardy from Montreal learned the transsphenoidal technique from Guiot and added the routine use of the operating microscope and the concept of the microadenoma together with its selective removal with respect to the normal pituitary gland [13]. This decreed for Hardy a fundamental role in the history of transsphenoidal surgery and the definitive success of the transsphenoidal technique for pituitary adenomas over the transcranial approach. Finally, credit should be given to Ed Laws for having studied the technique and the disease in all its aspects with a personal series of around 5,000 cases operated transsphenoidally.

It was Guiot in the 1960s who first used the endoscope for inspection of the sellar cavity at the end of a transsphenoidal procedure in order to further and deeper visualize the surgical dome [5]. Nevertheless, it was 1977 when Apuzzo et al. [14], referring to Perneczky's experience of 'minimally invasive neurosurgery', started to apply the concept of 'adjunctive endoscopy' during a conventional transsphenoidal procedures. They reported the use of a side viewing endoscope to control the angles hidden from the perspective of the microsurgical approach, even though the quality of vision achieved at that time by endoscopes still remained inferior when compared to the surgical microscope. Shortly thereafter, inspired by Guiot's pioneering application of the endoscope during transsphenoidal pituitary surgery in 1963, Bushe and Halves [15] actualized Apuzzo's concept, reporting their modified technique for transsphenoidal approaches to pituitary adenomas. Above all they stressed the role of the endoscope as: 'contributing considerably to complete tumor extirpation, especially with endocrine-active tumors'.

On the other hand, the confidence and experience gained by rhinologists during functional endoscopic sinus surgery (FESS) [16, 17] together with the accessibility of the sphenoid sinus encouraged them to sporadically explore the role of endoscopy in sellar lesions. Just as Dandy got the idea from urologists a long time ago and started to apply the endoscope in neuroendoscopic procedures, a neurosurgeon, Jho, following the great experience of the otorhinolaryngologists of the University of Pittsburgh Medical Center, namely Carrau et al. [18], started to apply the endoscope for pituitary adenomas [19] and fixed the guidelines of fully endoscopic transsphenoidal procedures. Cappabianca and de Divitiis [20–22] applied the approach to different sellar lesions and widely systematized the principles and steps of the endoscopic transsphenoidal technique, especially relative to reconstruction strategies [23, 24], complications [25], instrument development [26] and organizing since 2001 an annual international workshop on the topic. The present frontier is represented by the extended or expanded transnasal skull base approaches. Following the first report by Weiss [27], some sporadic reports, and recent anatomical studies and research, Kassam's group in Pittsburgh [28–32] is piloting a group of young surgeons to further advancements for an innovative, strictly anatomically based, endoscopic skull base surgery. Together with contributions from other teams, such as the Naples group [33–36], Frank and Pasquini [37, 38], Castelnuovo and Locatelli [39, 40], Laws [41, 42], Schwartz and Anand [43], and Stamm [44] they are dealing with areas like the cavernous sinus and pathologies like CSF leaks, tuberculum or olfactory groove meningiomas, intraventricular craniopharyngiomas and clival chordomas, once considered amenable to open transcranial surgery only.

The transsphenoidal approach should be considered an evolutionary process rather than a revolutionary one [10]. Its more recent progress is tied to endoscopy and endoscopic surgery of the skull base. It is gaining ground every day thanks to the interest of patients, cooperating surgeons from different specialties and technologic investors. Through the last two decades, an interesting interchange between the evolving approaches and the new technological advances has taken place. Concepts and further technological developments will enrich and define future scenarios [45].

References

1 Leonhard M, Cappabianca P, de Divitiis E: The endoscope, endoscopic equipment and instrumentation; in de Divitiis E, Cappabianca P (eds): Endoscopic Endonasal Transsphenoidal Surgery. Wien, Springer, 2003, pp 9–19.

2 Prevedello DM, Doglietto F, Jane JA Jr, Jagannathan J, Han J, Laws ER Jr: History of endoscopic skull base surgery: its evolution and current reality. J Neurosurg 2007;107:206–213.

3 Matula C, Tschabitscher M, Day JD, Reinprecht A, Koos WT: Endoscopically assisted microneurosurgery. Acta Neurochir (Wien) 1995;134:190–195.

4 Perneczky A, Fries G: Endoscope-assisted brain surgery. 1 Evolution, basic concept, and current technique. Neurosurgery 1998;42:219–24; discussion 224–225.

5 Guiot G, Rougerie J, Fourestier M, Fournier A, Comoy C, Voulmiere J, Groux R: Intracranial endoscopic explorations (in French). Presse Med 1963;71: 1225–1228.

6 Jankowski R, Auque J, Simon C, Marchal JC, Hepner H, Wayoff M: Endoscopic pituitary tumor surgery. Laryngoscope 1992;102:198–202.

7 Cappabianca P, de Divitiis E: Back to the Egyptians: neurosurgery via the nose – a five-thousand year history and the recent contribution of the endoscope. Neurosurg Rev 2007;30:1–7; discussion 7.

8 Artico M, Pastore FS, Fraioli B, Giuffre R: The contribution of Davide Giordano (1864–1954) to pituitary surgery: the transglabellar-nasal approach. Neurosurgery 1998;42:909–11; discussion 911–912.

9 Cappabianca P, de Divitiis O, Maiuri F: Evolution of transsphenoidal surgery; in de Divitiis E, Cappabianca P (eds): Endoscopic Endonasal Transsphenoidal Surgery. Wien, Springer, 2003, pp 1–7.

10 Kanter AS, Dumont AS, Asthagiri AR, Oskouian RJ, Jane JA Jr, Laws ER Jr: The transsphenoidal approach: a historical perspective. Neurosurg Focus 2005;18:e6.

11 Lanzino G, Laws ER Jr: Pioneers in the development of transsphenoidal surgery: Theodor Kocher, Oskar Hirsch, and Norman Dott. J Neurosurg 2001;95:1097–1103.

12 Liu JK, Das K, Weiss MH, Laws ER Jr, Couldwell WT: The history and evolution of transsphenoidal surgery. J Neurosurg 2001;95:1083–1096.

13 Hardy J: Transsphenoidal hypophysectomy. J Neurosurg 1971;34:582–594.

14 Apuzzo ML, Heifetz MD, Weiss MH, Kurze T: Neurosurgical endoscopy using the side-viewing telescope. J Neurosurg 1977;46:398–400.

15 Bushe KA, Halves E: [Modified technique in transsphenoidal operations of pituitary adenomas. Technical note (author's transl)]. Acta Neurochir (Wien) 1978;41:163–175.

16 Kennedy DW: Functional endoscopic sinus surgery. Technique. Arch Otolaryngol 1985;111:643–649.

17 Stammberger H, Posawetz W: Functional endoscopic sinus surgery. Concept, indications and results of the Messerklinger technique. Eur Arch Otorhinolaryngol 1990;247:63–76.

18 Carrau RL, Jho HD, Ko Y: Transnasal-transsphenoidal endoscopic surgery of the pituitary gland. Laryngoscope 1996;106:914–918.

19 Jho HD, Carrau RL, Ko Y: Endoscopic pituitary surgery; in Wilkins H, Rengachary S (eds): Neurosurgical Operative Atlas. Park Ridge, American Association of Neurological Surgeons, 1996, vol 5, pp 1–12.

20 Cappabianca P, Alfieri A, de Divitiis E: Endoscopic endonasal transsphenoidal approach to the sella: towards functional endoscopic pituitary surgery (FEPS). Minim Invasive Neurosurg 1998;41:66–73.

21 Cappabianca P, Cavallo LM, de Divitiis E: Endoscopic endonasal transsphenoidal surgery. Neurosurgery 2004;55:933–40; discussion 940–941.

22 de Divitiis E, Cappabianca P, Cavallo LM: Endoscopic endonasal transsphenoidal approach to the sellar region; in de Divitiis E, Cappabianca P (ed): Endoscopic Endonasal Transsphenoidal Surgery. Wien, Springer, 2003, pp 91–130.

23 Cavallo LM, Messina A, Esposito F, de Divitiis O, Dal Fabbro M, de Divitiis E, Cappabianca P: Skull base reconstruction in the extended endoscopic transsphenoidal approach for suprasellar lesions. J Neurosurg 2007;107:713–20.

24 Cappabianca P, Cavallo LM, Esposito F, Valente V, De Divitiis E: Sellar repair in endoscopic endonasal transsphenoidal surgery: results of 170 cases. Neurosurgery 2002;51:1365–1371; discussion 1371–1372.

25 Cappabianca P, Cavallo LM, Colao A, de Divitiis E: Surgical complications associated with the endoscopic endonasal transsphenoidal approach for pituitary adenomas. J Neurosurg 2002;97:293–298.

26 Cappabianca P, Alfieri A, Thermes S, Buonamassa S, de Divitiis E: Instruments for endoscopic endonasal transsphenoidal surgery. Neurosurgery 1999;45:392–395; discussion 395–396.

27 Weiss MH: The transnasal transsphenoidal approach; in Apuzzo MLJ (ed): Surgery of the Third Ventricle. Baltimore, Williams & Wilkins, 1987, pp 476–494.

28 Kassam A, Snyderman CH, Mintz A, Gardner P, Carrau RL: Expanded endonasal approach: the rostrocaudal axis. I. Crista galli to the sella turcica. Neurosurg Focus 2005;19:E3.

29 Kassam A, Snyderman CH, Mintz A, Gardner P, Carrau RL: Expanded endonasal approach: the rostrocaudal axis. II. Posterior clinoids to the foramen magnum. Neurosurg Focus 2005;19:E4.

30 Kassam AB, Gardner P, Snyderman C, Mintz A, Carrau R: Expanded endonasal approach: fully endoscopic, completely transnasal approach to the middle third of the clivus, petrous bone, middle cranial fossa, and infratemporal fossa. Neurosurg Focus 2005;19:E6.

31 Kassam AB, Snyderman C, Gardner P, Carrau R, Spiro R: The expanded endonasal approach: a fully endoscopic transnasal approach and resection of the odontoid process: technical case report. Neurosurgery 2005;57:E213.

32 Snyderman C, Kassam A, Carrau R, Mintz A, Gardner P, Prevedello DM: Acquisition of surgical skills for endonasal skull base surgery: a training program. Laryngoscope 2007;117:699–705.

33 de Divitiis E, Cappabianca P, Cavallo LM: Endoscopic transsphenoidal approach: adaptability of the procedure to different sellar lesions. Neurosurgery 2002;51:699–705; discussion 705–707.

34 Cappabianca P, Frank G, Pasquini E, de Divitiis O, Calbucci F: Extended endoscopic endonasal transsphenoidal approaches to the suprasellar region, planum sphenoidale and clivus; in de Divitiis E, Cappabianca P (eds): Endoscopic Endonasal Transsphenoidal Surgery. Wien, Springer, 2003, pp 176–187.

35 de Divitiis E, Cavallo LM, Cappabianca P, Esposito F: Extended endoscopic endonasal transsphenoidal approach for the removal of suprasellar tumors. Part 2. Neurosurgery 2007;60:46–58; discussion 58–59.

36 Cappabianca P, Cavallo LM, Esposito F, de Divitiis O, Messina A, de Divitiis E: Extended endoscopic endonasal approach to the midline skull base: the evolving role of transsphenoidal surgery; in Pickard JD (ed): Advances and Technical Standards in Neurosurgery. Wien, Springer, 2007, vol 33, pp 1–48.

37 Frank G, Pasquini E: Endoscopic endonasal approaches to the cavernous sinus: surgical approaches. Neurosurgery 2002;50:675.

38 Frank G, Pasquini E, Doglietto F, Mazzatenta D, Sciaretta V, Farneti G, Calbucci F: The endoscopic extended transsphenoidal approach for craniopharyngiomas. Neurosurgery 2006;59(suppl 1):ONS75–ONS83.
39 Castelnuovo P, Locatelli D, Mauri S: Extended endoscopic approaches to the skull base. Anterior cranial base CSF leaks; in de Divitiis E, Cappabianca P (eds): Endoscopic Endonasal Transsphenoidal Surgery. Wien, Springer, 2003, pp 137–158.
40 Locatelli D, Rampa F, Acchiardi I, Bignami M, De Bernardi F, Castelnuovo P: Endoscopic endonasal approaches for repair of cerebrospinal fluid leaks: nine-year experience. Neurosurgery 2006;58:ONS-246–256; discussion ONS-256–257.
41 Kaptain GJ, Vincent DA, Sheehan JP, Laws ER Jr: Transsphenoidal approaches for the extracapsular resection of midline suprasellar and anterior cranial base lesions. Neurosurgery 2001;49:94–101.
42 Laws ER, Kanter AS, Jane JA Jr, Dumont AS: Extended transsphenoidal approach. J Neurosurg 2005;102:825–827; discussion 827–828.
43 Laufer I, Anand VK, Schwartz TH: Endoscopic, endonasal extended transsphenoidal, transplanum transtuberculum approach for resection of suprasellar lesions. J Neurosurg 2007;106:400–406.
44 Stamm AC, Pignatari SS, Vellutini E: Transnasal endoscopic surgical approaches to the clivus. Otolaryngol Clin North Am 2006;39:639–656.
45 Cappabianca P, Decq P, Schroeder HW: Future of endoscopy in neurosurgery. Surg Neurol 2007;67: 496–498.

Paolo Cappabianca, MD
Department of Neurological Sciences, Division of Neurosurgery
Università degli Studi di Napoli Federico II
Via Pansini 5, IT–80131 Naples (Italy)
Tel. +39 081 7462 582, E-Mail paolo.cappabianca@unina.it

Kassam AB, Gardner PA (eds): Endoscopic Approaches to the Skull Base.
Prog Neurol Surg. Basel, Karger, 2012, vol 26, pp 7–20

Advantages of the Endoscope and Transitioning from the Microscope to the Endoscope for Endonasal Approaches

Jay Jagannathan[a] · Edward R. Laws[b] · John A. Jane Jr.[a]

[a]Department of Neurosurgery, University of Virginia Health Sciences Center, University of Virginia, Charlottesville, Va., and [b]Department of Neurosurgery, Brigham and Women's Hospital, Harvard Medical School, Boston, Mass., USA

Abstract

Although the transsphenoidal approach is well established, until recently the operating microscope was the primary visualization tool for the resection of pituitary tumors. More recently, the endoscope has gained popularity for the exposure of the anterior skull base. The endoscope allows a panoramic view of the sella, and the exploration of far lateral structures, such as the cavernous sinus, which are difficult to visualize using the microscope. In this paper, we describe the evolution of the endoscopic technique and its utility in approaching the sellar region.

Historical Evolution of the Endoscope for Transsphenoidal Surgery

Almost from its inception, the transsphenoidal approach has been minimally invasive. The initial procedure, as first performed by Schloffer [1] and modified by von Eiselsberg [2] and Kocher [3] required external rhinotomy incisions. Endonasal and sublabial approaches were introduced later by Hirsch [4] and Halstead [5] at the end of the 1st decade of the 20th century. These procedures were not transseptal and required some degree of middle or inferior turbinectomy, ethmoidectomy, and septectomy in order to provide illumination and room for the use of operative instruments. By 1914, however, Harvey Cushing [6] reported a less traumatic transsphenoidal technique using a sublabial transseptal approach. This was the avenue adopted by Norman Dott, Guiot [7], and later Jules Hardy [8]. Until the late 1960s, the primary obstacles to the transsphenoidal approach remained illumination and visualization of the operative field. These obstacles were overcome by the operating microscope, introduced by Hardy. The microscope proved superior magnification and illumination and facilitated the effective removal of large and small tumors alike. The recognition of this potential provided the basis for the renaissance of the transsphenoidal approach that has continued until today.

The endonasal microscopic transsphenoidal approach has several variations, including the transseptal submucosal technique, the septal pushover, and the direct sphenoidotomy [9–12]. Essentially, these approaches differ according to the location within the nose where the initial mucosal incision is made and to the width of sellar exposure. The more traditional transseptal submucosal approach is performed using a hemitransfixion incision located just within the nose. The initial incision using the septal pushover is at the junction of the cartilaginous and osseous septum, and the incision using the direct sphenoidotomy is made even farther back, at the rostrum of the sphenoid.

The trend in microscopic transsphenoidal surgery has been towards less invasive operations. Sublabial approaches have given way to endonasal approaches and endonasal transseptal approaches have been replaced by endonasal direct sphenoidotomies. The direct sphenoidotomy is associated with fewer anterior septal complications, and less postoperative discomfort [12]. In addition, the direct sphenoidotomy provides the most expeditious exposure of the sella. The decreased invasiveness however, comes with several costs, including more limited exposure, an off-midline trajectory and diminished working room for instruments.

The advantage of the endoscope is that it allows a magnified, panoramic view of the sella (like the sublabial approach, but wider), giving the surgeon enough working room to insert various types of surgical instruments while causing minimal post-operative patient discomfort. The evolution of the endoscope in brain surgery is complex.

Lespinasse was the first to use a cystoscope to perform fulguration of the choroid plexus, but Walter Dandy is widely recognized as the father of neuroendoscopy. He first attempted cauterization of the choroid plexus in 1922 for the treatment of hydrocephalus with little success [13, 14]; but, in 1932, succeeded in traveling along the axis of the ventricle to cauterize choroid plexus in the treatment of hydrocephalus, with outcomes similar to a craniotomy [14].

According to Duffner et al. [15], in 1923 William Mixter reported the first endoscopic third ventriculostomy. Therefore, the endoscope's initial impact in neurosurgery was in its use within the ventricular system. Intraventricular endoscopic surgery likely represented the most important initial influence of this technical adjunct in the field of neurosurgery [16].

The manner in which the endoscope is used in transsphenoidal surgery varies significantly. The basic divisions are procedures in which the endoscope is used as an adjunct to a microscopic resection (endoscope-assisted transsphenoidal surgery) versus those in which the endoscope is the sole tool employed (pure endoscopic transsphenoidal surgery).

Although this latter concept had been reported by others [17], the pure endoscopic transsphenoidal approach was introduced and popularized in the late 1990s by Jho and Carrau from the University of Pittsburgh Medical Center [18, 19]. Advances in endoscopic endonasal neurosurgical techniques at Pittsburgh continue in the work of

Kassam, Snyderman, Carrau, Gardner and colleagues [20–22], who have expanded the scope of complex skull base tumors accessible by the endoscope. In Europe, the neurosurgical groups of Cappabianca and de Divitiis [23–26] and Frank and Pasquini and coworkers [27, 28] have also made important contributions. There are several variations of the endoscopic technique, and over time we have drawn from these to establish the approach which we favor. In this chapter, we discuss the evolution of our current endoscopic technique and detail what we believe are the advantages and limitations of this approach as compared with the microscopic adenomectomy.

Endoscope-Assisted Microscopic Transsphenoidal Surgery

Our initial experience with the endoscope was as an adjunct to the endonasal transseptal microscopic transsphenoidal approach. When a transsphenoidal retractor is placed via a transseptal route and an anterior sphenoidotomy is made, an endoscope can provide heightened visualization and supply a panoramic view at the posterior wall of the sphenoid sinus. This enables the surgeon to clearly view the optic protuberances, opticocarotid recesses, carotid protuberances, cavernous sinuses, sella and clival indentation. Even if the sphenoid sinus is septated in a complex manner, the anatomical demonstration of the sinus provided by an endoscope is often so obvious that the use of intraoperative fluoroscopic C-arm is not necessary. When microscopic surgery is performed for removal of a pituitary tumor, an angled lens endoscope can be used to directly inspect the suprasellar region or lateral wall of the sella. Traditional pituitary surgeons use a mirror for this purpose; however, an endoscope allows a surgeon to visualize the anatomy more clearly and directly.

However, the rigid surgical corridor provided by a transsphenoidal retractor limits a neurosurgeon's ability to maneuver surgical instruments under endoscopic guidance. We found that this created the greatest limitation to the use of the endoscope. As our practice progressed, we began to adopt the direct sphenoidotomy for all of our microscopic approaches. With increased experience using the direct approach in conjunction with the endoscope, we found that we could remove the speculum and use the endoscope. The benefits surgeons can observe with this technique are a wider panoramic view of the sphenoidal sinus which provides distinct visualization of the anatomy at the posterior wall of the sphenoidal sinus, angled views at the lateral wall of the sella and the suprasellar region, and a close-up view of the junction of tumor and normal pituitary tissue.

Two-Nostril vs. One-Nostril Technique

Initial reports of the 'pure' endoscopic transsphenoidal technique involved the two-handed technique, only two patients required a two-nostril technique [19].

The advantage of a two-nostril technique is the elimination of the endoscope shaft from one of the surgeon's operating corridors, which provides more freedom for the maneuvering of surgical instruments. The disadvantage is the additional surgical trauma to the nasal mucosa of the other nasal cavity. During our initial experience with the pure endoscopic technique, we used a one-nostril technique. We found that this constrained our ability to maneuver instruments (endoscope, suction and dissector) within the nares. In order to create enough working room we found that a partial middle turbinectomy was helpful. However, this maneuver tended to create more nasal complications postoperatively.

Transition from Microscopic Transsphenoidal Surgery to Endoscopic Endonasal Transsphenoidal Surgery

Microscopic transsphenoidal surgery has been performed with good surgical outcomes and minimal morbidities [29]. Nevertheless, an endoscope carries advantages over the operating microscope such as its ability to visualize through a narrow surgical corridor and to provide angled, close-up views. As mentioned earlier, endoscope-assisted microscopic surgery is a reasonable first step taken when a neurosurgeon desires to adopt endoscopy into pituitary surgery. In this case, an endoscope can provide certain advantages in microscopic pituitary surgery by providing panoramic views as well as visualizing angled, close-up views. However, the surgeon should be aware that the speculum will restrict maneuverability of the endoscope, and create 'sword play' between the endoscope and other surgical instruments.

Endoscopic Endonasal Pituitary Surgery

Although the use of an endoscope during microscopic surgery can sometimes be a nuisance in this stage, this initial step will provide the neurosurgeon the opportunity to exercise the use of an endoscope without adding extra risks to the patient. A change in the surgical route from a conventional transseptal approach to an endonasal approach should be the next transition. Surgeons who already perform a microscopic direct sphenoidotomy will find that this is less of a dramatic departure than those who perform transseptal approaches.

Teamwork between an endoscopic rhinologist and a neurosurgeon can be an easy way to facilitate this transition. In these situations, the rhinologist performs an endonasal endoscopic anterior sphenoidotomy. A transsphenoidal retractor is placed through the endonasal route. The neurosurgeon then can perform either microscopic pituitary tumor surgery with the speculum in place or explore his or her ability to accomplish endoscopic pituitary tumor surgery without the use of a transsphenoidal retractor. If surgery does not progress well, a transsphenoidal retractor can always be placed through an endonasal route for microscopic surgery.

Evolution of the Current Surgical Technique

Endoscope Holder versus Hand

Early in our experience with the endoscopic technique, we attempted to recapitulate the microscopic approach. Just as the microscope is fixed in space, we felt that the endoscope should be as well. The endoscope holder seemed to provide the closest approximation of the microscopic technique. We soon found, however, the holder tends to negate the advantages of the endoscope. Current endoscopes have limited zoom capability; hence the surgery is generally performed with maximal zoom from the outset. The surgeon can obtain a pseudo-depth perception from the dynamic movement of the endoscope relative to the operative instruments that, when fixed, is absent. Placing the endoscope in a fixed position likens the technique to a microscopic adenomectomy during which the surgeon has a wide-angle view but has limited depth perception and zoom views. Also, if the endoscope becomes occluded by blood beyond the cleaning ability of the irrigation system, it must be removed from the holder, cleaned, and then brought back into the field. This interruption tends to disrupt the flow of the operation significantly and, in situations of significant bleeding, can be disconcerting. Even with a wide anterior sphenoidotomy, the endoscope occasionally restricts the maneuverability of instruments and access to the tumor. Using the three-hand technique as advocated by Kassam and others [20, 21], the benefits of the endoscope can be realized. This maneuver requires cooperation between the endoscopist and the surgeon. The endoscopist can move in during the tumor resection, and focus closely on areas of interest.

The pseudo-three-dimensional perspective is also greatly enhanced by the in-and-out movement of the endoscope. As instruments are moved in and out of the nose, the endoscope operator can follow the instruments, ensuring that they do not injure the nasal mucosa.

Patient Positioning

Over time, we have experimented with the supine and semirecumbent positions. We prefer the latter but recognize certain limitations. The supine position increases the venous pressure and can cause significant bleeding from the cavernous sinus and tumor. As with the microscopic adenomectomy, significant bleeding can be the pivotal factor separating an inadequate tumor resection from a successful operation. Nevertheless, the supine position is more comfortable for the surgeon and causes less arm and shoulder fatigue. The arm strain associated with the semirecumbent position can be alleviated by standing on step stools, which allows the endoscopist to maintain elbows at his or her side. Because of the advantages of decreased venous pressure and more facile tumor removal, we advocate a semirecumbent position, with the back and head elevated approximately 20°. The other keys to minimizing bleeding are adequate pre-operative decongestion and injection of vasoconstrictive agents, careful insertion and removal of instruments, and use of deliberate and efficient maneuvers in performing the operation. Most sellar, cavernous sinus, and bone bleeding can be quickly controlled using FloSeal (Baxter Health Care Corp., Deerfield, Ill., USA) [27]. Its disadvantage is that it does not fully wash away with irrigation and can make inspecting for tumor remnants more difficult.

An ideal bipolar instrument has not yet been introduced. We also do not advocate routine partial middle turbinectomy because it is mostly unnecessary in the adult patient, except for those with an unusually small nose and nasal cavity. If it is performed routinely, the minimally invasive nature of the endoscopic procedure as compared with its microscopic transsphenoidal counterpart becomes dubious. Difficulties with crusting and delayed epistaxis become more prominent, increasing patient discomfort and negating many of the advantages of the endoscopic approach.

Advantages and Limitations of the Pure Endoscopic Adenomectomy

To better understand the role of the pure endoscopic technique, it is helpful to understand the advantages and limitations of the microscopic adenomectomy. Among the important advantages of the microscope include its familiarity to the neurosurgeon. The operating microscope is standard equipment used for all types of neurosurgical procedures on the spine and brain. The benefit of the microscope's familiarity to the surgeon should not be underestimated. The microscopic view is three-dimensional, which is of enormous importance during tumor dissection, and it also has easily manipulated zoom and focus features. Once it is focused at maximum zoom, the surgeon can increase and decrease the zoom without needing to refocus. Furthermore, after the appropriate trajectory to the sella has been discerned, the operating microscope can easily maintain it, preventing unintentional breach of the anterior cranial fossa. Although a nasal speculum is used for a microscopic adenomectomy, it is not part of most pure endoscopic procedures. The speculum protects the nasal mucosa from injury by instruments during the operative procedure. Finally, the operating microscope (along with the nasal speculum) is out of the surgical field and does not obstruct the entry or maneuvering of instruments. Because it is out of the surgical field, the microscopic view does not suffer from 'red out' when bleeding fills the surgical field. For busy centers, the relative brevity of the microscopic adenomectomy (particularly if a direct endonasal sphenoidotomy approach is employed) allows for multiple cases to be addressed in a single day.

There are problems with the microscopic adenomectomy, however. Although the optics are excellent and changes in magnification can be performed easily, the field of view is narrow (fig. 1). This restriction necessarily means that some anatomical landmarks within the sphenoid sinus are not readily visualized. In our experience, it is quite rare to see the carotid or optic protuberances or the opticocarotid recesses microscopically. Although some may argue that because tumors (especially microadenomas) are centrally located it is unnecessary to see these landmarks, their visualization does orient the surgeon to the anatomical midline and to the limits of the sella.

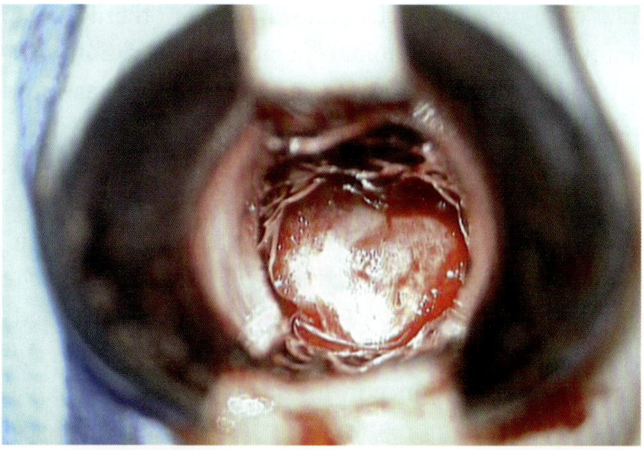

1

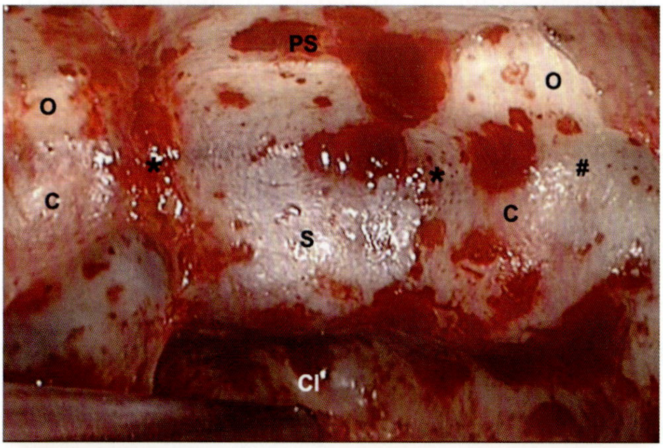

2

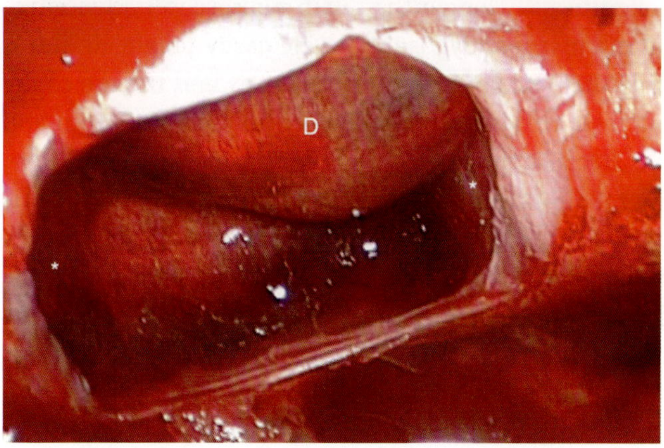

3

Fig. 1. Microscopic view of the anterior wall of the sella.
Fig. 2. Endoscopic view of the anterior wall of the sella. C = Carotid protuberance; Cl = clivus; O = optic protuberance; PS = planum sphenoidale; S = sella. # Lateral opticocarotid recess; * medial opticocarotid recess.
Fig. 3. Tumor cavity viewed using a 0° endoscope. D = Diaphragma sellae. * Cavernous sinus walls.

Therefore, it is our standard practice to use C-arm videofluoroscopy or other forms of image guidance for all of our microscopic transsphenoidal operations. In addition, visualization with the microscope is limited by line of sight. The surgeon cannot see around corners, either toward the cavernous sinus or the suprasellar space. Visualization of the optic chiasm, confirming its decompression during transdiaphragmatic dissection, is rarely possible microscopically. The standard sublabial or transseptal approaches can also be associated with sinonasal complications and with significant patient discomfort early on in the perioperative period. Nasal packing causes facial pain and headache in as many as 35% of patients, and the procedures can cause rhinological complaints including alveolar numbness, anosmia, saddle nose deformity, and nasal septal perforations [30]. These complications are less pronounced with the endonasal transseptal approach, but they do continue to occur. The more minimally invasive approaches of the septal pushover and direct sphenoidotomy do not require nasal packing and are associated with fewer sinonasal complications [10, 12, 31]. Nevertheless, these benefits come at the cost of a more limited exposure, an off-midline trajectory tending to lead to the carotid, and a confined working area.

The endoscopic approach also presents difficulties. Although many neurosurgeons perform ventriculoscopy, nasal endoscopy is much less familiar. This means that most neurosurgeons, who typically perform their own microscopic exposures, will need to find an interested and cooperative ENT surgeon. In many centers, the endoscopic approach requires the presence of an ENT surgeon throughout the operation. In microscopic cases, the ENT surgeon performs the transsphenoidal exposure and nasal closure but is not necessarily present for the tumor resection. When neurosurgeons perform endoscopic operations without ENT surgeons, the operative times during the learning curve are significantly longer than with microscopic adenomectomy. Whereas the transseptal microscopic exposure can be easily taught to junior neurosurgery residents, teaching them both the surgical anatomy and the use of the endoscope can be an imposing task. Other major limitations include the zoom and focus capacity of the endoscope. Because the endoscope has a relatively limited zoom capability, our tendency is to use it at maximum zoom at all times. To obtain magnification, the endoscope is brought closer to the region of interest, requiring frequent refocus maneuvers that are not as easily performed as with the microscope. Before the endoscopic surgeon fully understands the depth perception provided by the dynamic interaction between surgical instruments and the endoscope, it is possible to dissect into the posterior pituitary, cavernous sinus, and diaphragm over-aggressively and cause more complications, such as CSF leaks and diabetes insipidus. Because instruments enter the field out of the line of sight of the endoscope and because no nasal speculum is used, the nasal mucosa along the septum and the medial wall of the middle turbinate can be injured in the course of the operation.

This damage can be minimized by lateralizing the middle turbinates and by careful entry of surgical instruments into the nose. During the endoscopic sphenoidotomy, the posterior septal branches of the sphenopalatine artery are also at greater risk than

Table 1. Comparison of various transsphenoidal approaches

	Endoscopic binasal	Microscopic transseptal	Direct sphenoidotomy
Nasal packing	no	yes	no
Septum resection	posterior bone and mucosa	bone only	little or none
Sphenoidotomy	necessarily large	size varies with pathology	size varies with pathology
Middle turbinectomy	occasionally: requires serial ENT follow-up	never	rarely

during transseptal microscopic approaches. In these approaches, the mucosa containing this vessel are elevated from the sphenoid rostrum and are thereby protected. The direct sphenoidotomy places these vessels at greater risk of damage and of early postoperative epistaxis however, care must be taken with hemostasis, as over-cauterization of the mucosa of the rostrum can result in incisor and palate numbness.

It is perhaps an overstatement to assert that the endoscope is less invasive than the microscope (table 1). The endoscopic approach may seem so to the patient initially because there is no nasal packing, but the endoscopic approach, as we perform it, disturbs and removes more anatomical structures than the various standard microscopic approaches (sublabial, endonasal transseptal, and direct sphenoidotomy). The sphenoidotomy is larger so that the endoscope does not impede the necessary maneuvering of the operative instruments. To achieve the same maneuverability of the operative instruments as in the microscopic adenomectomy, a binasal technique is used that requires a posterior partial septectomy. Although not routine, a partial middle turbinectomy is also performed at times, an action never necessary when performing a microscopic adenomectomy. All of these maneuvers are undertaken in an effort to provide an exposure that allows the surgeon to use two instruments and the endoscope.

Indeed, it can be reasonably argued that these factors necessarily mean that the binasal endoscopic technique is more invasive than the microscopic adenomectomy. The mononostril approaches as advocated by Jho and Carrau [19] and Cappabianca and colleagues [23, 24, 32], however, can reasonably be considered less invasive. We simply have not been able to achieve the same operative maneuverability in most cases using a mononostril approach. Nevertheless, each of the microscopic approaches requires reflection of some portion of the nasal septum, an act that can lead to nasal septum deviation. The microscopic sublabial and transseptal approaches also require anterior septum dissection, creating the risks of nasal septal perforation, septal hematoma, alveolar numbness, and saddle nose deformity [33–35]. All of these risks are relatively low, and the choice to use the endoscopic in lieu of the microscopic technique should not be in the pursuit of a less invasive approach, but because of the advantages provided by the endoscopic procedure.

Because the endoscopic technique is relatively new, appropriate instruments are still in development. Still needed are a proper bipolar instrument and slotted suckers with angled tips to work in the regions visualized by the endoscope but inaccessible with direct suction. Because current angled suction devices are not slotted, problems can arise when placing the suction into the cavernous sinus or suprasellar region. Smaller endoscopes with more zoom range and focus capacity also need to be developed. To foster a wider application of this technique, a standardized set of instruments required to begin performing these operations must be developed.

The endoscope does afford significant advantages both during the surgical approach and during tumor resection. It provides panoramic views of areas outside of a microscope's line of sight and allows dynamic, magnified inspection of areas of interest. During the approach, the wide views of the nasal anatomy allow the surgeon to discern the appropriate level of entry into the sphenoid sinus more easily (either by visualizing the sphenoid ostia or the level of the superior turbinates). This wide-angle view and superior visualization of the sphenoid anatomy provides excellent information regarding superior and inferior limits of the sella and the anatomical midline (fig. 2). These factors obviate the use of intraoperative videofluoroscopy in most cases. Visualization of the carotid protuberances is rarely possible with the operating microscope, and confirmation of their precise location does at least improve the surgeon's comfort.

Not only have we found that the endoscopic approach is different from the microscopic approach, so too is the endoscopic tumor resection. In the microscopic resection of macroadenomas, tumor is often out of the surgeon's line of sight. Lateral and superior portions of the tumor are removed by feel, making surgeon experience a more important factor in successful adenomectomy. By contrast, with the endoscopic approach, the tumor is constantly in view, enabling the surgeon to directly visualize the tumor being removed from the sellar floor, cavernous sinus walls and suprasellar region. In cases where the tumor is adherent to the normal gland, the surgeon can also directly visualize the interface between the normal gland and the tumor. At the end of the resection, the surgeon can use angled endoscopes to confirm the thoroughness of tumor resection (fig. 3).

During tumor resection, particularly with microadenomas and sellar macroadenomas, exceptionally magnified views of the tumor/gland interface can be discerned and dissection enabled. Even with the 0° endoscope, the sellar floor, cavernous sinus walls, and diaphragm can be directly inspected. The exception is the proximal (anterior) portion of the medial cavernous sinus wall just posterior to the dural opening on the ipsilateral side to the endoscope. This portion of the cavernous sinus wall is more difficult to see, but it can be done by placing the endoscope within the other nostril (the 'cross-court' approach). During transdiaphragmatic dissection, the optic chiasm can be seen and chiasmal decompression, which is often the primary goal of surgery, can be confirmed. Using the microscope, the sellar floor, cavernous sinus walls, and chiasm are rarely fully visible. When the anatomy is not completely apparent, the 30° endoscope can be used. Angled endoscopes do tend to conflict with inferiorly placed operative instruments. We have found it more useful to place the 30° endoscope inferiorly, with the suction and operative instruments above it, or to place it in one nostril and introduce the operative instruments through the other. It is not yet known whether these advantages will result in higher remission rates for secretory adenomas and lower recurrence rates for nonfunctioning adenomas. The endoscopic complication rate does not appear to be increased, but longer follow-up periods are needed so that conclusions regarding efficacy can be drawn [36, 37]. The endoscopic adenomectomy rarely requires nasal packing unless there is a significant CSF leak. As has been shown by Zada et al. [12], foregoing nasal packing significantly decreases patient discomfort and affects patient satisfaction. Although we have not yet begun to assess this aspect systematically, our impression is that patients undergoing endoscopic surgery experience much less postoperative discomfort.

The endoscopic adenomectomy can be associated with alterations in the sense of smell, but it is not generally associated with the complications of alveolar numbness, nasal septal perforations and deviations, and saddle nose deformities that are more common with the traditional transsphenoidal sublabial or transseptal microsurgical approaches. The endoscopic exposure is most like the direct sphenoidotomy as described by Griffith and Veerapen [9], and now advocated by Zada, et al. [12]. The main anatomical difference is that the three- or four-hand binasal endoscopic approach requires a partial posterior septectomy. During the endoscopic approach, the nasal mucosa is at greater risk of injury because no nasal speculum is used. With the microscopic direct sphenoidotomy, the posterior septum is simply reflected laterally. Zada et al. [12] have reported that one fifth of patients undergoing the direct sphenoidotomy required a relaxing alar incision; such incisions are not necessary during endoscopic cases. In our view, the alar incision is a major drawback of the microscopic direct sphenoidotomy. The most significant deficiency of the direct microscopic adenomectomy, however, is the narrow exposure and slightly off midline trajectory. Cadaveric or clinical studies directly comparing these approaches would be helpful.

Reflections of the Past and Future of the Endoscope in Microneurosurgery

From the initial use of the endoscope to inspect the sphenoidal sinus in the 1960s, interest in the endoscope in microneurosurgery has blossomed [7, 38]. During conventional microscopic pituitary surgery, an endoscope has been used to inspect hidden anatomical corners. Now, many pituitary neurosurgeons have adopted an endoscope to take advantage of endoscopic angled and closely magnified views, while performing the main segment of an operation under three-dimensional microscopic visualization. Endoscope assisted microscopic surgery makes an excellent first step for neurosurgeons who desire to master endoscopy for pituitary surgery. However, adopting the use of endoscopic equipment in conjunction with the operating microscope is time consuming and can be an additional burden for neurosurgeons who are well accustomed to microscopic surgery. The rapid patient recovery with short hospital stays observed with endoscopic pituitary surgery is mainly due to the surgeon's choice of a paraseptal endonasal route, rather than the use of the endoscope itself. This endonasal surgical route has been well established in its use for microscopic pituitary surgery [9, 39]. When microscopic pituitary surgery is performed via an endonasal direct sphenoidotomy, its immediate postoperative outcome will be very similar to endoscopic pituitary surgery. Patients do not require nasal packing, do not experience much postoperative discomfort and do not require prolonged hospital stays for reasons related to the surgical approach itself.

Likewise, if endoscopic surgery was performed via a conventional transseptal approach, nasal packing would be required as it would be with microscopic surgery.

Conclusions

The endoscope offers a safe and effective approach to the anterior skull base, which circumvents many of the limitations of the microscope. It provides an excellent wide-angle and magnified view of the operative anatomy, and although it requires more anatomical exposure it remains within the group of minimally invasive approaches to the sella. New instruments and smaller endoscopes with more focus and zoom capacity still need to be developed. Unbiased understanding of the endoscopic limitations and advantages will better allow the pure endoscopic adenomectomy to realize its place in transsphenoidal surgery.

References

1 Schloffer H: Erfolgreiche operationen eines hypophysentumors auf nasalem wege. Wien Klin Wochenschr 1907;20:621–624.
2 von Eiselsberg A: The operative cure of acromegaly by removal of a hypophysial tumor. Ann Surg 1908; 48:781–783.
3 Kocher T: Ein fall von hypophysis-tumor mit operativer heilung. Dtsch Z Chir 1909;100:13–37.
4 Hirsch O: Endonasal method of removal of hypophyseal tumors: with a report of two successful cases. JAMA 1910;5:772–774.
5 Halstead A: Remarks on the operative treatment of tumors of the hypophysis. With the report of two cases operated on by an oronasal method. Trans Am Surg Assoc 1910;28:73–93.
6 Cushing H: Partial hypophysectomy for acromegaly: with remarks on the function of the hypophysis. Ann Surg 1909;50:1002–1017.
7 Guiot J, Rougerie J, Fourestier M, Fournier A, Comoy C, Vulmiere J, Groux R: Intracranial endoscopic explorations. Presse Med 1963;71:1225–1228.
8 Hardy J: Transsphenoidal microsurgery of the normal and pathological pituitary. Clin Neurosurg 1969;16:185–217.
9 Griffith HB, Veerapen R: A direct transnasal approach to the sphenoid sinus. Technical note. J Neurosurg 1987;66:140–142.
10 Jane JA Jr, Thapar K, Alden TD, Laws ER Jr: Fluoroscopic frameless stereotaxy for transsphenoidal surgery. Neurosurgery 2001;48:1302–1307; discussion 1307–1308.

11 Wilson WR, Laws ER Jr: Transnasal septal displacement approach for secondary transsphenoidal pituitary surgery. Laryngoscope 1992;102:951–953.

12 Zada G, Kelly DF, Cohan P, Wang C, Swerdloff R: Endonasal transsphenoidal approach for pituitary adenomas and other sellar lesions: an assessment of efficacy, safety, and patient impressions. J Neurosurg 2003;98:350–358.

13 Abbott R: History of neuroendoscopy. Neurosurg Clin N Am 2004;15:1–7.

14 Dandy W: Cerebral ventriculoscopy. Johns Hopkins Hosp Bull 1922;33:189.

15 Duffner F, Freudenstein D, Wacker A, Straub-Duffner S, Grote EH: 75 years after Dandy, Fay and Mixter – looking back on the history of neuroendoscopy. Zentralbl Neurochir 1998;59:121–128.

16 Harris LW: Endoscopic techniques in neurosurgery. Microsurgery 1994;15:541–546.

17 Apuzzo ML, Heifetz MD, Weiss MH, Kurze T: Neurosurgical endoscopy using the side-viewing telescope. J Neurosurg 1977;46:398–400.

18 Gondim J, Schops M, Tella OI Jr: Transnasal endoscopic surgery of the sellar region: study of the first 100 cases. Arq Neuropsiquiatr 2003;61:836–841.

19 Jho HD, Carrau RL: Endoscopic endonasal transsphenoidal surgery: experience with 50 patients. J Neurosurg 1997;87:44–51.

20 Kassam A, Snyderman CH, Mintz A, Gardner P, Carrau RL: Expanded endonasal approach: the rostrocaudal axis. I. Crista galli to the sella turcica. Neurosurg Focus 2005;19:E3.

21 Kassam A, Snyderman CH, Mintz A, Gardner P, Carrau RL: Expanded endonasal approach: the rostrocaudal axis. II. Posterior clinoids to the foramen magnum. Neurosurg Focus 2005;19:E4.

22 Carrau RL, Kassam AB, Snyderman CH: Pituitary surgery. Otolaryngol Clin North Am 2001;34:1143–1155, ix.

23 Cappabianca P, Cavallo LM, Esposito F, de Divitiis E: Endoscopic endonasal transsphenoidal surgery: procedure, endoscopic equipment and instrumentation. Childs Nerv Syst 2004;20:796–801.

24 Cappabianca P, Cavallo LM, Colao A, de Divitiis E: Surgical complications associated with the endoscopic endonasal transsphenoidal approach for pituitary adenomas. J Neurosurg 2002;97:293–298.

25 Koren I, Hadar T, Rappaport ZH, Yaniv E: Endoscopic transnasal transsphenoidal microsurgery versus the sublabial approach for the treatment of pituitary tumors: endonasal complications. Laryngoscope 1999;109:1838–1840.

26 Prevedello DM, Thomas A, Gardner P, Snyderman CH, Carrau RL, Kassam AB: Endoscopic endonasal resection of a synchronous pituitary adenoma and a tuberculum sellae meningioma: technical case report. Neurosurgery 2007;60:E401; discussion E401.

27 Frank G, Pasquini E, Doglietto F, Mazzatenta D, Sciarretta V, Farneti G, Calbucci F: The endoscopic extended transsphenoidal approach for craniopharyngiomas. Neurosurgery 2006;59:ONS75–83.

28 Sciarretta V, Pasquini E, Farneti G, Frank G, Mazzatenta D, Calbucci F: Endoscopic sinus surgery for the treatment of vascular tumors. Am J Rhinol 2006;20:426–431.

29 Jagannathan J, Prevedello DM, Ayer VS, Dumont AS, Jane JA Jr, Laws ER: Computer-assisted frameless stereotaxy in transsphenoidal surgery at a single institution: review of 176 cases. Neurosurg Focus 2006;20:E9.

30 Sherwen PJ, Patterson WJ, Griesdale DE: Transseptal, transsphenoidal surgery: a subjective and objective analysis of results. J Otolaryngol 1986;15:155–160.

31 Jane JA Jr, Vance ML, Woodburn CJ, Laws ER Jr: Stereotactic radiosurgery for hypersecreting pituitary tumors: part of a multimodality approach. Neurosurg Focus 2003;14:e12.

32 Cannavo S, Venturino M, Curto L, De Menis E, D'Arrigo C, Tita P, Billeci D, Trimarchi F: Clinical presentation and outcome of pituitary adenomas in teenagers. Clin Endocrinol (Oxf) 2003;58:519–527.

33 Sharma K, Tyagi I, Banerjee D, Chhabra DK, Kaur A, Taneja HK: Rhinological complications of sublabial transseptal transsphenoidal surgery for sellar and suprasellar lesions: prevention and management. Neurosurg Rev 1996;19:163–167.

34 Sharma R, Tyagi I, Banerjee D, Pandey R: Nasoethmoid schwannoma with intracranial extension: case report and review of literature. Neurosurg Rev 1998;21:58–61.

35 Spencer WR, Levine JM, Couldwell WT, Brown-Wagner M, Moscatello A: Approaches to the sellar and parasellar region: a retrospective comparison of the endonasal-transsphenoidal and sublabial-transsphenoidal approaches. Otolaryngol Head Neck Surg 2000;122:367–369.

36 Cavallo LM, Dal Fabbro M, Jalalod'din H, Messina A, Esposito I, Esposito F, de Divitiis E, Cappabianca P: Endoscopic endonasal transsphenoidal surgery. Before scrubbing in: tips and tricks. Surg Neurol 2007;67:342–347.

37 Orlando R, Cappabianca P, Tosone G, Esposito F, Piazza M, de Divitiis E: Retrospective analysis of a new antibiotic chemoprophylaxis regimen in 170 patients undergoing endoscopic endonasal transsphenoidal surgery. Surg Neurol 2007;68:145–148; discussion 148.
38 Gamea A, Fathi M, el-Guindy A: The use of the rigid endoscope in trans-sphenoidal pituitary surgery. J Laryngol Otol 1994;108:19–22.
39 Cooke RS, Jones RA: Experience with the direct transnasal transsphenoidal approach to the pituitary fossa. Br J Neurosurg 1994;8:193–196.

John A. Jane Jr., MD
Department of Neurosurgery, University of Virginia Health System
PO Box 800212
Charlottesville, VA 22908–0711 (USA)
Tel. +1 434 243 5749, Fax +1 434 243 5204, E-Mail johnjanejr@virginia.edu

Kassam AB, Gardner PA (eds): Endoscopic Approaches to the Skull Base.
Prog Neurol Surg. Basel, Karger, 2012, vol 26, pp 21–26

Principles of Endoneurosurgery

Amin B. Kassam[a] · Paul A. Gardner[b] · Daniel M. Prevedello[d] · Carl H. Snyderman[b,c] · Ricardo L. Carrau[e]

[a]Division of Neurological Surgery, University of Ottawa, The Ottawa Hospital Civic Campus, Ottawa, Ont., Canada; Departments of [b]Neurological Surgery, and [c]Otolaryngology, Head and Neck Surgery, University of Pittsburgh Medical Center, Pittsburgh, Pa.; Departments of [d]Neurological Surgery, and [e]Otolaryngology, Head and Neck Surgery, The Ohio State University Medical Center, Columbus, Ohio, USA

Abstract

The usage and role of endoneurosurgery using three different techniques are described: (1) keyhole surgery, (2) endoport surgery, and (3) endoscopic endonasal surgery. The technical approach for endonasal surgery is discussed followed by the principles of surgical resection using bimanual dissection. Emphasis is place on the reconstruction of the skull-base, case selection and cross-specialty development and application of endoscopic endonasal surgery is emphasized.

Endoneurosurgery is cranial neurosurgery performed with an endoscope as the primary or sole form of visualization. There are three different techniques that fit this description: (1) keyhole surgery, (2) endoport surgery, and (3) endoscopic endonasal surgery.

Keyhole surgery is surgery through a miniature craniotomy, designed to limit the skin incision and bony opening. Endoport surgery is surgery for deep white matter or intraventricular lesions; a small, clear cylinder is introduced over a stereotactic needle and dilator and the surgery is performed through this port or cannula. The endoscopic endonasal approach (EEA) is surgery through the nostrils that uses the paranasal sinuses to access the skull base. All of these techniques rely on and take advantage of the unique characteristics of the endoscope.

Microsurgery was a significant advance as a visualization tool because it allowed surgeons to access deeper areas with improved visualization and detail. This, in turn, led to improvement in and development of new surgical techniques and approaches. The endoscope has similar potential. The microscope as a tool is kept at a distance from the target, casting a cone of light on the surgical field. As a result, it is necessary to create a larger opening that allows light to funnel down to deeper structures. This creates limitations on the exposure and approach based on intervening superficial structures. This access often determines the approach, rather than critical neurovascular structures associated with a tumor. The endoscope, however, acts like a flashlight held next to the target. The superficial access can be minimal as long as there is sufficient maneuverability and access in the depth. The flashlight effect allows for the endoscope to subtend a wide viewing angle, thereby creating a divergent view as opposed to the convergent view provided by the microscope. However, it should be noted that because the endoscope itself takes physical space within the nose it requires a greater working corridor within the sinonasal cavity.

With any surgical technique, especially one involving the skull base, there are three phases of surgery: approach, resection and reconstruction. There are unique principles associated with each phase of surgery when the endoscope is applied. Never is this more true than with the EEA.

Finally, any new technique has to be applied carefully and selectively. It may provide a new corridor for accessing tumors, but this does not mean that it replaces existing techniques. There is a learning curve for each surgeon who adapts it. There are also many patient factors that may make it useful or undesirable depending on the case. All of this must be taken into account.

Approach

The EEA begins with the sinonasal phase. There are two main goals of this phase that are critical to the technique. Bimanual access and dissection are first and foremost. Without this, endonasal techniques become inferior to microscopic approaches. In fact, we believe that the inability to create bimanual access represents a relative contraindication to proceeding. Secondly, wide exposure is necessary to allow bimanual access as well as to make room for the endoscope as a tool that takes up physical space in the surgical field. The goal of the approach is therefore to create a 'cavity and a half'. The working cavity allows for the bimanual dissection while the half cavity provides for physical space for the endoscope thus optimizing visualization.

Bimanual access begins with the use, in most cases, of a binarial approach. Using one nostril to access the paranasal sinuses and skull base inherently limits the surgeons' freedom of movement by limiting the initial orifice. Throughout the exposure, steps must be taken to ensure continued bimanual freedom. If there are areas in which this is not possible, the approach should be reconsidered. Hemostasis and application of proper resection techniques are critically dependent on it. A critical initial consideration is removal of the lower third of the middle turbinate in the patient's right naris. While this may not be absolutely necessary in all cases, in cases of expanded endonasal surgery this will facilitate movement of the endoscope and suction. This maneuver is performed only in the right naris as two instruments (the scope and suction) are employed. The contralateral turbinate is not removed but only outfractured. This provides adequate room as only one instrument (dissection tool, bipolar or drill) is passed through the patient's left naris. There are other steps that must be taken during the exposure to continuously allow visualization while bimanual and binarial techniques are used. The most critical of these is a limited, semicircular posterior septectomy. A small amount of the posterior nasal septum must be trimmed to allow an instrument to be introduced from one nostril while the endoscope is introduced through the other without obscuring the endoscopic view.

Binarial access also allows additional width of exposure. An endoscopic approach is much different than a microscopic approach. Even when addressing a simple pituitary lesion, a much wider exposure is needed to allow room for the endoscope and take advantage of the close, dynamic visualization it provides. If the goal is to merely park a static endoscope in the nostril and utilize the same exposure and resection techniques as a microscopic approach, then there is no advantage to it. If, however, a wide sphenoidotomy, lateral to the parasellar internal carotid arteries (ICAs), is used, the endoscope can be introduced all the way into the sphenoid, with its tip working next to the dissecting instruments. This allows for dynamic movement of the endoscope during the case, visualizing instruments as they are introduced and providing a close, magnified view of finer intrasellar and intracranial dissections.

Another key benefit of bimanual exposure is the ability to maintain proprioception. It is argued that a fundamental disadvantage of endoscopy is the loss of 3-dimensional perception from monocular optics. While this may be a factor, it is easily compensated for by proprioception. Therefore, it is critical to create a bimanual exposure that allows for continuous palpation of bony landmarks with the operators left hand, while working instruments are maneuvered with the right. This creates 3-dimensional perception through proprioception. The learning curve associated with this is relatively short, especially for experienced microsurgeons who are used to bimanual technique.

Resection

The overriding principle in any endoscopic approach must be maintenance of standard microsurgical techniques. If this is not possible, either due to inadequate instrumentation or access, another approach should be considered. When applied to the EEA, this means that two surgeons must work together. During resection, one surgeon constantly moves the endoscope, both to provide visual cues to substitute for the lack of binocular vision and to keep the endoscope clear of working instruments yet as close as possible to provide adequate detail and visualization as the resection deepens. Both surgeons need to read the case together.

The entire approach segment described above is designed to facilitate bimanual dissection to allow the application of microsurgical technique. Tumor resection begins with careful internal debulking and is followed by extracapsular dissection using blunt and sharp microsurgical dissection techniques. Debulking allows the tumor to be 'light' enough so that only gentle countertraction with a slotted suction is needed for dissection. Debulking can be achieved with two suctions working together, one suction and an extended pistol-grip rotatable microscissor, one suction and one ultrasonic aspirator or one suction and a bipolar. All of these variations are identical to those used for microsurgical debulking. Indeed, any technique used during microsurgical resection should be able to be and should be applied to endosurgical resection.

Extracapsular dissection requires even closer cooperation between the endoscopist and dissecting surgeon. As the anatomy deepens and becomes more delicate, instrumentation must be followed into the cavity with a dynamic endoscope. Dissecting microvasculature or cutting arachnoid bands require placement of the endoscope in close proximity with the anatomy in concert with two dissecting instruments. This requires a team that is well-versed and practiced in these techniques.

Finally, hemostasis must be possible in all settings, handling both venous and arterial bleeding both intra- and extradurally. Proper instrumentation, including bipolars, as well as many different hemostatic techniques, are critical for controlling the endoscopic, minimal access surgical field. All techniques are, again, extrapolations of microsurgical techniques.

Reconstruction

As with open skull base approaches, endoscopic endonasal skull base approaches went through an evolution with respect to reconstruction. Many different multilayered, nonvascularized techniques have been described, with varying degrees of success. However, CSF leak rates were unacceptably high and threatened to destroy the applicability of EEA until the development of vascularized flaps, most notably the Hadad-Bassagasteguy-Carrau nasal septal mucosal flap [1]. The development of this flap and its refinement has been critical in endonasal surgery. Several variations of this and other vascularized flaps are discussed at length in later sections of this text, but the concept remains the same. Just as vascularized pericranial flaps provided a huge improvement in reconstructive outcomes for open approaches, these mucosal flaps have led to very acceptable CSF leak rates (in the range of 5%) and robust repairs even for patients who may require high-dose radiation.

This truly has been the Holy Grail in the evolution of EEA techniques. As such, skull base repair and reconstruction with vascularized tissue has become our preferred approach for all but the simplest defects.

Case Selection

Corridor Surgery

EEA provides unparalleled access to the ventral skull base. The introduction of the endoscope has allowed the paranasal sinuses to become a gateway. However, this remains only one approach. The overarching principle in selecting the approach is to avoid crossing the plane of a cranial nerve. Cranial nerves represent the least tolerant structures to manipulation and are responsible for the vast majority of the morbidity in skull base surgery. EEA is an extremely versatile and applicable approach because the majority of tumors arise from the ventral, midline skull base. An anterior, midline approach allows direct access to the tumor without the need for manipulation of critical neurovascular structures. As a result, EEA is *not* a panacea for skull base disease, but rather a tool that greatly expands the anterior corridor options for treating this disease.

Learning Curve

Any new approach or technique has an inherent learning curve. This is especially true when adding a new, often unfamiliar technology. The endoscope is not a familiar instrument to most neurosurgeons. Learning to use it as a visualization device while understanding its position within the often-restricted surgical field presents a unique challenge. In addition, the 'dance' that takes place when two surgeons are operating endoscopically together, in a dynamic fashion, requires even greater practice.

During this time period, it is critical that cases be chosen at the level of the team. Overextending the technique too early in the learning curve can have disastrous consequences. There are clear levels for endoscopic techniques, starting with extradural work, proceeding through intradural work and ending with the 'lateral' coronal plane approaches and vascular lesions. We believe strongly that incremental and stepwise progression is critical to the evolution of endoscopic skill sets. The underlying foundation of all skull base surgery, not just endoscopy, is the principles of cerebrovascular surgery and the management of the Circle of Willis and the large vessels supplying it. This will be covered more in-depth in later chapters.

Patient Comorbidities

In the practice of medicine, nothing is more important than understanding each individual patient's wishes and comorbidities. An approach is only 'minimally invasive' if it limits the impact on that person's life. For example, a chef with a small olfactory groove meningioma may not be a good candidate for an EEA, but rather may prefer an open craniotomy with incomplete resection in favor of preservation of olfaction. Conversely, an elderly patient with a giant olfactory groove meningioma who may not tolerate an open approach and who also does not require a complete resection to relieve his/her symptoms and live out their natural lifespan is an excellent candidate for an EEA, even if the tumor extent reaches beyond what the approach can access. In the end, it is not the radiographic appearance, but rather the patient's appearance and satisfaction that are paramount.

Cross-Specialty Development

Neurosurgery has lagged behind other specialties in the application of endoscopy. The lessons from these other specialties have been slowly applied to allow ventricular endoscopy and keyhole approaches. Without the collaboration of well-trained otolaryngologists and neurosurgeons, the EEAs would have never been developed. This cross-fertilization is the key to the rapid and safe development of new techniques and the application of new technologies.

Reference

1 Hadad G, Bassagasteguy L, Carrau RL, Mataza JC, Kassam A, Snyderman CH, Mintz A: A novel reconstructive technique after endoscopic expanded endonasal approaches: vascular pedicle nasoseptal flap. Laryngoscope 2006;116:1882–1886.

Dr. Amin B. Kassam
Chief, Division of Neurosurgery
The Ottawa Hospital – Civic Campus
1053 Carling Avenue, Box 615
Ottawa, ON K1Y 4E9 (Canada)
E-Mail kassamab@gmail.com

Kassam AB, Gardner PA (eds): Endoscopic Approaches to the Skull Base.
Prog Neurol Surg. Basel, Karger, 2012, vol 26, pp 27–40

Otolaryngology Head and Neck Surgery Approaches

Arif Janjua · Iman Naseri · Ian Witterick · Allan Vescan

Department of Otolaryngology Head and Neck Surgery, University of Toronto, Toronto, Ont., Canada

Abstract

Decisions are made on the fundamental sinus approaches for endonasal access to the skull base and the technical adjuncts that are necessary to optimize the procedure. These include discussions on patient positioning, mucosal decongestion and techniques for improving access including middle turbinate resection, inferior turbinate reduction and septoplasty. Other methods for wider access to the cranial base are also described such as maxillary antrostomy and transpterygoid approach, ethmoidectomy and frontal sinusotomy while emphasizing preservation of sinonasal structures when possible. The necessary technical features are described to facilitate a minimally invasive endonasal approach to the skull base.

The advent of rod-lens endoscopic technology for illumination and visualization of various body cavities via narrow access portals has led to considerable advances in the field of minimally invasive surgery. Several otolaryngologists embraced this technology early in its development and pioneered its use in the field of endoscopic sinonasal surgery. Their work has revolutionized the diagnosis and treatment of rhinologic diseases. In the early-to-mid 1980s, Wigand, Messerklinger, Stammberger and Kennedy developed special instruments and refined many techniques for endoscopic approaches to the paranasal sinuses [1–6]. In the mid-to-late 1990s, otolaryngologists began collaborative efforts with neurosurgeons interested in employing this technology to explore novel, and less invasive approaches to the skull base. Such collaborations marked the beginning of the field of endoscopic skull base surgery [7–10]. Initial clinical application of these endoscopic skills to accessing pituitary lesions allowed for refinements in operative technique. Subsequent integration of modern neuro-navigation systems and creative experimentation with expanded use of this endoscopic technique has led to an extension of the regions of the cranial base which are accessible via the nasal cavities.

Endoscopic exposure of the ventral skull base via the nasal cavities involves the use of sequential intranasal endoscopic dissections to provide adequate visualization and access to the area(s) of interest. We will examine each step separately, and indicate how they may be utilized in conjunction to provide adequate exposure of the skull base for subsequent neurosurgical resection.

Endoscopic Approaches to the Skull Base

General Considerations

There is a fundamental difference between endoscopic sinonasal surgery and dissection within the nasal cavities for endoscopic access to the skull base. The central concept in endoscopic opening of the paranasal sinuses in the setting of chronic sinus disease is the use of minimal tissue dissection to achieve functional sinus aeration. With this in mind, endoscopic sinus surgery involves the removal of the minimal amount of nasal mucosa and bony framework to aerate the sinus while maintaining its native function. When endoscopic access to the skull base is planned, the otolaryngologist within the skull base team must shed this notion and realize that a more extensive dissection and tissue removal is required to obtain appropriate visualization and access for subsequent dual-surgeon ablation of the cranial base lesion. Nonetheless, basic endoscopic principles must be employed to minimize unnecessary mucosal trauma in order to ensure a blood free visualization.

The use of an irrigating sheath may aid in keeping the lens of the endoscope clean without having to remove it from the nasal cavity. This is particularly useful during the sensitive tumor removal stage of the case during which a stable and clear image is essential. Should more substantial bleeding occur that may compromise proper visualization, warm saline irrigation may be employed to irrigate the nasal cavities and to promote hemostasis and improved visualization.

Patient Positioning

During endoscopic skull base surgery, patients are positioned supine on the operating table with their head rigidly stabilized using a Mayfield head holder. The head may be slightly rotated to the right to improve access for the primary surgeon who is positioned to the right of the patient. Depending on the area of the skull base that is to be accessed, the neck may be slightly flexed or extended (fig. 1). Access to the frontal sinuses and the most rostral areas of the cranial base is further achieved via the use of angled endoscopes.

Injection and Mucosal Decongestion

Prior to starting any endoscopic dissection, it is important to decongest the nasal mucosal lining. This may be achieved with the topical application of 1:1,000 epinephrine on ribbon gauze or small neurosurgical patties. Topical epinephrine soaked

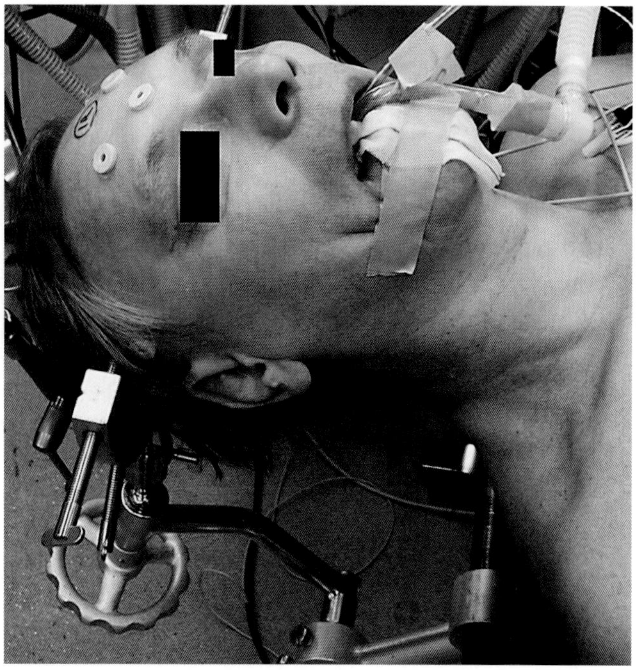

Fig. 1. Patient head positioning and stabilization.

gauze may be inserted into each nasal cavity with a nasal speculum and bayonet forceps prior to immobilizing the patient's head, scrubbing, prepping and draping. In doing so, the topical epinephrine has adequate time to decongest the nasal mucosa. After draping, the ribbon gauze is removed and the nasal cavities inspected with a 0° endoscope.

In preparation for the dissection, the lateral nasal wall, septum and/or middle turbinate(s) are injected with local anesthetic. Several local anesthetic and decongestant regimes have been employed with success. In our institution, the use of 1% lidocaine with 1:200,000 epinephrine has been associated with optimal visualization while minimizing adverse hemodynamic effects on the patient's heart rate and blood pressure [11]. The lateral nasal wall is injected in 2–3 locations just anterior to the attachment of the uncinate process (fig. 2). The area superior to the insertion of each middle turbinate may be separately injected if there are plans to resect them during the course of the procedure. The purpose of middle turbinate resection may be either oncologic or for improved access for instrumentation or exposure. Following injection, topical epinephrine-soaked neurosurgical patties may be placed under endoscopic visualization into the middle meatus for further decongestion of the lateral nasal wall prior to uncinectomy and maxillary antrostomy (if required). Additional patties may be placed on the injection sites or used throughout the case to achieve adequate hemostasis and maintain optimal visualization.

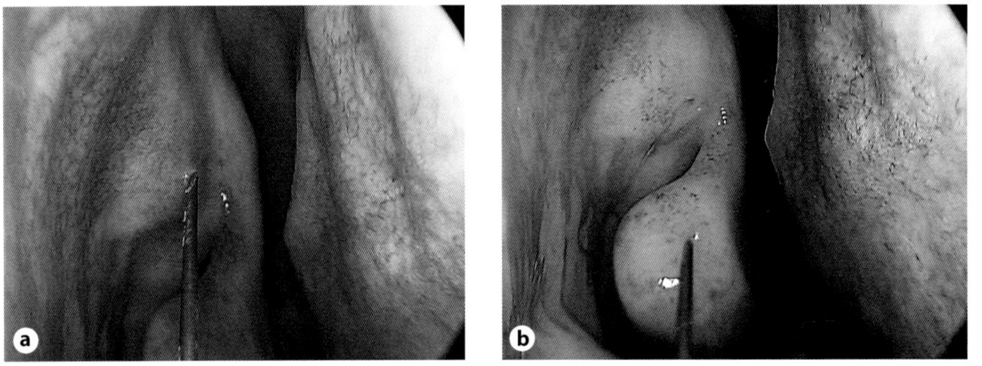

Fig. 2. **a** Local injection of the right lateral nasal wall near the insertion of the middle turbinate. **b** Injection of the right middle turbinate. Note the blanching of the surrounding nasal mucosa indicating infiltration of the vasoconstrictor.

Inferior Turbinate Reduction

The first surgical step is inferior turbinate reduction, a fast and simple way to achieve a significant improvement in access to all sinonasal cavities. Additionally, it allows the use of multiple instruments, providing improved angles of approach through one or both nares. Using a freer elevator, the lateral mucosal side of the inferior turbinate is moved medially with careful consideration to avoid mucosal trauma. Elevation of the inferior turbinate serves to partially destabilize the insertion of the turbinate to the lateral nasal wall. The back side of the freer elevator is then used on the medial mucosal surface of the inferior turbinate to lateralize the structure. Adequate visualization is achieved once one is able to visualize the choana with the endoscope placed anteriorly within the vestibule.

Endoscopic Septoplasty

Deviations in the bony or cartilaginous septum may provide obstruction to instrumentation or visualization throughout the case. If the deflected portions of the septum are posterior, they may be removed during the posterior septectomy section of the skull base access procedure. Several techniques have been previously described for the purpose of achieving functional results [12–14]. For the purpose of our approach to the skull base, deviated segments of the anterior cartilaginous septum are specifically cumbersome if not properly addressed, as they may create a challenge with instrumentation and visualization throughout the case (fig. 3).

In the setting of an anterior cartilaginous deviation, removal of the deviated portion of cartilage may be performed relatively quickly using the endoscope and sinus instruments. The first step in performing an endoscopic septoplasty is the injection of the septal mucosa on the side of the deflection with approximately 1–2 ml of local anesthetic with epinephrine. Decongestion with topical epinephrine-soaked patties is

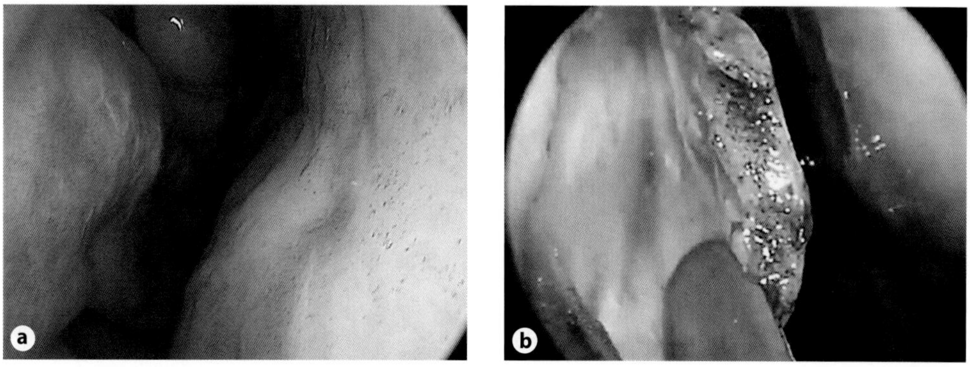

Fig. 3. **a** Left inferior septal deviation with a spur, requiring an endoscopic septoplasty for appropriate visualization and proper use of instrumentation. **b** Elevation of the mucoperichondrial layer during endoscopic septoplasty.

recommended for at least 1 min prior to incision. Using a No. 15 scalpel blade, a vertical incision is made immediately anterior to the deviated segment of septal cartilage. A suction freer is then used to elevate the mucoperichondrium and mucoperiostium off of the deviated portions of cartilage and bone. The sharp edge of the freer elevator is then used to traverse the cartilaginous septum immediately anterior to the deflection. The suction freer is again used to elevate the mucoperichondrium and mucoperiostium off of the contralateral side of the deviated cartilage. Care must be taken to ensure that the elevation occurs in the correct plane as the perichondrium and periostium provides the blood supply to the overlying mucosa. As a result, the correct plane of elevation is relatively avascular. Once the mucoperichondrial and mucoperiosteal layers have been elevated off of both sides of the deviated cartilage and bone, thru-cutting forceps or double-action rongeurs are used to remove the deviated segments of cartilage and/or bone. The flaps may be redraped to determine whether adequate resection has been achieved to appropriately improve visualization. At the conclusion of the case, the two mucosal flaps may be redraped in position, held together by an absorbable suture (e.g. chromic) using a 'quilted' suturing technique or nasal packing may be used depending on surgeon preference.

Resection of the Middle Turbinate

Routinely, the middle turbinate on the side where most of the endoscopic dissection will occur is removed to provide improved access during two-surgeon skull base resections. Some surgeons advocate maintaining both middle turbinates during endoscopic pituitary surgery [15] but many others believe the added visualization and access in the setting of unexpected bleeding or difficult dissection outweighs the benefit. There are several ways to remove the middle turbinate. The important considerations during its removal are the blood supply which enters posteriorly and

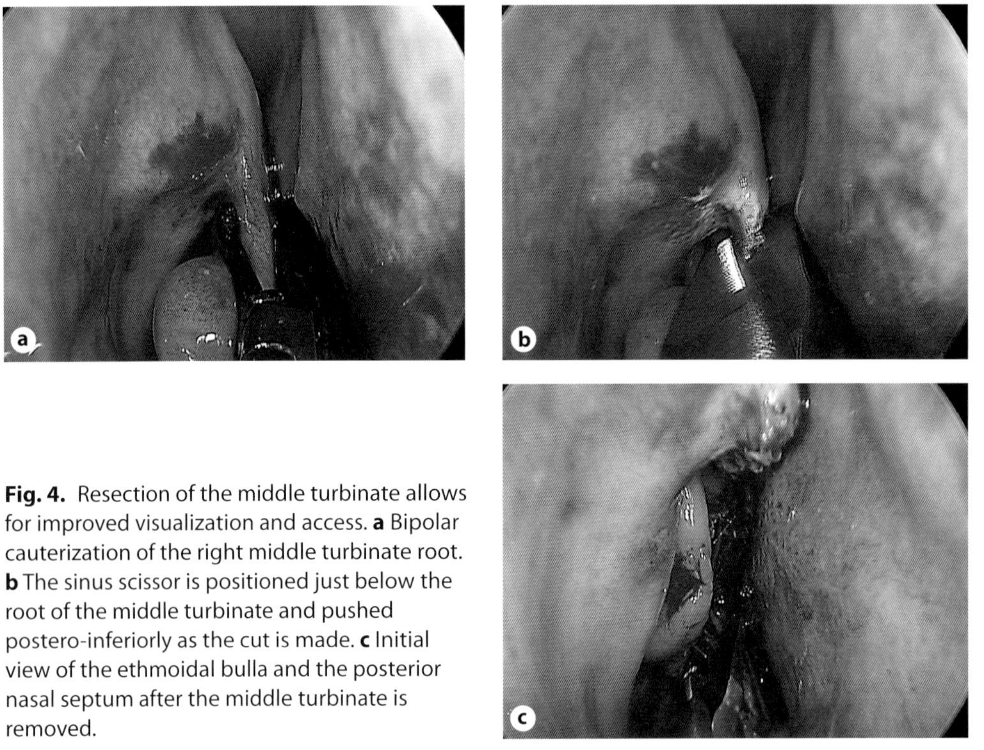

Fig. 4. Resection of the middle turbinate allows for improved visualization and access. **a** Bipolar cauterization of the right middle turbinate root. **b** The sinus scissor is positioned just below the root of the middle turbinate and pushed postero-inferiorly as the cut is made. **c** Initial view of the ethmoidal bulla and the posterior nasal septum after the middle turbinate is removed.

the orientation of the attachment of the different portions of the middle turbinate to the skull base and lateral nasal wall. In our centre, bipolar cautery is used prior to resection of the turbinate to minimize mucosal bleeding and potential compromise of visualization. Care must be taken to maintain a short stump of the turbinate anteriorly so it can be used as a surgical landmark during the remainder of the dissection. Following cauterization, endoscopic scissors can be used to resect the turbinate. After the initial cut, the scissors may be held partially open and dragged posteriorly and inferiorly (fig. 4). Upon doing so, the middle turbinate usually detaches itself from its insertion along the lateral nasal wall and becomes pedicled on a narrow stalk posteriorly, which includes its arterial supply from a branch of the sphenopalatine artery. This stalk is then cauterized with the bipolar, and the turbinate removed. Care should be taken to ensure that the turbinate is resected with minimal mucosal damage so the mucosa may be removed from the underlying bony framework and utilized as subsequent graft material, if needed.

Maxillary Antrostomy

Although rarely required for access to the cranial base, a maxillary antrostomy may be routinely performed as it provides exposure to several surgical landmarks. In addition, impairment of normal sinus function may occur postoperatively if the maxillary

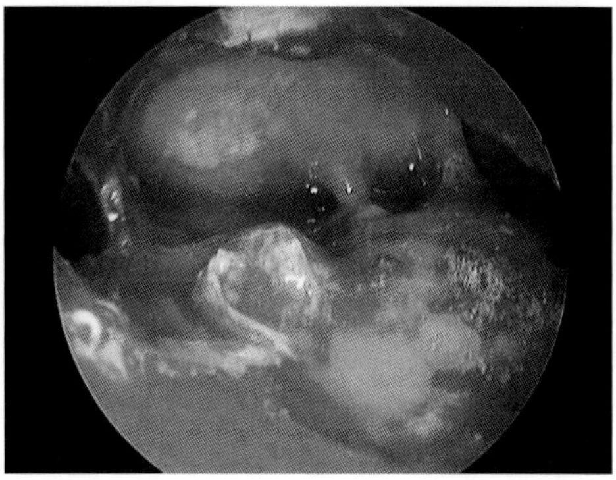

Fig. 5. Angled endoscopic visualization of the frontal sinus after a Draf 3 procedure.

sinus is not adequately aerated. Furthermore, in the setting of a clival lesion, an antrostomy may be used to house a posteriorly pedicled septal mucosal flap, which may be harvested at the beginning of the procedure. During the tumor extirpation phase of the surgery, the flap may be temporarily stored either in the maxillary sinus or pushed into the nasopharynx, thereby allowing protection from instrument damage. Harvest of this septal flap is not described here, as it is the major focus of the reconstruction chapter found later in this volume.

The first step in performing the antrostomy is identification of the margins of the uncinate process. This may be removed in several ways. One method involves identification of the anterior margin of the vertical uncinate process and dissection along this anterior border, performed with a freer elevator or sickle knife. Careful attention should be given to the orientation of the vertical segment of the uncinate process as the dissection is carried inferiorly. The uncinate process is sickle-shaped and thus the anterior border of the inferior portion extends posteriorly into a horizontal plane. A straight pair of Wilde's forceps may then be used to divide the superior and inferior attachments such that the uncinate can be removed in one piece. A second method uses a backbiter to remove the uncinate process. With any method, but particularly with the sickle knife, care is required not to lacerate the adjacent periorbita.

Removal of the uncinate process normally reveals the natural maxillary ostium, in addition to an anterior accessory ostium along the lateral nasal wall. Back-biting forceps and straight thru-cut forceps may then be used to enlarge the antrostomy as required to visualize the orbital floor and posterior wall of the maxillary sinus, which are important landmarks for the remainder of the dissection.

At this point, one must start to tailor the subsequent dissection steps to the location of the mass lesion. Should a frontal sinusotomy or extended Draf procedure [16] be required (fig. 5), it is often advantageous to identify the frontal sinus ostia with the ethmoid bulla in place. If the lesion is located further posteriorly within the cranial base, and does not require frontal sinus work, an ethmoidectomy is recommended. We will review each of these steps in detail and allow the reader to employ them in the correct order as the situation dictates.

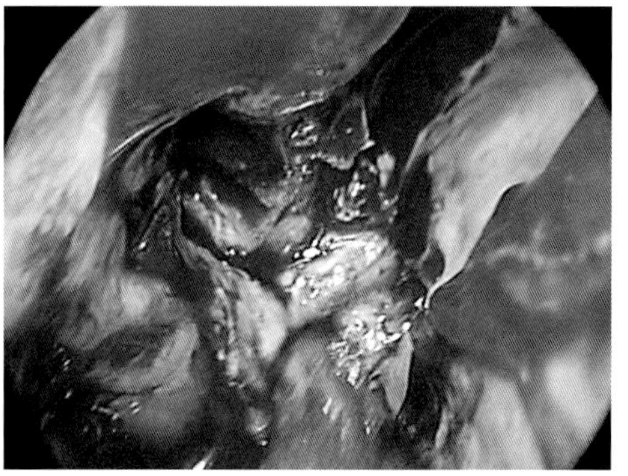

Fig. 6. Ligation of the left sphenopalatine artery by cauterization and/or clip application.

Ethmoidectomy

A straight curette is used to enter the ethmoid bulla via its anterior or inferior face. A pair of up-biting Wilde's forceps is used to remove the bony walls of the ethmoid bulla. Once the posterior wall of the bulla is removed, one will encounter the basal lamella of the middle turbinate. This oblique portion of the middle turbinate attaches laterally to the lamina and separates the anterior and posterior ethmoid air cells. The basal lamella can be traversed with a straight curette and a dissection of the posterior ethmoid air cells may be undertaken in a similar fashion. Removal of all of the bony walls of the posterior ethmoid air cells should allow visualization of the superior turbinate and the anterior face of the sphenoid sinus. Additionally, it is important to follow the ethmoid septations superiorly to the skull base and ensure their complete removal. In doing so, the entirety of the ethmoid roof is exposed for subsequent dissection along the slope of the skull base.

Sphenopalatine Artery Ligation

In performing a wide sphenoidotomy, one may encounter the posterior septal branch of the sphenopalatine artery (SPA) as it crosses the anterior face of the sphenoid sinus, at a level between the choana and the natural sphenoid ostium (fig. 6). After an adequate maxillary antrostomy, the anterior-posterior position of the SPA can often be located immediately behind the posterior wall of the maxillary sinus. Its superior-inferior position is between the roof of the inferior turbinate and the remaining stump of the posterior attachment of the middle turbinate to the lateral nasal wall. A sharp freer elevator is used to make a vertical incision in the mucosa of the lateral wall of the nose immediately anterior to the position of the posterior wall of the maxillary sinus. The freer can then be utilized to elevate the mucosa off of the bony lateral nasal wall. At this point, a small bony projection called the crista ethmoidalis can be routinely identified. The SPA may be a single trunk or have a variable branching in this position. The branch(es) of the SPA are located immediately posterior and inferior to the crista ethmoidalis. Elevation of the mucosa, superior and inferior to this structure

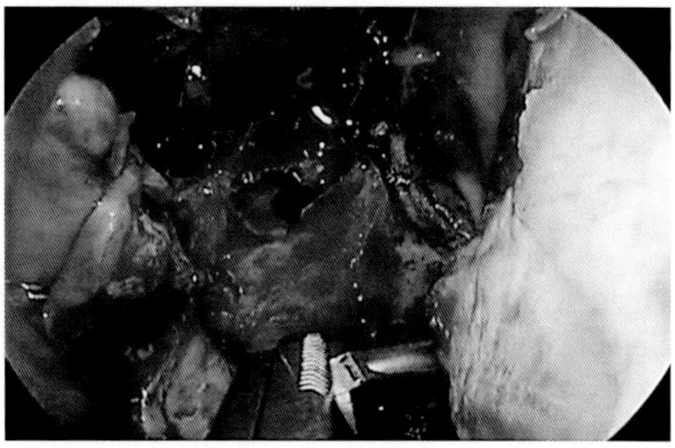

Fig. 7. Bimanual instrumentation access is significantly improved after removal of the posterior nasal septum.

allows for adequate exposure of the artery and often makes the visibility of these arteries easier as they may be stretched by subsequent manipulation. Prior to cautery or clip ligation, the crista ethmoidalis may be removed with a fine Kerrison punch. This improves visualization and access for ligation/cauterization. A bipolar cautery is often used to control the branches of the SPA or alternatively, an endoscopic clip applicator may be used. Should a bipolar be solely used, it is best to first bipolar the vessel, and then cut half of its circumference, followed by a final bipolar cauterization of the vessel prior to its complete transection. This maneuver will minimize resultant bleeding.

Posterior Septectomy and Sphenoidotomy

Access to sellar, parasellar or clival lesions requires a wide, common sphenoidotomy. The first step in creating a wide common sphenoid opening is disarticulating the posterior margin of the bony nasal septum from the rostrum of the sphenoid (fig. 7). A freer elevator is used to traverse the bony septum just anterior to the rostrum of the sphenoid. Upon moving the posterior margin of the septum, one will be able to visualize both sphenoid ostia separated by the rostrum. Back-biting forceps may then be used to remove the posterior portion of the nasal septum. Routinely, approximately 1–2 cm of the posterior septum must be removed. This step is essential to ensure adequate visualization and room for instrumentation during the two-surgeon skull base dissection.

Prior to enlarging the individual sphenoid ostia, care must be taken cauterize the mucosa of the anterior face of the sphenoid sinus (between the ostium and choana) to prevent bleeding from the posterior septal branch. Subsequently, a pair of thru-cutting forceps may be used to remove the superior turbinate(s) on each side and widely expose the anterior face of the sphenoid sinus, separated at the midline by the rostrum. Wide opening of the natural sphenoid ostia inferiorly on each side is recommended. The lateral aspect of the anterior wall of the sphenoid may also be removed to allow visualization of the optico-carotid recess. Removal of the rostrum may require the use of a high speed drill. Upon removal of the sphenoid rostrum, a

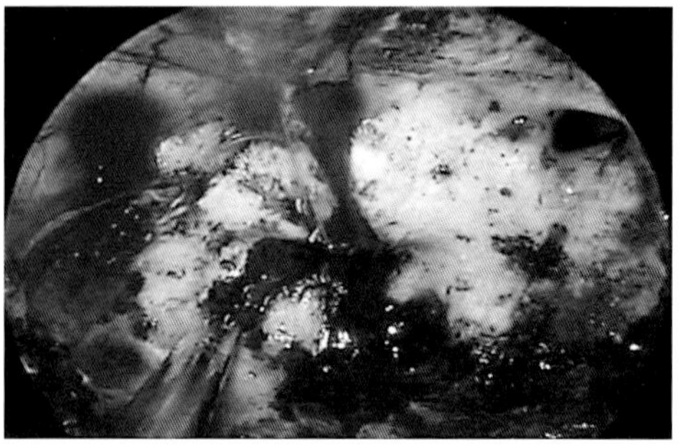

Fig. 8. Endoscopic view of the sphenoid sinus demonstrating the wide access spanning from each orbital wall, with the sella, optic and optico-carotid recess.

common sphenoid cavity is created. Thru-cutting forceps or the drill may be used to remove the inter-sinus septations such that they are flush with the posterior wall of the sphenoid sinus (fig. 8). Attention should be given to the position of the sphenoid inter-sinus septations on preoperative imaging. Para-sagittal septations can run posteriorly onto the carotid arteries. Exposure and identification of the carotid arteries, optic nerves and the sella is imperative prior to instrumentation of the posterior wall of the sphenoid sinus.

If there is a need to gain access to a lesion involving the clivus, removal of the floor of the sphenoid sinus will be required and may be accomplished with the use of a high-speed drill. The floor is removed such that posterior wall of the sphenoid is continuous with the nasopharynx. Further removal of the nasopharyngeal soft tissues may be achieved with a microdebrider or a large Kerrison rongeur. Such an exposure of the sphenoid sinus cavity for clival lesions allows for safe identification of the carotids superiorly.

Transpterygoid Approach

In cases involving pathology within the lateral recess of the sphenoid sinus, a transpterygoid approach is often required to achieve adequate visualization and access. The transpterygoid exposure is also the initial step in accessing the pterygopalatine fossa and the infra-temporal fossa (fig. 9).

The first step in gaining access to the lateral recess of the sphenoid sinus is removal of the medial aspect of the posterior wall of the maxillary sinus. This may be accomplished with Kerrison forceps or a high-speed drill. Removal of the posterior wall of the maxillary sinus will expose the vascular origin of the SPA, and the internal maxillary artery. Exposure posterior to the internal maxillary artery reveals the pterygoid canal and the anterior surface of the pterygoid processes. Endoscopic surgical access to the lateral recess of the sphenoid requires removal of the medial root of the pterygoid plates, also known as the pterygoid 'wedge' [17–19]. This forms the infero-lateral boundary of the previously established common sphenoid opening. Removal of this thick bony wedge of bone provides direct access to the lateral recess of the sphenoid

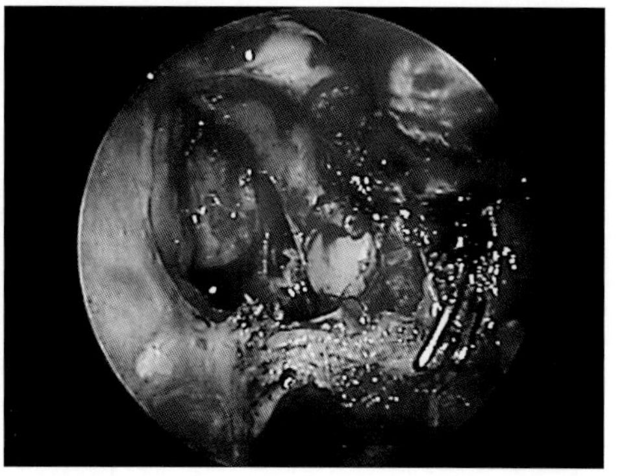

Fig. 9. A left transpterygoid access showing the clips on the ligated sphenopalatine artery.

sinus. Of particular note, the vidian nerve and artery pass through the pterygoid canal. The vidian artery originates from the lacerum (horizontal) segment of the internal carotid artery and runs through the pterygoid canal en route to the pterygopalatine fossa. Proper care must be taken to control possible bleeding from the vidian artery during removal of the pterygoid wedge and one must remember its important relationship to the carotid artery.

Expanded Frontal Sinusotomies

Access to lesions involving the more anterior portions of the skull base may involve identification and enlargement of the frontal sinus ostia. Combined with the resection of the superior aspect of the nasal septum, widening the frontal sinus ostia creates a common frontal sinus opening accessible from both nares (fig. 5). This creates a surgical corridor for endoscopically assisted visualization and instrumentation of the posterior wall of the frontal sinus in continuity with the cribriform plates.

Because of the anatomic variability and complexity of the frontal sinus surgical anatomy, careful review and knowledge of the preoperative imaging is vital for identification of the drainage pattern of the frontal sinuses and the location of the various air cells lining its outflow tract [20–24]. The most common arrangement involves an agger nasi cell that forms the anterior boundary of the frontal recess accompanied by a variable number of fronto-ethmoidal air cells lining the path to the frontal sinus ostium.

Identification of the native frontal sinus ostium is performed using angled nasal endoscopes using various techniques [25–30]. A 30, 45 or 70° endoscope may be used to provide visualization of the anterior-superior region of the nasal cavity. The ethmoid bulla, if it has not been previously removed, may be used as useful landmark for identification of the frontal sinus ostium. The mucosa on the anterior surface of the ethmoid bulla forms the posterior margin of the frontal sinus outflow tract. With this knowledge, a frontal sinus probe or curved image-guided suction, may be placed immediately anterior to the bulla and used to seek superiorly to allow identification of the natural ostium of the frontal sinus. Upon identification of this ostium, a curette may be used to dissect the anteriorly located agger nasi cell(s), and potentially the other fronto-ethmoidal cells. This allows better visualization of the native frontal sinus ostium. Upon removal of the agger nasi and fronto-ethmoidal cells lining the anterior aspect of the frontal recess, visualization of the floor of the frontal sinus improves. This dissection constitutes a simple, or Draf type 1, frontal sinusotomy [16].

For mass lesions involving the anterior-most portions of the skull base, expansion of the bilateral simple frontal sinusotomies into a common frontal sinus drainage pathway is required (Draf type 3; fig. 5). The initial step in the creation of this common pathway is the creation of a superior septal window between the anterior ends of the middle turbinate. Care must be taken to ensure that the septal window extends anterior to the anterior ends of the middle turbinate and low enough that the area of the insertion of each turbinate (axilla) may be accessed from either nare. This septal window may be created with a microdebrider to remove the mucosa and a freer elevator to remove the bony and cartilaginous portions of the septum.

The subsequent steps in the dissection require the use of a high-speed drill. First, the frontal process of the maxillary bone can be drilled superiorly such that the axilla does not hood the frontal sinus ostia. Upon removal of the bone superior to the axilla, a cutting or coarse drill burr may be used to enlarge each frontal sinus ostium anteriorly. The hard bone encountered when attempting to extend the frontal sinusotomy anteriorly is known as the frontal 'beak'. The aim at this stage is to bring the anterior wall of the frontal sinus flush with the anterior portion of the nasal cavity, such that the frontal 'beak' is eliminated. The limit of the anterior dissection is the soft tissues of the nasal dorsum. Some surgeons routinely expose a small area of skin on either side to ensure they are achieving the widest anterior-posterior dimension of the new common frontal sinus drainage pathway. Once completely extended anteriorly, drilling of the medial floor of the frontal sinuses is undertaken until such time as the frontal intersinus septum is reached. The drill, or Kerrison punch, may be used to remove the inter-sinus septum as high as possible.

Careful note must be made of the direction of enlargement of the frontal sinus openings. The two frontal sinusotomies are not simply joined by drilling in a medial direction. The natural ostia of the frontal sinuses are located postero-medially within the floor of the sinuses and simply joining these through medial dissection would like result in the violation of the lateral lamella of the cribriform plate and resultant entry in the anterior cranial fossa. The shape of the common frontal sinus opening is that of a crescent. Prior to completion of the procedure, the anterior-posterior dimension of the common opening may be maximized by using a high-speed drill to carefully smooth any forward projections of the posterior wall of the frontal sinuses.

At the conclusion of the dissection, one has attained a contiguous view of the bilateral posterior walls of the frontal sinuses and the adjacent cribriform areas (fig. 5). This view provides adequate exposure for an anterior skull base osteotomy with an appropriate margin from the anterior extent of the mass lesion in question.

Conclusion

Endoscopic access for lesions involving the skull base requires a systematic surgical technique, coupled with careful planning and the proper instrumentation. This expanded endonasal approach uses many of the techniques and principles used by many otolaryngologists in functional endoscopic sinus surgery. In contrast, one encounters greater anatomic variability and a higher risk in such expanded approaches to the skull base. Therefore, careful consideration must be given to the creation of adequate space for dual-surgeon instrumentation, in addition to exposure of the relevant sinonasal landmarks with associated neurovascular structures. Endoscopic opening of the frontal sinus, exposure of the ethmoid roof and wide common sphenoid access provide corridors through which to access the cribriform region, planum sphenoidale and sella turcica. Furthermore, access to the lateral sphenoid recess and the petrous apex may be achieved through a transpterygoid dissection. Access to clival lesions may be achieved through removal of the nasopharyngeal soft tissue. The lower limit of this clival dissection is limited only by endoscopic visualization and lack of access for instrumentation below the posterior margin of the hard palate. The surgical techniques and principles described above may serve as a blueprint to guide and encourage otolaryngologists through a systematic process allowing an unprecedented minimally invasive endonasal approach to lesions involving the skull base.

References

1 Kennedy DW: Functional endoscopic sinus surgery: technique. Arch Otolaryngol 1985;111:643–649.
2 Messerklinger W: Diagnosis and endoscopic surgery of the nose and its adjoining structures. Acta Otorhinolaryngol Belg 1980;34:170–176.
3 Stammberger H: Endoscopic endonasal surgery – concepts in treatment of recurring rhinosinusitis. I. Anatomic and pathophysiologic considerations. Otolaryngol Head Neck Surg 1986;94:143–147.
4 Stammberger H: Endoscopic endonasal surgery – concepts in treatment of recurring rhinosinusitis. II. Surgical technique. Otolaryngol Head Neck Surg 1986;94:147–156.
5 Stammberger H, Posawetz W: Functional endoscopic sinus surgery: concept, indications and results of the Messerklinger technique. Eur Arch Otorhinolaryngol 1990;247:63–76.
6 Wigand ME: Transnasal ethmoidectomy under endoscopical control. Rhinology 1981;19:7–15.
7 Carrau RL, Jho HD, Ko Y: Transnasal-transsphenoidal endoscopic surgery of the pituitary gland. Laryngoscope 1996;106:914–918.
8 Jho HD, Carrau RL: Endoscopy assisted transsphenoidal surgery for pituitary adenoma: technical note. Acta Neurochir (Wien) 1996;138:1416–1425.
9 Jho HD, Carrau RL, Ko Y, Daly MA: Endoscopic pituitary surgery: an early experience. Surg Neurol 1997;47:213–222; discussion 222–223.

10 Jho HD, Carrau RL, McLaughlin MR, Somaza SC: Endoscopic transsphenoidal resection of a large chordoma in the posterior fossa. Acta Neurochir (Wien) 1997;139:343–347; discussion 347–348.
11 Cohen-Kerem R, Brown S, Villasenor LV, Witterick I: Epinephrine/lidocaine injection vs. saline during endoscopic sinus surgery. Laryngoscope 2008;118: 1275–1281.
12 Bothra R, Mathur NN: Comparative evaluation of conventional versus endoscopic septoplasty for limited septal deviation and spur. J Laryngol Otol 2009;123:737–741.
13 Castelnuovo P, Pagella F, Cerniglia M, Emanuelli E: Endoscopic limited septoplasty in combination with sinonasal surgery. Facial Plast Surg 1999;15:303–307.
14 Hwang PH, McLaughlin RB, Lanza DC, Kennedy DW: Endoscopic septoplasty: indications, technique, and results. Otolaryngol Head Neck Surg 1999;120:678–682.
15 de Divitiis E, Cappabianca P, Cavallo LM: Endoscopic transsphenoidal approach: adaptability of the procedure to different sellar lesions. Neurosurgery 2002; 51:699–705; discussion 706–707.
16 Draf W, Weber R, Keerl R, Constantinidis J: Current aspects of frontal sinus surgery. I. Endonasal frontal sinus drainage in inflammatory diseases of the paranasal sinuses. HNO 1995;43:352–357.
17 Kassam A, Thomas AJ, Snyderman C, et al: Fully endoscopic expanded endonasal approach treating skull base lesions in pediatric patients. J Neurosurg 2007;106:75–86.
18 Kassam AB, Vescan AD, Carrau RL, et al: Expanded endonasal approach: vidian canal as a landmark to the petrous internal carotid artery. J Neurosurg 2008;108:177–183.
19 Vescan AD, Snyderman CH, Carrau RL, et al: Vidian canal: analysis and relationship to the internal carotid artery. Laryngoscope 2007;117:1338–1342.
20 Wang Y, Zhang K: Applied anatomy of the ostium of frontal sinus and the nasofrontal duct. Lin Chuang Er Bi Yan Hou Ke Za Zhi 1998;12:164–167.
21 McLaughlin RB, Jr., Rehl RM, Lanza DC: Clinically relevant frontal sinus anatomy and physiology. Otolaryngol Clin North Am 2001;34:1–22.
22 Lothrop HA VI: The anatomy and surgery of the frontal sinus and anterior ethmoidal Cells. Ann Surg 1899;29:175–217.
23 Kew J, Rees GL, Close D, Sdralis T, Sebben RA, Wormald PJ: Multiplanar reconstructed computed tomography images improves depiction and understanding of the anatomy of the frontal sinus and recess. Am J Rhinol 2002;16:119–123.
24 Iinuma T, Ikeda T, Kase Y, Kuriyama J, Yamane M, Ichimura K: Surgical anatomy of the so-called dangerous frontal sinus (Boenninghaus). Nippon Jibiinkoka Gakkai Kaiho 1990;93:18–22.
25 Carrau RL, Snyderman CH, Curtin HB, Weissman JL: Computer-assisted frontal sinusotomy. Otolaryngol Head Neck Surg 1994;111:727–732.
26 Close LG, Lee NK, Leach JL, Manning SC: Endoscopic resection of the intranasal frontal sinus floor. Ann Otol Rhinol Laryngol 1994;103:952–958.
27 Har-El G, Lucente FE: Endoscopic intranasal frontal sinusotomy. Laryngoscope 1995;105:440–443.
28 Loury MC: Endoscopic frontal recess and frontal sinus ostium dissection. Laryngoscope 1993;103: 455–458.
29 Moriyama H: The technique of endoscopic surgery and diagnosis of frontal recess and sinus disease under local anesthesia. J Otolaryngol 1991;20:382–384.
30 Schaefer SD, Close LG: Endoscopic management of frontal sinus disease. Laryngoscope 1990;100:155–160.

Dr. Allan D. Vescan
Department of Otolaryngology Head and Neck Surgery
Mount Sinai Hospital, 600 University Avenue, Suite 401
Toronto, ON M5G 1X5 (Canada)
Tel. +1 416 586 4439, E-Mail avescan@mtsinai.on.ca

Kassam AB, Gardner PA (eds): Endoscopic Approaches to the Skull Base.
Prog Neurol Surg. Basel, Karger, 2012, vol 26, pp 41–59

Sellar/Tuberculum Approach

Paolo Cappabianca · Luigi Maria Cavallo ·
Isabella Esposito · Domenico Solari

Università degli Studi di Napoli Federico II, Division of Neurosurgery, Napoli, Italy

Abstract

Background: Extending the transsphenoidal approach has allowed its increasing use for suprasellar pathologies. The addition of the endoscope has further advanced this approach. **Methods:** To describe the endoscopic transsphenoidal approach to the sella and suprasellar regions from nasal phase to reconstruction. **Results:** The endoscopic endonasal transsphenoidal transtuberculum-transplanum approach to the suprasellar area provides direct access for large or fibrotic pituitary adenomas, suprasellar Rathke's cleft cysts and meningiomas and craniopharyngiomas. The use of two surgeons allows for bimanual dissection and thereby maintains the advantages of a craniotomy while employing a less invasive approach to this region. This and other techniques for safely performing this approach are presented and reviewed. **Conclusions:** The endoscopic endonasal transsphenoidal approach to the suprasellar region provides direct access for many tumor types. Bleeding and reconstruction concerns can be overcome by an experienced team.

The transsphenoidal technique is currently the most used procedure for the treatment of lesions involving the sellar area especially pituitary adenomas. The endoscopic transsphenoidal approach represents a minimally invasive route commonly used in many centers throughout the world, under the same indications as the conventional microsurgical technique [1]. The endoscopic approach provides some advantages from the use of the endoscope itself and from the absence of the transsphenoidal retractor. As a matter of fact, the endoscope provides the surgeon with an increased panoramic, close-up view of the surgical area [2], thus reducing surgical trauma and complication rates [3]. Two main procedures can be considered: the standard approach to the sellar area and the extended or expanded transtuberculum-transplanum approach to the suprasellar compartment, both with their respective peculiarities.

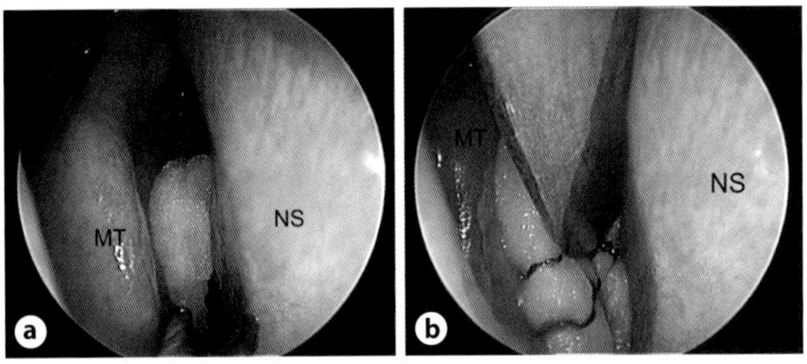

Fig. 1. Right nostril approach. Nasal phase of the procedure. **a** Positioning of a cottonoid between the middle turbinate and the nasal septum. **b** Lateralization of the middle turbinate with an elevator and exposure of the spheno-ethmoid recess. NS = Nasal septum; MT = middle turbinate.

Standard Endoscopic Endonasal Transsphenoidal Approach to the Sella

The standard endoscopic endonasal transsphenoidal approach to the sella requires different instrumentation from that used during microsurgical procedures, from the endoscope with its related components to dedicated straight, non-bayonet instruments.

The patient is under general anesthesia with orotracheal intubation in the supine position with the trunk elevated 10° and the head turned 10° toward the surgeon fixed with tape on a horseshoe headrest. Just before introducing the endoscope, the nasal cavities are packed with pledgets soaked in a diluted solution of 5% chlorhexidine gluconate; the face and the nose are prepped with the same agent and then the patient is aseptically draped.

The procedure consists of three main aspects, i.e. exposure of the lesion, removal of the relevant pathology and reconstruction of the sella, that are addressed through three different steps: the nasal, the sphenoid and the sellar phases. In the first two steps, the corridor to the lesion and the room to work comfortably are created and adapted to the need of each single case. In the sellar phase, the lesion is removed and the tailored reconstruction of the sellar area is realized.

Nasal Phase

As soon as a rigid 0° endoscope, 18 cm in length, 4 mm in diameter (Karl Storz® & Co, Tuttlingen, Germany) is introduced through the chosen nostril (usually the right), it becomes possible to identify the main anatomic landmarks such as the inferior turbinate laterally and the nasal septum medially. Moving deeper, following the tail of the inferior turbinate, it is possible to reach the choana, limited medially by the vomer (a midline landmark) and superiorly by the floor of the sphenoid sinus. Cottonoid pledgets soaked with diluted adrenaline (1:100,000) or with xylometazoline hydrochloride are positioned between the middle turbinate and the nasal septum (fig. 1a, b) and once the nasal mucosa seems to be decongested and bloodless (the

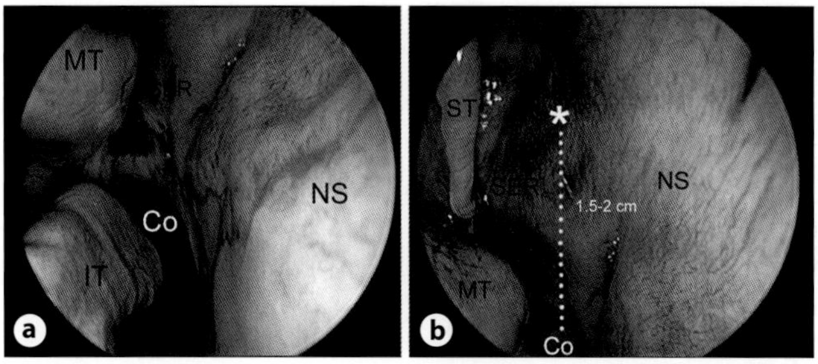

Fig. 2. Right nostril approach. Nasal phase of the procedure. **a** Exploration of the posterior part of the nasal cavity and identification of the choana. **b** Localization of the sphenoid sinus. Starting from the choana and ascending the endoscope along the spheno-ethmoid recess for about 1.5–2 cm, the sphenoid sinus is reached. The asterisk represents the key point to enter into the sphenoid sinus. NS = Nasal septum; MT = middle turbinate; SER = spheno-ethmoid recess; Co = choana; ST = superior turbinate; SO = sphenoid ostium.

anesthesiologists could play a significant role), the middle turbinate is gently pushed laterally to enlarge the surgical corridor between the nasal septum and the middle turbinate (fig. 2a). Looking superiorly with the endoscope, the sphenoid ostium, usually located approximately 1.5 cm above the roof of the choana, can be identified. If the sphenoid ostium is covered by either the superior or the supreme turbinate these can be gently lateralized or removed, protecting the lateral lamella of the cribriform plate on which they are inserted (fig. 2b). Much care should be taken during the removal or the lateral luxation of these turbinates in order to avoid ethmoidal plate injuries resulting in cerebrospinal fluid (CSF) leak. It is not mandatory to see the sphenoid ostium; once the choana is identified after ascending along the sphenoethmoid recess for approximately 1–1.5 cm, access to the sphenoid cavity can be achieved using a blunt instrument.

Sphenoid Phase

This part of the procedure starts with the coagulation of the sphenoethmoid recess and the area around the sphenoid ostium in order to avoid arterial bleeding from septal branches of the sphenopalatine artery (fig. 3a, b). By means of a microdrill with a cutting and/or a diamond burr (Ø: 4–5 mm), the nasal septum is detached from the sphenoid rostrum (fig. 3c). Subsequently, the anterior wall of the sphenoid sinus is widely opened with microdrill and/or bone punches, proceeding circumferentially taking care to not overextend the opening in the inferolateral direction where the sphenopalatine artery or its major branches lie (fig. 3c, d). Sometimes, the removal of the posterior part of the nasal septum is performed to obtain a wider working space, thus facilitating a two-nostril, four-handed approach [4]. Finally, the removal of all of the sphenoid septae is required to expose the anatomical landmarks inside the sphenoid cavity. After such a maneuver, the posterior and lateral walls of the sphenoid sinus, with the sellar floor at the center, the sphenoethmoid planum above it, and the

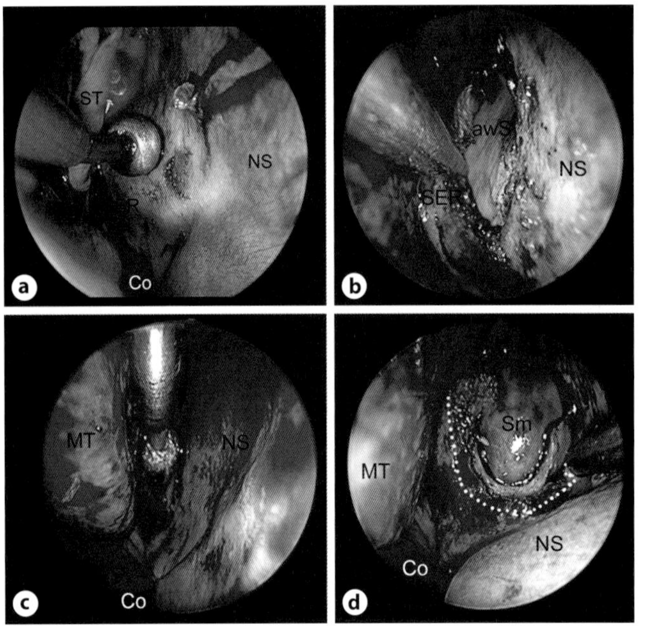

Fig. 3. Right nostril approach. Sphenoid phase of the procedure. **a** Coagulation of the spheno-ethmoid recess by means of a monopolar electrode. **b** Elevation of the mucosa and exposure of the anterior wall of the sphenoid sinus. **c** Elevation of the nasal septum from the sphenoid rostrum by means of a microdrill with diamond burr. **d** Exposure of the anterior wall of the sphenoid sinus. The white dotted line shows the border of the mucosa that has to be coagulated with bipolar forceps to prevent bleeding from nasopalatine branch of the sphenopalatine artery. NS = Nasal septum; MT = middle turbinate; SER = spheno-ethmoid recess; ST = superior turbinate; SO = sphenoid ostium; awS = anterior wall of the sphenoid sinus: Sm = sphenoid mucosa; Co = choana.

clival indentation below, become visible (fig. 4). Lateral to the sellar floor, the bony prominences of the intracavernous carotid artery, the optic nerve and, between them, the optico-carotid recess can be observed. Although in some cases the identification of each anatomical landmark is not possible, at least the bony protuberances of the intracavernous carotid artery should be recognized to define the sellar floor boundaries. Furthermore, in the presence of a presellar or a conchal sphenoid sinus, where there will be a paucity of anatomic landmarks, the image-guidance neuronavigation system could be very useful to guide the procedure.

Sellar Phase

From this phase of the procedure, the endoscope can be fixed to the holder, in order to free both of the surgeon's hands and allow comfortable introduction of two instruments under the endoscope without coming into conflict with it. However, it is our practice to continue using the endoscope free-hand, held dynamically by an assistant, while the surgeon moves the two instruments through one or both nostrils. In the case of a bilateral approach, the removal of a limited portion of the posterior nasal

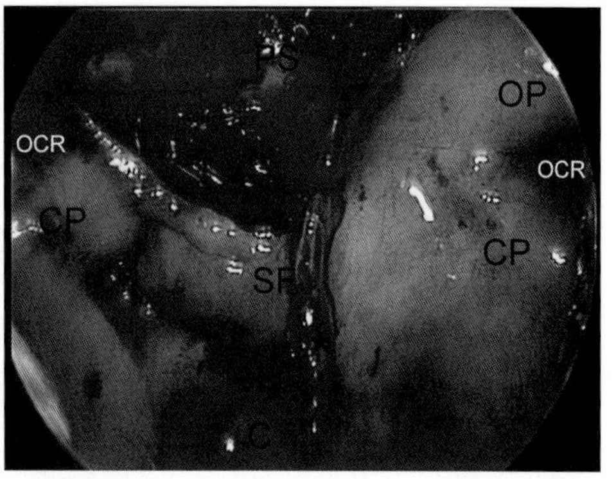

Fig. 4. Right nostril approach. Sphenoid phase of the procedure. Identification of the landmarks inside the sphenoid sinus. SF = Sellar floor; CP = carotid protuberance; C = clivus; PS = planum sphenoidale; OP = optic protuberance; OCR = opto-carotid recess; * sphenoid septum partially removed.

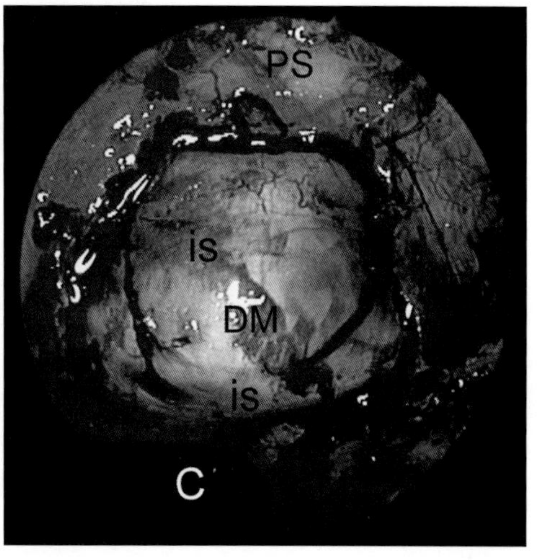

Fig. 5. Sellar phase of the procedure. Identification of the superior and inferior intercavernous sinus after the opening of the sellar floor in a case of a microadenoma. DM = Dura mater; is = intercavernous sinus; C = clivus; PS = planum sphenoidale.

septum could ease the introduction and maneuverability of the instruments through both nostrils.

The sellar phase of the procedure follows the same rules as the microsurgical transsphenoidal approach. Sellar floor opening is performed using a high-speed microdrill and Kerrison rongeur or Stammberger circular cutting punch® as needed according to the sellar floor thickness. Bone removal is usually extended from one cavernous sinus to the other and from the tuberculum to the floor of the sella, although its shape and size could be tailored depending on lesion removal needs (fig. 5). During such maneuvers, an ultrasound Doppler probe could be helpful for the identification of the carotid arteries [5], thus allowing a safer opening of the dura that thereafter is incised in a midline position in a linear, rectangular, or cruciate fashion. A small dural incision is initially performed in order to avoid damaging the superior and/or inferior intercavernous sinuses; once such venous structures become visible they

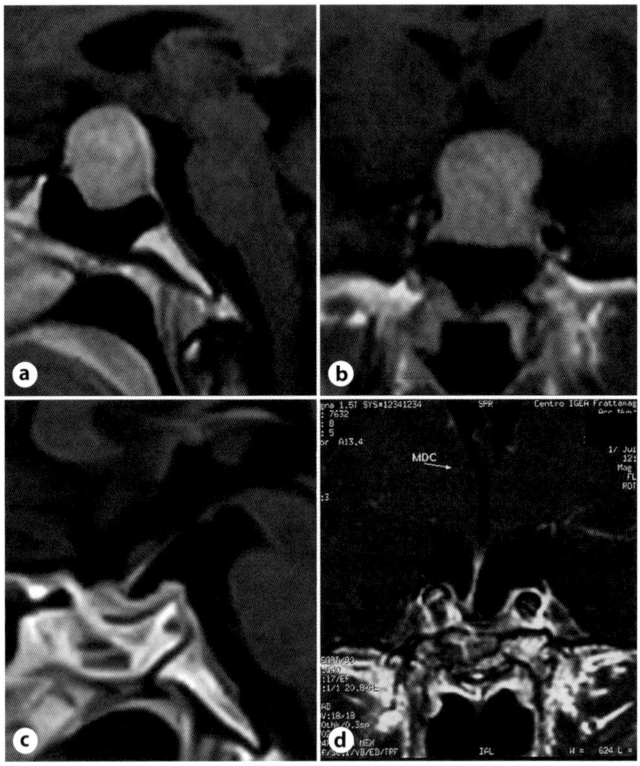

Fig. 6. a, b Preoperative MRI showing a case of intra-suprasellar nonfunctioning macroadenoma. **c, d** Postoperative MRI demonstrating the gross total removal of the lesion.

will be sealed with bipolar coagulation forceps and the dural incision can continue. Further dural bleeding, if any, can be controlled by gentle pressure or with hemostatic agents and the dural edges should be coagulated with bipolar forceps. It is now safe to begin lesion removal. In the case of macroadenoma (fig. 6), the inferior and lateral components of the lesion should be removed before the superior aspect. Indeed, the removal of the superior part first will prematurely let the suprasellar cistern and the redundant diaphragma fall into the operative field, thus reducing the possibility to expose and remove the lateral portions of the lesion (fig. 7). Nevertheless, if the descent of the suprasellar portion of the lesion is not observed, a Valsalva maneuver could be useful, providing the protrusion of the suprasellar cistern into the sellar cavity. Lesions involving the medial wall of the cavernous sinus can be removed as well under endoscopic control (fig. 8); as a matter of fact, the potential venous bleeding can be easily controlled by positioning hemostatic agents and cottonoids, by gentle compression of the medial wall of the cavernous sinus and irrigation with saline for a few minutes. In cases of microadenoma, dissecting the tumor pseudocapsule from pituitary gland tissue, in order to achieve an en bloc removal, is preferable when possible rather than performing an internal debulking [6]. Finally, after lesion removal, an endoscopic exploration of the tumor cavity, by means of a 0° and/or angled scope, is performed to assess the presence of any tumor remnants.

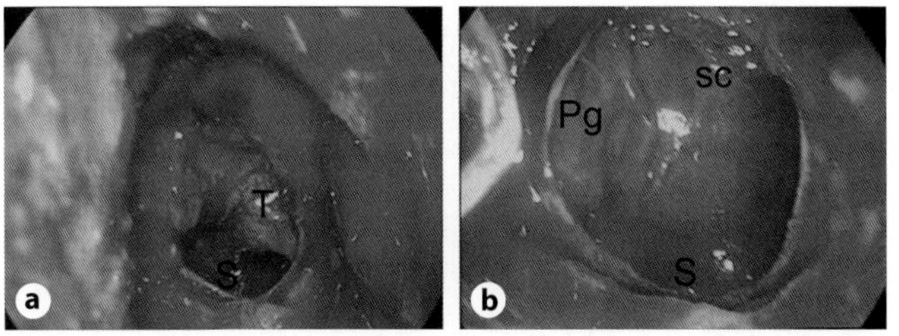

Fig. 7. Intraoperative pictures of the case showed in figure 6. Sellar phase of the procedure. **a** The inferior aspect of the tumor has been removed at first. **b** Close up view of the sellar cavity following complete tumor removal. The suprasellar cistern prolapsed after tumor removal and the pituitary gland is identified on its right side. T = Tumor; S = sella; Pg = pituitary gland; sc = suprasellar cistern.

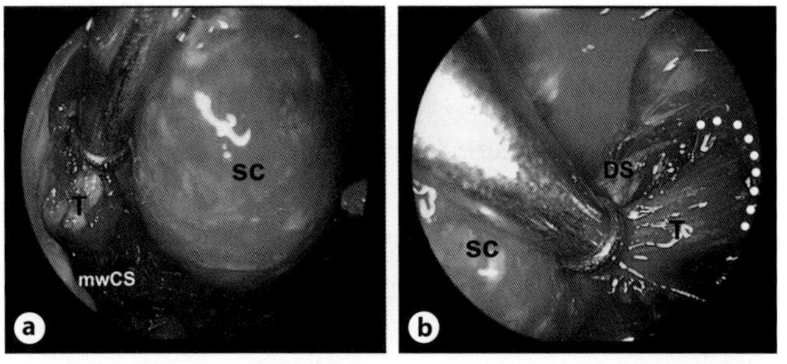

Fig. 8. Intraoperative pictures of an intra- and parasellar macroadenoma after removal of the intrasellar component. **a** The right intracavernous component of the tumor is removed through the medial wall of the cavernous sinus. **b** The left parasellar component of the tumor is mobilized with an atraumatic curved suction cannula through the medial wall of the cavernous sinus. T = Tumor; sc = suprasellar cistern; mwCS = medial wall of the cavernous sinus; DS = dorsum sellae; white dotted line = C-shaped tract of the intracavernous carotid artery that delimits the defect through the wall of the cavernous sinus.

Sellar Reconstruction

At the end of the procedure, mainly when an intraoperative CSF leak has occurred, sellar repair is required. Various techniques are used (intra- and/or extradural closure of the sella and packing of the sella with or without packing of the sphenoid sinus) depending on the size of the osteo-dural defect and 'dead space' inside the sella [7]. Since the standard endoscopic procedure does not need any skin incision and/or dissection of the oral or nasal mucosa, autologous bone or cartilage are not readily available. Therefore, eterologous or synthetic, either resorbable or nonresorbable materials, if necessary, are used to achieve a safe and effective sellar reconstruction. The aim of such a repair is to guarantee a watertight closure, reduce the dead space, and prevent the descent of the chiasm into the sellar cavity. Nonetheless, over-packing must be avoided to prevent compression of the optic system. In our experience, lumbar drainage is not employed anymore except in case of a minimal, unexpected postoperative CSF leak. At the end of the procedure, bipolar hemostasis is obtained and final irrigation of the nasal cavities is performed; then, the endoscope is removed gradually, and the middle turbinate is gently put back in a medial direction. Packing the nasal cavity is not necessary.

Extended or Expanded Transsphenoidal Transtubeculum-Transplanum Approach to the Suprasellar Compartment

The extended or expanded transsphenoidal transtubeculum-transplanum approach to the suprasellar compartment is the result of the evolution of endoscopic surgical techniques and technological developments in the last decade that have boosted the progressive reduction of the invasiveness of the transcranial approaches and provided new stimulation to transsphenoidal surgery. In 1987, Weiss [8] termed and originally described the extended transsphenoidal approach, intending a transsphenoidal approach with removal of additional bone along the tuberculum sellae and posterior planum sphenoidale between the optic canals, with subsequent opening of the dura mater above the diaphragma sellae. This approach, initially performed with microsurgical technique [8–10] through either an endonasal or sublabial route, provides midline access and direct visualization of the suprasellar space without brain manipulation, thus offering the possibility of treating small, midline suprasellar lesions traditionally approached transcranially. In order to achieve a more comfortable route to the supradiaphragmatic space and provide enough exposure for the removal of suprasellar/supradiaphragmatic tumors, other authors [10–21] described a modified transsphenoidal microsurgical approach, the so-called transsphenoidal transtuberculum approach. This technique, thanks to additional bone removal from the anterior cranial base (tuberculum and posterior planum sphenoidale), provides excellent, direct access to the suprasellar/supradiaphragmatic area, regardless of sellar size (even a nonenlarged sella), and avoids the risk of injury to the pituitary tissue.

The endoscopic endonasal transsphenoidal transtuberculum-transplanum procedure is performed using a rigid 0° endoscope, 18 cm in length 4 mm in diameter (Karl Storz Endoscopy, Tuttlingen, Germany), as the sole visualizing instrument of the surgical field (like the standard transsphenoidal operation). Sometimes, angled scopes are used to further explore the suprasellar area after lesion removal. Dedicated surgical instruments with different angled tips are needed in order to permit movement in all the visible corners of the surgical field.

To increase the working space and the instruments' maneuverability during such an approach, some additional steps are required [13]: (1) the removal of the middle turbinate on one or both sides; (2) complete posterior ethmoidectomy on one or both sides, and (3) the removal of the posterior portion of the nasal septum. These surgical maneuvers allow the use of both nostrils so that two or three instruments plus the endoscope can be inserted.

The use of some additional tools could be useful to render the extended endoscopic transsphenoidal transtuberculum-transplanum approach more safe and effective.

A detailed, complete preoperative planning, even integrated with three-dimensional computerized reconstruction of MRI and/or CT scans, has to be the backbone of the surgical procedure.

An image-guided system (neuronavigation) is also required as it provides information about midline and trajectory and offers more precision in defining the bony boundaries and neurovascular spatial relationships. Finally, it is extremely important to use dedicated instruments, among them a bipolar forceps with angled tips, both in the sagittal and coronal plane.

The patient is placed supine or in slight reverse Trendelenburg with the head turned 10–15° in the horizontal plane, towards the surgeon, fixed in a rigid three-pin Mayfield-Kees skeletal fixation device in order to allow the use of the neuronavigation system. In the sagittal plane, the head is extended about 10–15° to achieve a more anterior trajectory, keeping either the endoscope or the surgical instruments from hitting the thorax of the patient. The surgeon is on the patient's right side, in front of him. The endoscopic equipment and the neuronavigation system are positioned behind the head of the patient and in front of the surgeon.

Nasal Phase

The procedure begins by removing the right middle turbinate and performing an ipsilateral posterior ethmoidectomy. The head of the middle turbinate is cut with nasal scissors and pushed downward to expose its tail. After hemostasis has been performed, the turbinate is removed and stored to harvest a mucoperichondrial flap for reconstruction of the osteo-dural defect after lesion removal. It is not mandatory to remove the tail of the middle turbinate because it does not affect the surgical trajectory and furthermore its removal could increase the risk of sphenopalatine artery bleeding. Recently, the Pittsburgh group [22] reported the use of a vascularized nasal septal flap used for more effective reconstruction at the end of the procedure. This latter flap is made by cutting the septal mucosa along the inferior edge of the septum from the choana to the cartilaginous portion of the septum and superiorly at the level of the rostral portion of the middle turbinate. After it has been detached from the septal bone, it is pedicled laterally around the sphenopalatine foramen and stored in the choana during the surgical procedure. Then, the posterior nasal septum is detached from the sphenoid prow with a microdrill and removed with a retrograde bone punch; the mucosal edges are accurately coagulated with bipolar forceps. Finally, the middle turbinate of the opposite nostril is pushed laterally or removed depending on the width of the nasal cavities. Such maneuvers provide a wider view since other instruments, i.e. a suction tip, could be inserted through the other nostril.

The Sphenoid Phase

In the extended endoscopic endonasal transsphenoidal approach, the anterior sphenoidotomy needed is wider than in the standard approach; therefore, it is useful to remove the superior turbinate and the posterior ethmoid air cells (bilaterally) to

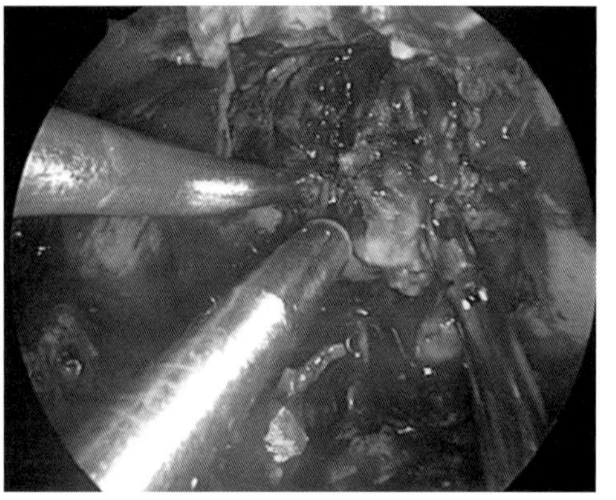

Fig. 9. Binostril approach. During tumor dissection and removal three instruments can be inserted within the operative field without any conflict. From the right to the left, the suction cannula, the bipolar forceps and the grasping forceps are recognized.

create enough space. All the septae inside the sphenoid sinus are removed including those attached to the bony protuberances and depressions on the posterior wall of the sphenoid sinus cavity. It is important that every irregularity of the bone and mucosa between the sphenoidal and ethmoidal planum be flattened to allow better maneuverability of the endoscope and surgical instruments while working above the sella. Once the complete exposure of the posterior wall of the sphenoid sinus is achieved, a series of protuberances and depressions (depending on the degree of pneumatization) becomes visible; precise knowledge of such anatomic landmarks is of great importance for correct orientation and bone opening.

From this point on, the surgeon can perform bimanual dissection while a coworker holds the endoscope and, if needed, another surgical instrument [4] (fig. 9). The '3–4 hands technique' requires good collaboration between two surgeons that should be tuned as if they were running a rally car race: one holds the endoscope and could be considered the 'navigator' while the other, the 'pilot', handles two surgical instruments inside the surgical field, as in the traditional microsurgical technique [17]. The 'pilot' surgeon actively manipulates the instruments whereas the 'navigator' dynamically follows such in and out movements with the endoscope, being responsible for keeping them under direct endoscopic view. Sometimes it could be that the first surgeon holds the endoscope in the non dominant hand and an instrument in the dominant hand, while the second surgeon helps with suction and/or other tools. Different from the fixed microsurgical view, the 'pilot' and the 'navigator' continuously pass between the close-up view, such as during dissecting maneuvers, and a panoramic view of the neurovascular structures.

The Sellar-Suprasellar Phase

Bone removal starts with drilling of the upper half of the sella in order to expose and isolate the superior intercavernous sinus. In case the sinus is accidentally damaged during the bone resection, the bleeding can be controlled with different hemostatic

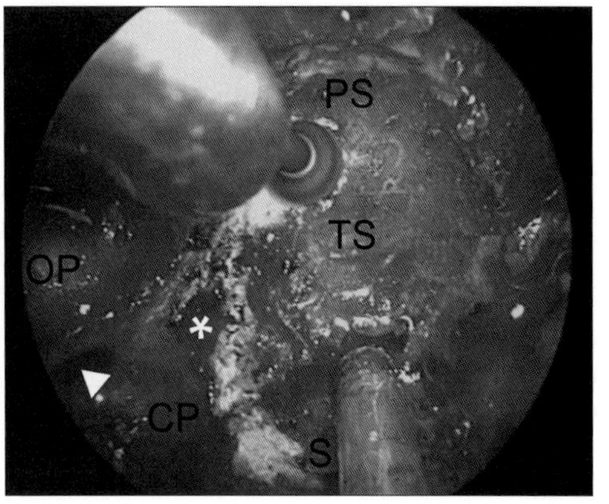

Fig. 10. Using a thin diamond burr the skull base is opened from the superior half of the sella to the planum sphenoidale. PS = Planum sphenoidale; TS = tuberculum sellae; OP = optic protuberance; CP = carotid protuberance; S = sella; white arrow head = lateral optocarotid recess; white asterisk = medial optocarotid recess.

agents, such as Floseal® (Baxter BioSciences, Vienna, Austria) and temporary, gentle compression with cottonoids.

The tuberculum sellae, observed from below by the endoscope through the sphenoid sinus cavity, corresponds to the angle formed by the planum sphenoidale with the anterior surface of the sella: it is thinned with a high speed microdrill moving from the center towards both medial opticocarotid recesses, which represent the lateral limits of the approach at this level (fig. 10).

Once the tuberculum sellae is drilled out from the two medial optico-carotid recesses and from the planum sphenoidale, it is gently dissected from the dura and periosteum and removed. Using a Kerrison rongeur, the bone removal can be extended anteriorly up to the falciform ligament or beyond according to the anterior extension of the lesion. Neuronavigation is quite useful to better define the limit. In the upper part, just above the medial optico-carotid recesses, the bone removal can be extended more laterally so that the opening resembles a 'chef's hat' [17]. This particular shape is due to the fact that the inferior part of the osteodural opening is narrower since it is limited by the parasellar portion of both the intracavernous carotid arteries and the optic nerves at their entrance in the optic canals, whereas it can be extended laterally in its superior half since the optic nerves converge from the orbital apex.

After the bone has been removed, bleeding from the superior intercavernous sinus, especially in cases of suprasellar craniopharyngioma, is not uncommon and therefore should be managed. The use of hemostatic agents, such as Floseal® (Baxter BioSciences, Vienna, Austria), may be effective or the sinus should be closed with bipolar forceps instead of using hemoclips which narrow the dural opening. The dura is incised horizontally a few millimeters above and below the superior intercavernous sinus in order to coagulate the sinus between the two tips of the bipolar forceps in its median portion. It is then incised with microscissors and the two resulting dural flaps are coagulated (fig. 11) achieving their retraction and the consequent enlargement of the dural opening, which over the planum can be easily extended using a Kerrison punch.

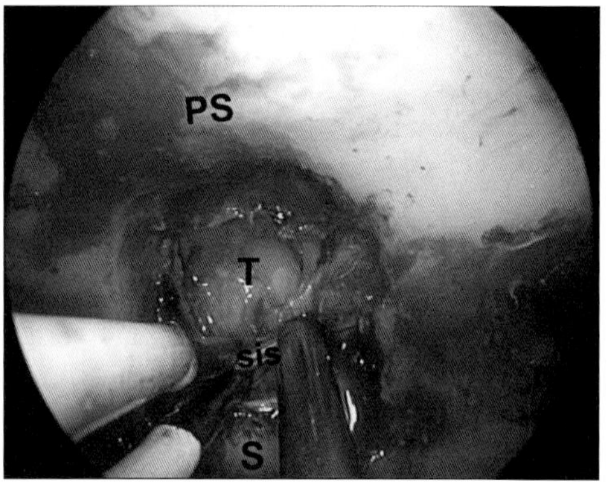

Fig. 11. Superior intercavernous sinus coagulation in a case of suprasellar craniopharyngioma. Two parallel incisions are made above and below the sinus which is then coagulated and resected in a midline position. Care should be taken to avoid a too lateral bipolar coagulation over the cavernous sinus medial walls. PS = Planum sphenoidale; T = tumor; sis = superior intercavernous sinus; S = sella.

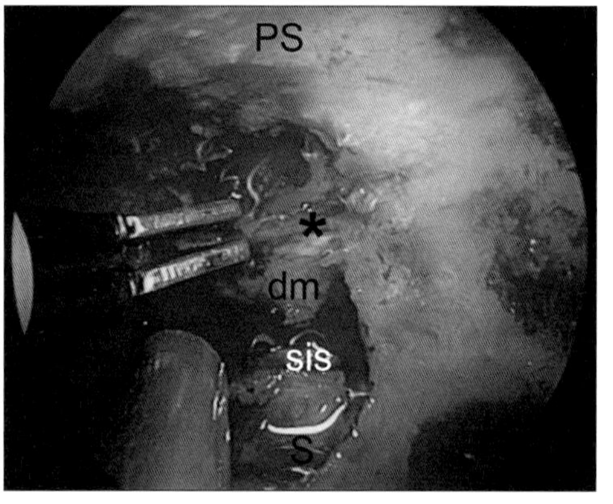

Fig. 12. A branch of the posterior ethmoidal artery is coagulated in a case of tuberculum sellae meningioma, allowing its early devascularization. Epidural diffuse bleeding can make vessels identification difficult. PS = Planum sphenoidale; dm = dura mater; sis = superior intercavernous sinus; S = sella; asterisk = branch of the posterior ethmoidal artery.

Dissection and removal maneuvers are tailored to each lesion following the same principles as transcranial microsurgery. To facilitate this, before entering the intradural space, any bleeding coming from the sphenoidotomy into the surgical field has to be controlled.

In the case of prechiasmatic lesions, i.e. a tuberculum sellae meningioma, the tumor immediately becomes visible after dural opening so that its base could be easily devascularized (fig. 12–14), whereas in cases of retrosellar lesions, like craniopharyngiomas (fig. 15), the tumor appears behind the pituitary stalk (fig. 16) and should therefore be first dissected using a surgical corridor lateral to such a structure (fig. 17, 18).

Thereafter, the internal debulking of the solid part and/or cystic evacuation in our experience is performed with suction and radiofrequency monopolar wire electrodes (SurgiMax, Ellman International, Inc., Hewlett, N.Y., USA) (fig. 14a). This last device emits minimal collateral heat dispersion thus minimizing the risk of heat injury to neurovascular structures during such maneuvers. Once the internal decompression

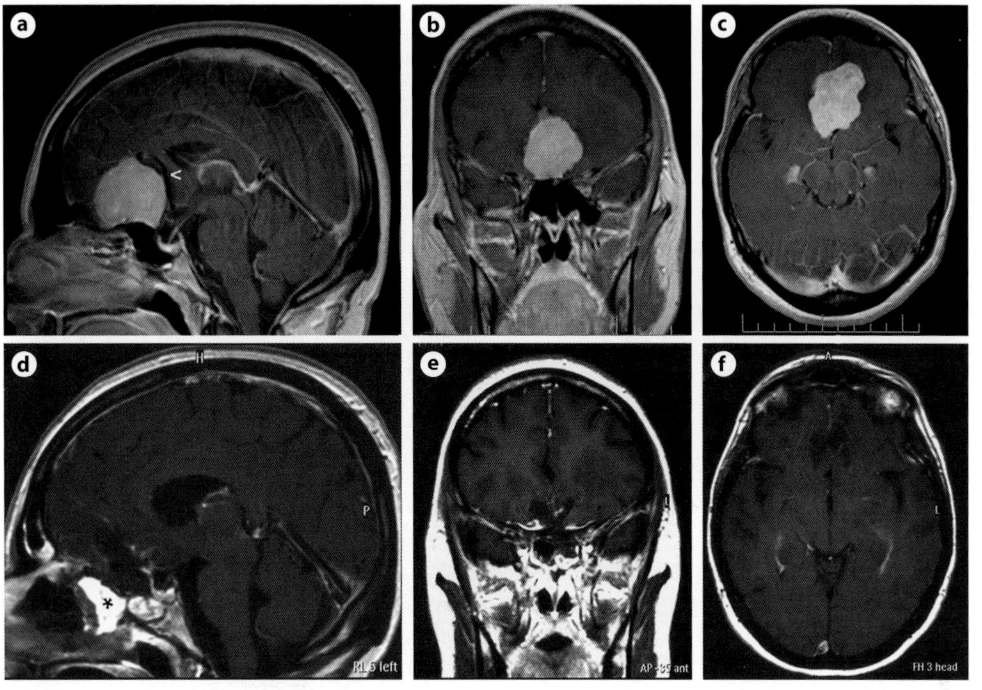

Fig. 13. **a–c** Preoperative MR images showing a case of planum sphenoidale meningioma and its relationship with the anterior cerebral arteries. **d–f** postoperative MRI reveals the gross total removal of the tumor. The sphenoidal packing and the piece of fat (asterix) buttressing the osteodural reconstruction are recognized in figure **d**. Arrowhead = Anterior cerebral arteries.

has been completed, the surrounding arachnoid is dissected away from the tumor capsule. During such maneuvers, the pituitary stalk, the dorsal aspect of the pituitary gland, the chiasm and both the superior hypophyseal arteries need to be identified and respected. Continuous irrigation and blunt and sharp dissection with the instruments under a close-up view are required to avoid injury to neurovascular structures and, moreover, the sacrifice of small arterial perforators. Dissection thus goes on taking continuous care to respect the arachnoidal plane. Once it has been freed from any adherence, the tumor is removed in either a piecemeal fashion or 'en bloc'. Finally, accurate hemostasis is performed since a clear, bloodless operating field is required.

In the final step of the procedure the operative field is inspected, even with angled endoscopes, and irrigated.

Reconstruction of the Skull Base Defect

Due to the consistent intraoperative CSF leakage resulting from a wider dural opening, an accurate reconstruction of the skull base defect is mandatory after lesion

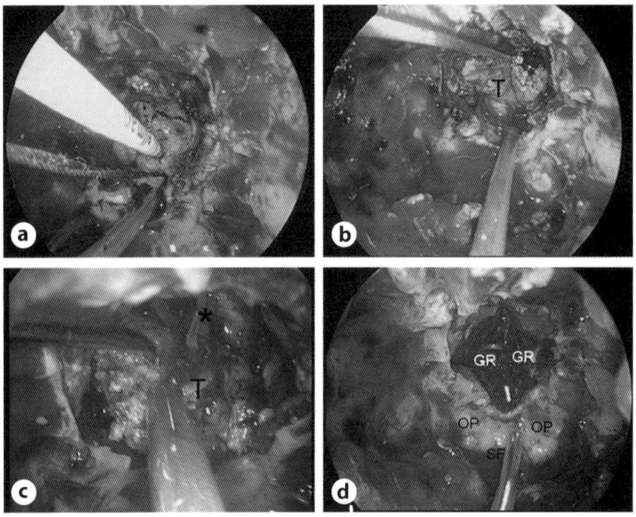

Fig. 14. Intraoperative pictures of the case showed in figure 13. **a** Internal debulking with radiofrequency monopolar. **b** Posterior pole dissection. Before the posterior pole elevation, graded dissection with a dedicated blunt hockey stick dissector and cottonoids has been performed. **c** Superior pole dissection of the tumor from a branch of the pericallosal artery. Close-up endoscopic view during these dissection maneuvers is mandatory. **d** Panoramic view after tumor removal. T = Tumor; asterisk = branch of the pericallosal artery. SF = sellar floor; OP = optic protuberance; GR = gyra recta.

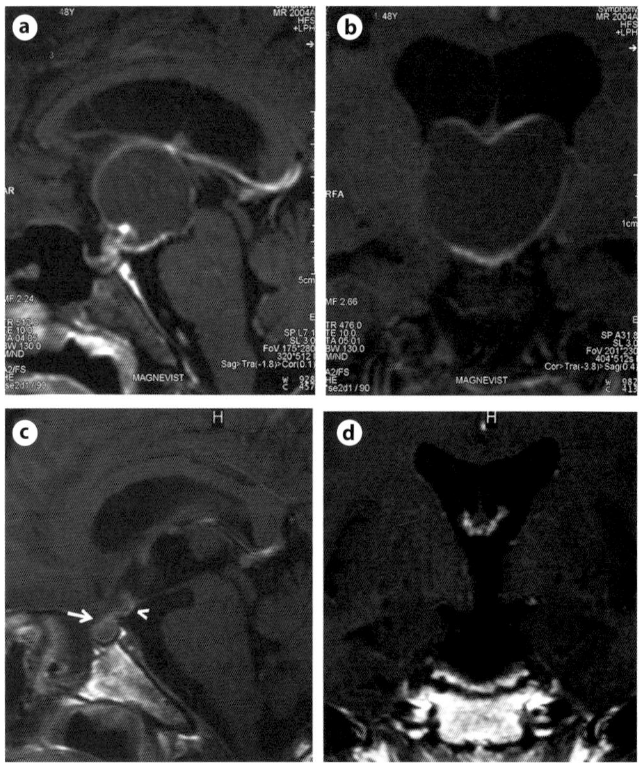

Fig. 15. a, b Preoperative MR images showing a case of third ventricle craniopharyngioma extending up to the foramens of Monro and causing hydrocephalus. **c, d** Postoperative MRI reveals cystic component evacuation, capsule removal, and hydrocephalus resolution. The pituitary stalk has been preserved. A small remnant of the tumor is visible at the level of the infundibular recess. Arrow = Pituitary gland; arrowhead = infundibular recess

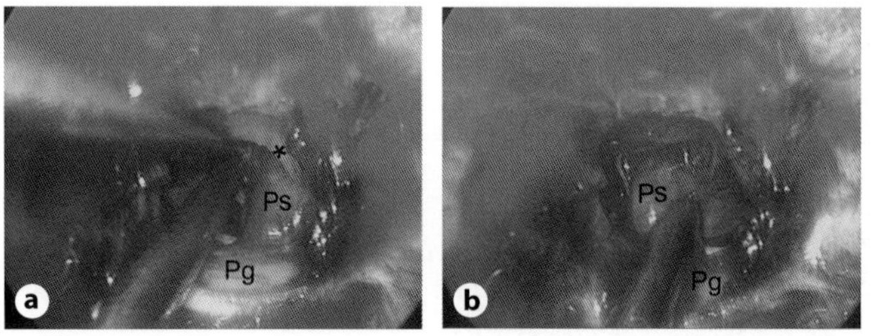

Fig. 16. Intraoperative pictures of the case showed in figure 15. **a, b** After the dural opening the lesion is not visible since is located behind the pituitary stalk. The lesion pushing downwards the inferior wall of the third ventricle is identified using two corridors laterally to the pituitary stalk. Ps = Pituitary stalk; Pg = pituitary gland; asterisk = arachnoid.

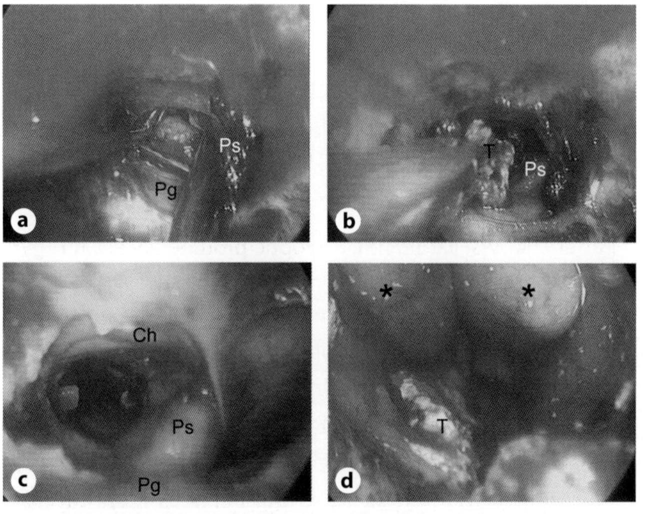

Fig. 17. Intraoperative pictures of the case showed in figure 15. **a** Evacuation of the cystic content and dissection. **b** After its complete dissection the tumor is piecemeal removed. **c** View of the anatomic landmarks of the surgical corridor created laterally to the pituitary stalk. **d** Endoventricular exploration showing calcifications adherent to the floor of the third ventricle. Such calcifications have to be carefully removed specially along the posterior part of the floor where the two mammillary bodies are located. It is also visible a partially prolapsed tumor capsule which covers the third ventricle walls. T = Tumor; Ps = pituitary stalk; Pg = pituitary gland; Ch = chiasm; asterisk = tumor capsule.

removal. The reconstruction should be watertight to prevent postoperative CSF leak, which could occur especially if lesion removal has required a large opening of the arachnoid cisterns or third ventricle.

Conventional sellar floor reconstruction techniques are inadequate during such extended approaches for several reasons: (1) the size of the defect; (2) the irregular shape of the defect due to the close distance of the osteo-dural defect to the optic nerves and carotid arteries, and (3) the wide intradural dead space lacking arachnoidal barriers.

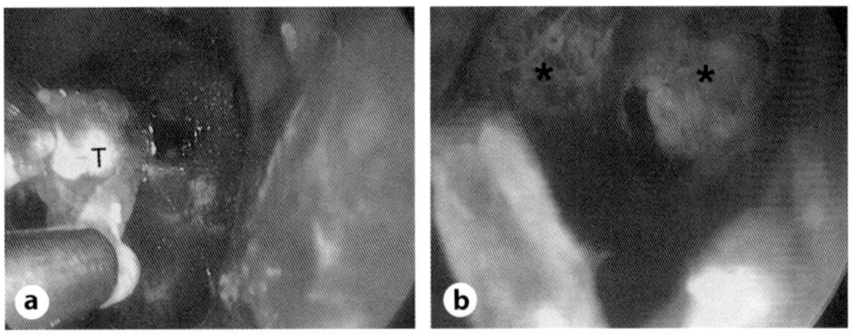

Fig. 18. Intraoperative pictures of the case showed in figure 15. **a** After its dissection the tumor capsule is removed. **b** After lesion removal the endoventricular exploration shows both choroid plexus and the restored CSF circulation. The ventricular ependyma has been partially abraded due to the close adhesion of the tumor. T = Tumor; asterisk = choroid plexus.

Our last policy is to position a thin layer of fibrin glue in the intradural space as a first barrier to CSF and moreover to fill the dead space (fig. 19a). Next, a solid or semisolid buttress made of an easy-to-shape material such as a synthetic copolymer, i.e. LactoSorb (Walter Lorenz Surgical, Inc., Jacksonville, Fla., USA), is combined with a dural substitute, i.e. Tutoplast® (Tutogen Medical GmbH). The reconstruction could be performed in different manners according to the osteodural defect: nevertheless, the most effective closure seems to be the extradural one [23]. In this technique, a single large layer of dural substitute is positioned in the extradural space, covering the dural opening and a conformed sheath of resorbable solid material (LactoSorb, Lorenz Surgical, Jacksonville, Fla., USA) is then overlapped on the dural substitute and embedded in the extradural space [23] (fig. 19b). Once a watertight barrier has been achieved, multiple layers of dural substitute are placed over it to support the reconstruction. Finally, the mucoperichondrium of the middle turbinate or the septal flap is used to cover the posterior wall of the sphenoid sinus. Periumbilical fat and fibrin glue (Tisseel®, Baxter, Vienna, Austria) are used to fill the sphenoid cavity, thus reducing 'dead space' and holding the materials in place [24].

Two or even three Foley catheters (usually 12–14 Fr) are inserted through both nostrils into the posterior nasal cavity and inflated in a triangular shape just in front of the opened sphenoid sinus. These hold the reconstruction materials and are left in place for 5 days.

No lumbar drainage is employed at the end of the procedure.

Different from the transcranial route, the extended transsphenoidal approach provides a direct view of the neurovascular structures of the suprasellar region from below, avoiding any brain manipulation; furthermore, the exposure provided by the endoscope through such an approach is median and bilateral. This route minimizes the risk of postoperative visual loss, which is strictly related to the integrity of the vascularization of the optic chiasm. In fact, at this level, most of the blood supply to the optic system comes from its superior surface, from the branches of the anterior cerebral and anterior communicating arteries, thus rendering the inferior approaches less dangerous than the transcranial routes.

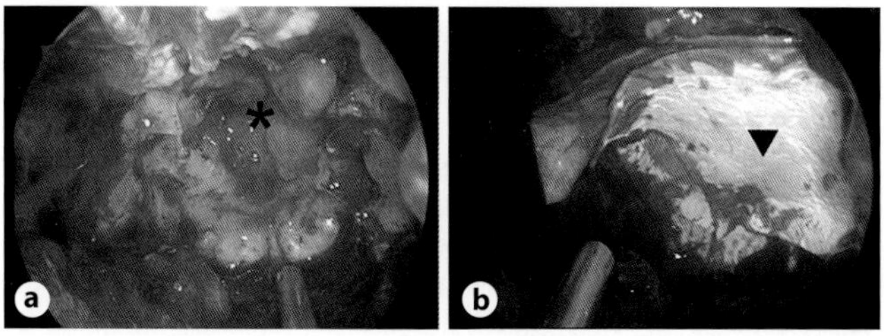

Fig. 19. Osteodural defect reconstruction after the removal of a planum meningioma. **a** A film of fibrin glue is positioned to create a first barrier to the CSF inside the osteodural defect. **b** Different layers of dural substitute are overlapped over the skull base defect. Asterisk = Fibrin glue; arrowhead = dural substitute.

The endoscopic endonasal approach to the supradiaphragmatic area is quite similar to the microscopic transsphenoidal transtuberculum approach; nevertheless, it offers some advantages due to the properties of the endoscope itself. Such an approach provides a wider, close-up view of the surgical field that permits better identification of many surgical landmarks, either in the sphenoid sinus and even intradurally, in the suprasellar area, thus allowing safer dissection of the tumor from the neurovascular structures without any brain retraction and optic apparatus manipulation. This direct approach from below offers also the possibility in some cases, i.e. tuberculum sellae meninigoma, to perform an early devascularization thus achieving an easier and almost bloodless tumor debulking.

Furthermore, using the endonasal endoscopic technique, oro-nasal complications, often related to the use of a nasal speculum and/or its overspreading, can be reduced or even completely avoided [3]. Also, this technique carries better cosmetic results associated with increased patient comfort.

It should be mentioned that the problems concerning bleeding control from main vessels in such a narrow space and the higher risk of postoperative CSF leak, as compared with the transcranial approaches, are still a challenging matter. Nevertheless, improvements in closure techniques and the use of new materials and dedicated instruments seem to significantly reduce such risks [22–24].

The transsphenoidal transtuberculum approach seems to be the less invasive and more direct route to the suprasellar area; therefore, it could be adopted in cases of suprasellar midline lesions, such as craniopharyngiomas [25], tuberculum sellae meningiomas [26], suprasellar Rathke's cleft cysts, or large fibrotic pituitary adenomas in which extracapsular dissection is required. This procedure can be proposed, as well, for the treatment of recurrent lesions already operated on transcranially.

However, it should be kept in mind that adequate endoscopic equipment, image-guidance systems, dedicated instruments and above all an increased experience with the endoscopic transsphenoidal technique are essential skills for the realization of the extended transsphenoidal approach to the suprasellar area.

References

1 Cappabianca P, Cavallo LM, de Divitiis E: Endoscopic endonasal transsphenoidal surgery. Neurosurgery 2004;55:933–40, discussion 940–941.

2 de Divitiis E, Cappabianca P, Cavallo LM: Endoscopic endonasal transsphenoidal approach to the sellar region; in de Divitiis E, Cappabianca P (eds): Endoscopic Endonasal Transsphenoidal Surgery. New York, Springer, 2003, pp 91–130.

3 Cappabianca P, Cavallo LM, Colao A, de Divitiis E: Surgical complications associated with the endoscopic endonasal transsphenoidal approach for pituitary adenomas. J Neurosurg 2002;97:293–298.

4 Castelnuovo P, Pistochini A, Locatelli D: Different surgical approaches to the sellar region: focusing on the 'two nostrils four hands technique'. Rhinology 2006;44:2–7.

5 Dusick JR, Esposito F, Malkasian D, Kelly DF: Avoidance of carotid artery injuries in transsphenoidal surgery with the Doppler probe and micro-hook blades. Neurosurgery 2007;60:322–328, discussion 328–329.

6 Oldfield EH, Vortmeyer AO: Development of a histological pseudocapsule and its use as a surgical capsule in the excision of pituitary tumors. J Neurosurg 2006;104:7–19.

7 Cappabianca P, Cavallo LM, Esposito F, Valente V, De Divitiis E: Sellar repair in endoscopic endonasal transsphenoidal surgery: results of 170 cases. Neurosurgery 2002;51:1365–71, discussion 1371–1372.

8 Weiss MH: The transnasal transsphenoidal approach; in Apuzzo MLJ (ed): Surgery of the Third Ventricle. Baltimore, Williams & Wilkins, 1987, pp 476–494.

9 Mason RB, Nieman LK, Doppman JL, Oldfield EH: Selective excision of adenomas originating in or extending into the pituitary stalk with preservation of pituitary function. J Neurosurg 1997;87:343–351.

10 Kato T, Sawamura Y, Abe H, Nagashima M: Transsphenoidal-transtuberculum sellae approach for supradiaphragmatic tumours: technical note. Acta Neurochir (Wien) 1998;140:715–719.

11 Cook SW, Smith Z, Kelly DF: Endonasal transsphenoidal removal of tuberculum sellae meningiomas: technical note. Neurosurgery 2004;55:239–244.

12 de Divitiis E, Cappabianca P, Cavallo LM: Endoscopic transsphenoidal approach: adaptability of the procedure to different sellar lesions. Neurosurgery 2002;51:699–705, discussion 705–707.

13 Kassam A, Snyderman CH, Mintz A, Gardner P, Carrau RL: Expanded endonasal approach: the rostrocaudal axis. I. Crista galli to the sella turcica. Neurosurg Focus 2005;19:E3.

14 Couldwell WT, Weiss MH, Rabb C, Liu JK, Apfelbaum RI, Fukushima T: Variations on the standard transsphenoidal approach to the sellar region, with emphasis on the extended approaches and parasellar approaches: surgical experience in 105 cases. Neurosurgery 2004;55:539–550.

15 Kim J, Choe I, Bak K, Kim C, Kim N, Jang Y: Transsphenoidal supradiaphragmatic intradural approach: technical note. Minim Invasive Neurosurg 2000;43:33–37.

16 Kouri JG, Chen MY, Watson JC, Oldfield EH: Resection of suprasellar tumors by using a modified transsphenoidal approach: report of four cases. J Neurosurg 2000;92:1028–1035.

17 de Divitiis E, Cavallo LM, Cappabianca P, Esposito F: Extended endoscopic endonasal transsphenoidal approach for the removal of suprasellar tumors. Part 2. Neurosurgery 2007;60:46–58; discussion 58–59.

18 Dusick JR, Esposito F, Kelly DF, Cohan P, DeSalles A, Becker DP, Martin NA: The extended direct endonasal transsphenoidal approach for nonadenomatous suprasellar tumors. J Neurosurg 2005;102: 832–841.

19 Kaptain GJ, Vincent DA, Sheehan JP, Laws ER Jr: Transsphenoidal approaches for the extracapsular resection of midline suprasellar and anterior cranial base lesions. Neurosurgery 2001;49:94–101.

20 Cappabianca P, Frank G, Pasquini E, de Divitiis O, Calbucci F: Extended endoscopic endonasal transsphenoidal approaches to the suprasellar region, planum sphenoidale and clivus; in de Divitiis E, Cappabianca P (eds): Endoscopic Endonasal Transsphenoidal Surgery. New York, Springer, 2003, pp 176–187.

21 Laufer I, Anand VK, Schwartz TH: Endoscopic, endonasal extended transsphenoidal, transplanum transtuberculum approach for resection of suprasellar lesions. J Neurosurg 2007;106:400–406.

22 Hadad G, Bassagasteguy L, Carrau RL, Mataza JC, Kassam A, Snyderman CH, Mintz A: A novel reconstructive technique after endoscopic expanded endonasal approaches: vascular pedicle nasoseptal flap. Laryngoscope 2006;116:1882–1886.

23 Cavallo LM, Messina A, Esposito F, de Divitiis O, Dal Fabbro M, de Divitiis E, Cappabianca P: Skull base reconstruction in the extended endoscopic transsphenoidal approach for suprasellar lesions. J Neurosurg 2007;107:713–720.

24 Kassam A, Carrau RL, Snyderman CH, Gardner P, Mintz A: Evolution of reconstructive techniques following endoscopic expanded endonasal approaches. Neurosurg Focus 2005;19:E8.
25 de Divitiis E, Cappabianca P, Cavallo LM, Esposito F, de Divitiis O, Messina A: Extended endoscopic transsphenoidal approach for extrasellar craniopharyngiomas. Neurosurgery 2007;61(suppl 2): 219–227.
26 de Divitiis E, Cavallo LM, Esposito F, Stella L, Messina A: Extended endoscopic transsphenoidal approach for tuberculum sellae meningiomas. Neuosurgery 2007;61(5 suppl 2):229–237.

Paolo Cappabianca, MD
Department of Neurological Sciences, Division of Neurosurgery
Università degli Studi di Napoli Federico II
Via Pansini 5
IT–80131 Naples (Italy)
Tel. +39 081 7462582, E-Mail paolo.cappabianca@unina.it

Kassam AB, Gardner PA (eds): Endoscopic Approaches to the Skull Base.
Prog Neurol Surg. Basel, Karger, 2012, vol 26, pp 60–75

Endoscopic Approach for Pituitary Tumors

Robert G. Louis · Nader Pouratian · John A. Jane Jr.

Department of Neurological Surgery, University of Virginia, Charlottesville, Va., USA

Abstract

The goals of pituitary surgery are threefold: normalization of secretion of excess hormones, alleviation of compression related to mass effect and preservation of normal pituitary function. All of this must be accomplished while preserving sinonasal function and avoiding cerebrospinal fluid leak and damage to critical surrounding structures including the carotid arteries and optic nerves. The transsphenoidal route provides the safest and most effective route for surgical access to the sellar region for the overwhelming majority of pituitary tumors. While there are advantages and disadvantages to both the endoscopic and microscopic transsphenoidal approaches, the endoscopic technique provides wider field of view and improved line of sight, which may be particularly beneficial during resection of large macroadenomas. Overall, in experienced hands, the morbidity and mortality associated with the endoscopic endonasal transsphenoidal approach is low and the common complications (postoperative CSF rhinorrhea, endocrinopathy, vascular injury, and sinonasal complications) are usually mild and transient. Important predictors of outcome include size of the tumor, degree of extension and experience of the surgeon.

Overall, pituitary tumors account for 10–15% of all intracranial neoplasms with an overall prevalence of 16.7% [1]. Although the vast majority of these are asymptomatic, those that do come to clinical attention can be associated with a high morbidity. Pituitary tumors generally present either from a hypersecretory syndrome or due to mass effect. Secretory adenomas usually present with syndromes related to the specific hormone being overproduced. Conversely, nonsecreting tumors are classified as nonfunctioning adenomas and usually do not come to clinical attention until they cause symptoms related to mass effect. As access to imaging has increased, a growing percentage of patients present incidentally during evaluation for unrelated processes. Besides the mode of presentation, tumors can also be classified by size: tumors <1.0 cm are classified as microadenomas while those measuring 1 cm or larger are designated as macroadenomas. Nonfunctioning tumors generally cause compression of surrounding structures (e.g. optic apparatus or the normal pituitary gland) before they come to clinical attention. On the other hand, tumors that secrete biologically active hormones are more likely to cause symptoms and thus be diagnosed at a smaller size.

Prolactinomas are the most common of the functioning adenomas and account for approximately 40% of all pituitary tumors [2]. The clinical presentation of prolactinomas varies with gender. Whereas females present with amennorhea/galactorrhea, males usually present with impotence and decreased libido. Prolactin (PRL)-secreting tumors remain the only subtype of pituitary adenoma for which the medical therapy is first-line treatment. Surgery should be performed in cases of apoplexy and may be considered for those patients who are either intolerant of or resistant to medical therapy (having either persistent hyperprolactinemia or mass effect).

Growth hormone (GH)-secreting adenomas account for approximately 20% of all pituitary adenomas and are more common in males. The overproduction of GH in these patients results in acromegaly in adults and gigantism in children. In addition to the typical and often striking cosmetic changes, the development of diabetes, hypertension and organomegaly places these patients at a significantly increased risk for morbidity and mortality. Although there have been recent reports favoring medical therapy, surgical resection is considered first-line treatment in all patients with GH-secreting adenomas [3].

Adrenocorticotropic hormone (ACTH)-secreting adenomas account for 10–12% of pituitary adenomas. Their clinical presentation is secondary to the effects of hypercortisolemia, characterized by weight gain, hypertension, purple striae, hyperglycemia, amenorrhea, thin skin, osteoporosis and cognitive and psychiatric disturbances. The most common source of endogenous overproduction of cortisol is ACTH-secreting pituitary adenomas (Cushing's disease), accounting for 60–80% of cases. As with GH-secreting adenomas, surgical resection is indicated in all patients with ACTH secreting adenomas and has an overall remission rate of 74% after initial surgery [4].

Thyrotropin-secreting adenomas are rare, accounting for approximately 1% of pituitary adenomas. These tumors may grow to be rather large by the time of diagnosis and may either present with symptoms of hyperthyroidism or with symptoms of mass effect including headaches and visual disturbances. Primary treatment is surgical resection.

Nonfunctioning adenomas are characterized by the absence of clinical and biochemical evidence of hormone overproduction. However, the majority will stain for pituitary hormones, with the most common being gonadotrophins (40–65%). In fact, only 20–40% of all nonfunctioning adenomas are true 'null-cell' tumors. While nonfunctioning adenomas account for approximately 30% of all pituitary tumors they comprise greater than 80% of macroadenomas. Patients with macroadenomas most commonly present with symptoms of mass effect, including headache, visual field disturbances (bitemporal hemianopsia), pituitary insufficiency and cranial nerve palsies from extension into the cavernous sinus. Up to 10% of patients with nonfunctioning macroadenomas may present with pituitary apoplexy. As with all other pituitary tumors (excluding prolactinomas) the primary treatment remains surgical.

Nonfunctioning adenomas tend to be large upon diagnosis and thus more likely than secretory adenomas to extend into the cavernous sinuses and suprasellar region. Accordingly, complete resection may be significantly more challenging, requiring a much wider exposure and possibly resulting in higher morbidity.

Surgical Approach to Pituitary Adenomas

Successful resection of pituitary tumors amidst the confines of the carotid arteries, optic nerves, hypothalamus, normal pituitary gland and cavernous sinuses can present a significant technical challenge. Moreover, the sellar region is relatively centrally located within the head, meaning any approach requires not only precise surgical technique but also the use of relatively long instruments through a deep and narrow corridor.

The transsphenoidal route provides the safest and most efficacious route for surgical access to the sellar region. While complete removal can be achieved in most patients, subsequent craniotomy may be of additional benefit in those with substantial residual tumor, particularly within the anterior and middle cranial fossae in cases of giant adenomas. Significant predictors of successful resection include size of the tumor, degree of extension and experience of the surgeon [5]. Overall, in experienced hands, the morbidity and mortality associated with the transsphenoidal approach is low and the common complications (diabetes insipidus and cerebrospinal fluid leakage) are usually mild and transient [6]. Successful transsphenoidal surgeons have high rates of gross total resection, often with corresponding improvements in function with both visual and endocrine disturbances. Young et al. [7], for example, demonstrated 70–80% improvement in visual symptoms of those patients with compression of the optic chiasm. Furthermore, preservation of normal pituitary function is usually possible and up to 65% may even recover lost function [8, 9].

Evolution of the Transsphenoidal Approach

While the first transsphenoidal surgeries by Schloffer, von Eiselsberg, and Kocher required external rhinotomy incisions, techniques quickly developed which decreased the invasiveness of this approach [10]. In 1910, Hirsch [11] introduced the endonasal approach by reporting 2 cases and, nearly simultaneously, Halstead pioneered the sublabial approach [12]. While these both required some degree of turbinectomy or ethmoidectomy, these represent the earliest versions of the two most common approaches used for transsphenoidal surgery today. By 1914, Cushing described successful use of the sublabial transseptal approach [13]:

> 'The usual sublabial, transsphenoidal approach was conducted without great difficulty. The membrane on the right side was torn but the other remained intact. The median septum was cleared away down to the anterior wall of the sphenoid cells. An unusually good exposure of the

cells was made. The anterior wall of the cells was removed, exposing the base of a large sella turcica. The bony floor of which was intact and was removed piecemeal. The bulging dura was incised in a linear direction.' Cushing H: Operative Note April 28, 1914.

The technique described by Cushing was recognized as less invasive and providing better visualization and was subsequently adopted by Norman Dott and then Guiot and eventually Hardy [10].

Since the time of Cushing, advances in technology have significantly improved the transsphenoidal approach. Of particular importance are advances in illumination capability as well as the development of the operative microscope. The development of advanced magnification and illumination have allowed for increasingly improved exposure with minimal disruption of normal anatomy. The introduction of the endoscope has added another powerful tool which can be used either in conjunction with the microscope or on its own as in the pure endoscopic endonasal approach, which was first popularized by Jho and Carrau [14] in the late 1990s.

Advantages and Limitations of Pure Endoscopic Approach

The goals of pituitary surgery are threefold: normalization of secretion of excess hormones, alleviation of compression related to mass effect and preservation of normal pituitary function. All of this must be accomplished while avoiding damage to critical surrounding structures.

The advantages of the endoscopic approach can best be appreciated in comparison to the microscopic approach. While both the endoscopic and microscopic techniques have been used successfully on a variety of sellar and parasellar tumors (fig. 1) our evolving experience suggests that the endoscope may have several distinct advantages in certain situations. Perhaps most importantly, by providing a panoramic picture, the endoscope may provide superior visualization compared to the microscopic approach (fig. 4, 5). This is of particular importance when addressing tumors with extension beyond the sella, including suprasellar, cavernous sinus and anterior cranial fossa, as can often be seen with nonfunctioning pituitary adenomas (fig. 2, 3). The limited field of view provided by the microscope rarely allows for visualization of the opticocarotid protuberances, or the opticocarotid recess [10]. While not necessarily important during resection of small, midline tumors, visualization of these important landmarks can be critical to avoid catastrophic injury, particularly during resection of larger and more expansive tumors. An additional advantage of the endoscope is the ability to manipulate the line of sight. Once set in place, the operative microscope provides a clear three dimensional view of the sellar region. The endoscope is mobile and may provide the ability to 'see around corners'. This can be a particular advantage when removing tumor from the region of the optic chiasm and in close inspection of the tumor/gland interface (fig. 6). Visualization can be further improved by the addition of angled cameras such as the 30° or 45° scope (fig. 7, 8).

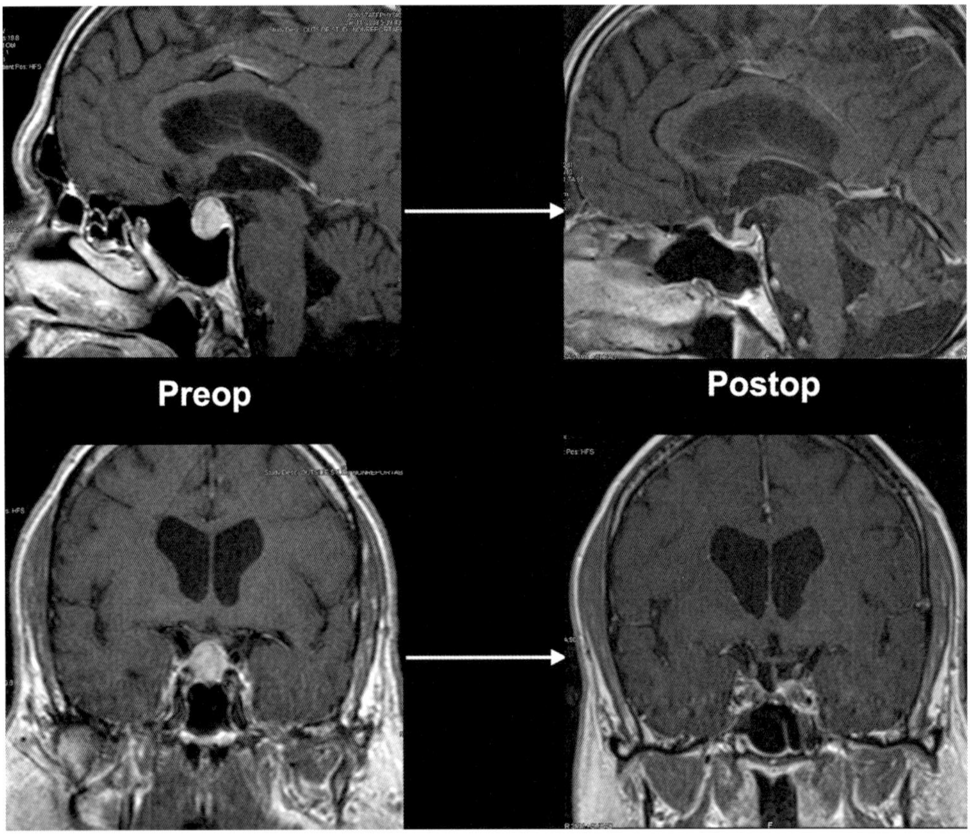

Fig. 1. Pre- and postoperative sagittal and coronal postcontrast MRI images demonstrating pure endoscopic resection of a non-functioning macroadenoma contained within the sella.

The pure endoscopic approach also obviates the need for and therefore the complications associated with sublabial or trans-septal approaches. In addition to the facial pain and headache caused by nasal packing, patients may suffer from anosmia, alveolar numbness, saddle nose deformity and nasal septal perforations [15]. Although these complications do still occur with endonasal approaches, they are less common and may be further reduced by techniques such as the septal pushover and direct sphenoidotomy [16].

The advantages of the endoscopic approach are not without cost. The endoscopic approach introduces an entirely new system for neurosurgeons, who are usually more accustomed to the operating microscope. The importance of surgeon familiarity with instruments and camera systems cannot be overstated and there is a significant learning curve when attempting endonasal endoscopy. This is underscored by the fact that operator experience is associated with better outcomes and lower complication rate [5]. Besides the new technology, the presence of the endoscope within the operative

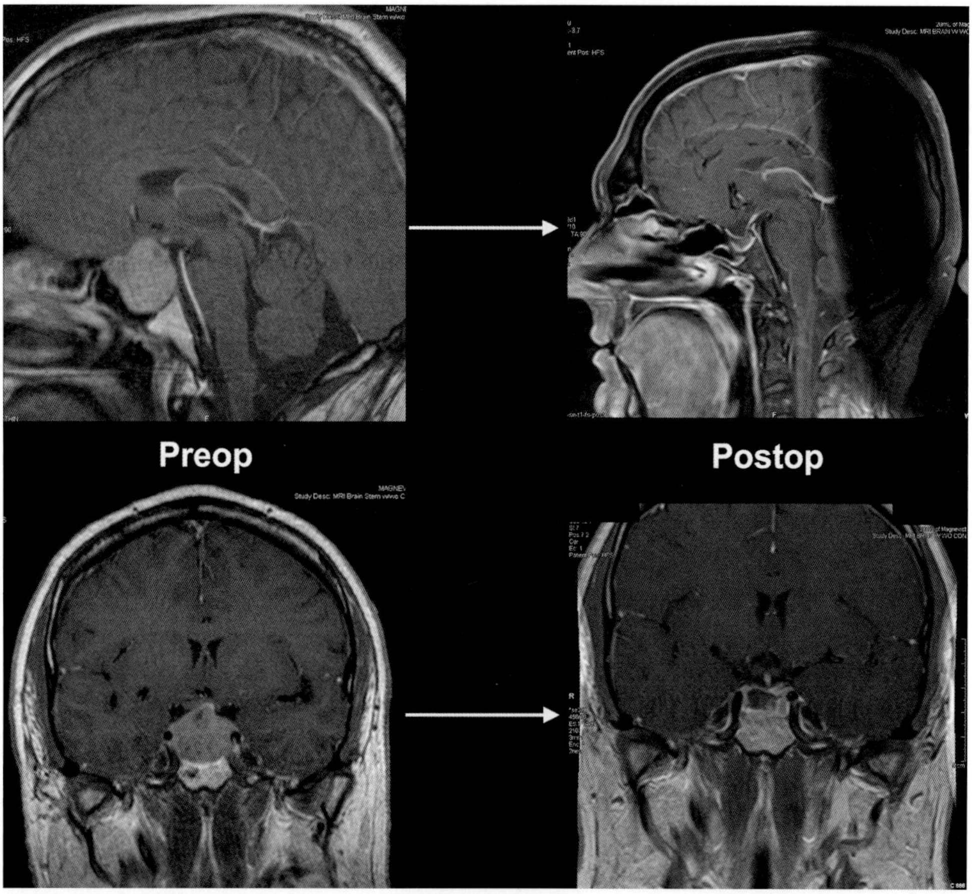

Fig. 2. Pre- and postoperative sagittal and coronal postcontrast MRI images demonstrating endoscopic resection of a non-functioning macroadenoma with suprasellar extension and chiasmal compression.

field introduces a unique challenge, representing a physical obstacle that must be accommodated and worked around. The addition of the endoscope itself further limits the maneuverability of the surgical instruments. This is further complicated by the limited zoom capacity of the endoscope, which necessitates advancing the scope deep into the operative field and often results in collisions with surgical instruments. Because of the presence of multiple simultaneous instruments, the nasal mucosa is at greater risk of being injured and thus care must be taken to sufficiently lateralize the middle turbinates to minimize damage. Finally, in order to manipulate the scope and still have two hands to operate, this technique requires an additional assistant in order to perform the 'three hand technique'.

Another limitation of endoscopy is that despite a larger field of view, the endoscope provides only a two-dimensional image as compared to the three-dimensional

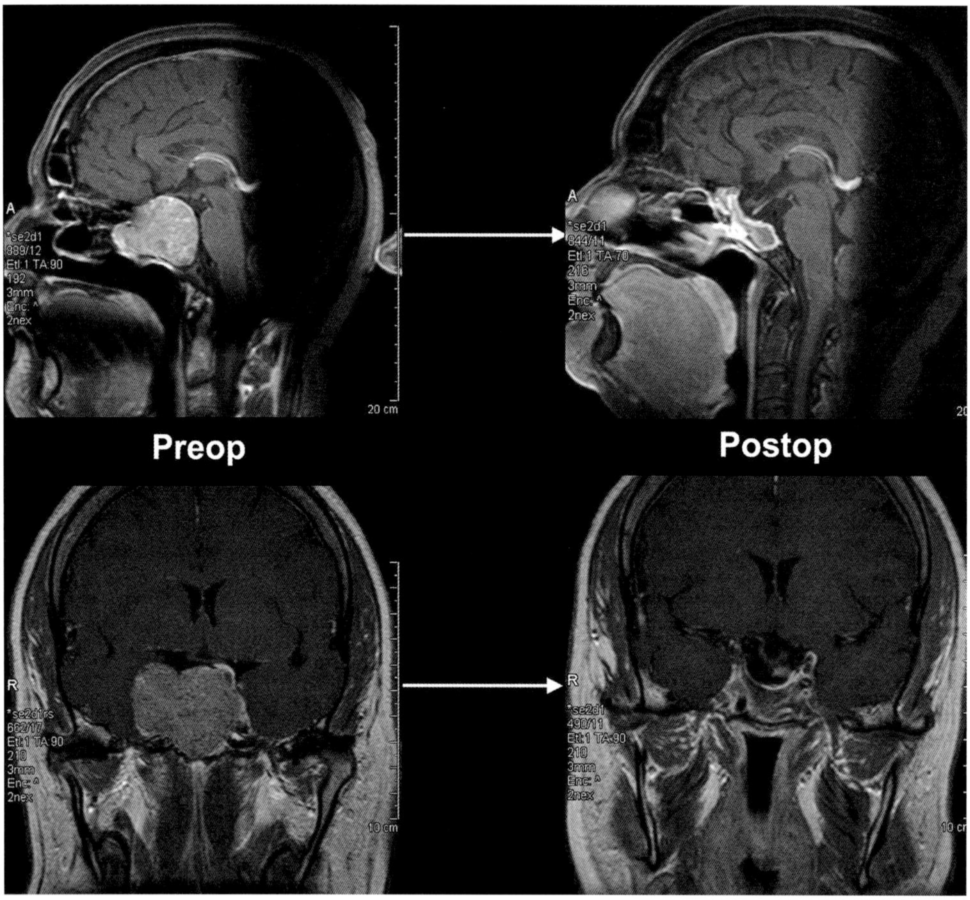

Fig. 3. Pre- and postoperative sagittal and coronal postcontrast MRI images demonstrating endoscopic resection of a giant nonfunctioning macroadenoma with bilateral cavernous sinus invasion. The postoperative images show the degree of resection afforded by the endoscopic approach to this large tumor.

microscopic visualization (fig. 9). This places the inexperienced surgeon at risk for overdissection and complications, including CSF leak. Nevertheless, with operative experience the endoscopic surgeon does eventually achieve a 'pseudo-3D' perspective.

Surgical Technique

Patient Positioning

The patient is placed in a modified beach chair position with the back elevated to approximately 20° and the head supported by a horseshoe headrest in a standard

Mayfield frame. The use of the horseshoe headrest has two advantages. First, it avoids the pain and complications associated with pin fixation. Second, it allows for slight movements of the head from side to side during surgery to increase visualization. Still, in those cases where intraoperative image guidance is required, rigid fixation with pins may be necessary. By convention, the surgeon is positioned on the patient's right side. The right shoulder is placed at the upper right hand corner of the bed. From the neutral position, the patient's neck is laterally flexed toward the left shoulder and then the head is turned to the right. The angle of the bed is then adjusted such that the bridge of the nose is parallel to the floor. Finally, the bed is turned so that the ears are parallel to the walls of the operating room. In our experience, this allows the surgeon to stand closest to the patient and have the straightest route to the rostrum of the sphenoid sinus.

Patient Prep and Draping
Starting in the preoperative waiting area, the patient is given Afrin (oxymetazoline) nasal spray and instructed to instill two sprays per nostril every 5 min times three on call to the OR. Once in the operating room, the patient is anesthetized and intubated in a standard fashion. The endotracheal tube is taped to the left side of the patient's mouth so we can access the nose from the right. In addition, we routinely place an oro-gastric tube to allow for evacuation of blood from the stomach and esophagus prior to extubation, reducing the amount of postoperative nausea and emesis. The nose and upper lip are then prepped with Sure-Clens. Next oxymetazoline-soaked patties are placed in each nostril, between the nasal septum and middle turbinate. These are left in place until draping is complete and then removed. Next, the periumbilical region is prepped with iodine, toweled off and covered with Ioban. A clamp is secured to the towels in the umbilical region to facilitate localization of the prepped area should it become necessary to harvest an abdominal fat graft. A split drape is secured in place with the base at the upper lip and coming to rest on either side of the nose. Finally, a top drape is placed at the forehead.

Nasal Anatomy
The 18 cm, 0° endoscope is first introduced and used to inspect both nasal cavities. Taking into account individual variations in anatomy, the nares with more working room is chosen for the initial dissection. We first begin by identifying the endonasal anatomy, starting inferiorly with the inferior and middle turbinates and choana. Under endoscopic visualization 0.2% ropivicane with 1:200,000 is injected into the nasal mucosa, including the middle turbinates, nasal septum and rostrum of the sphenoid. A suction-freer is used to lateralize the middle turbinates, taking care not to disrupt the mucosa. This should be done carefully to avoid excessive bleeding which will obscure the lens of the endoscope and make the remainder of the approach unnecessarily challenging. Furthermore, it is important not to place excessive force

4
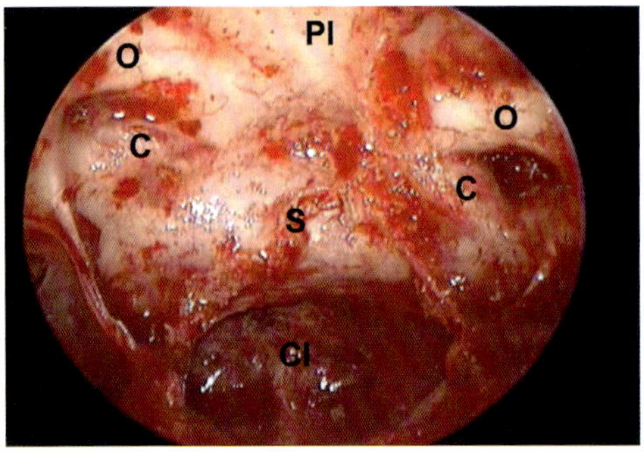

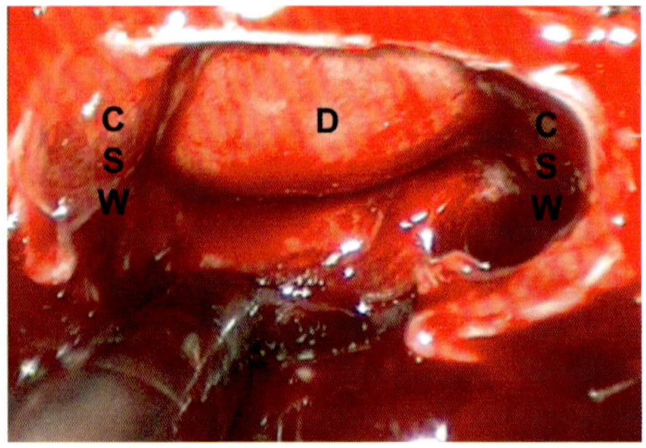

5

6
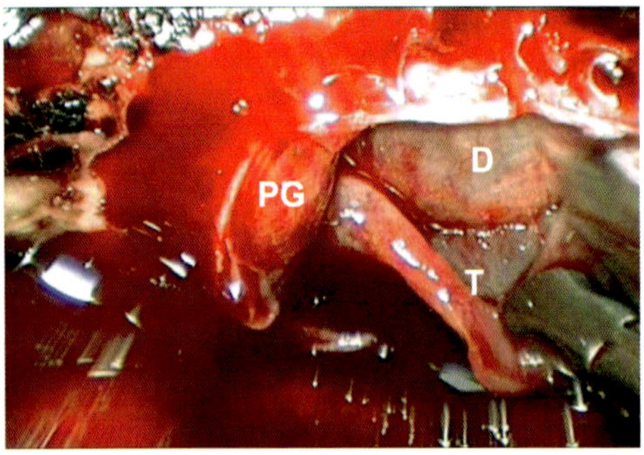

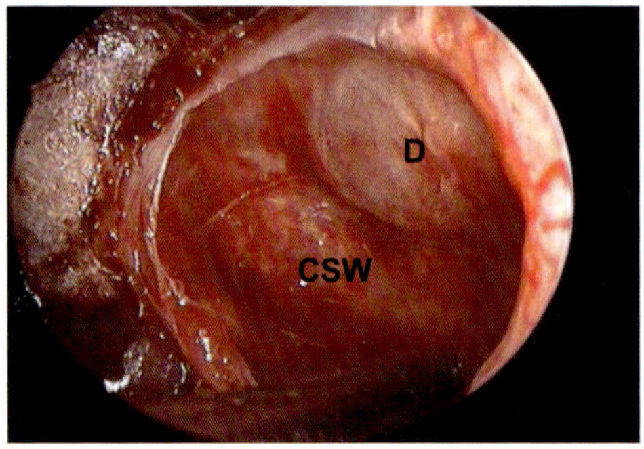

7

8
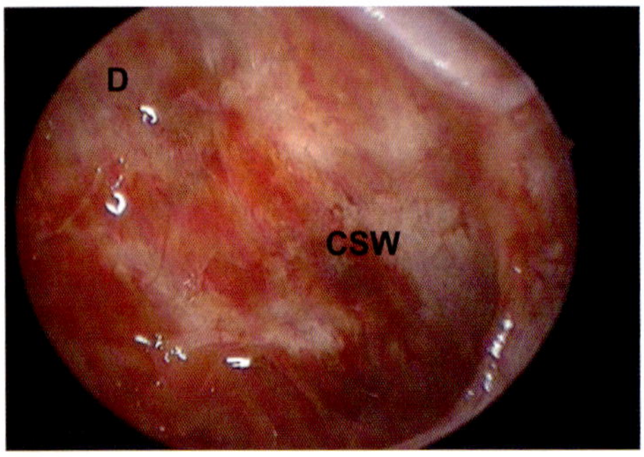

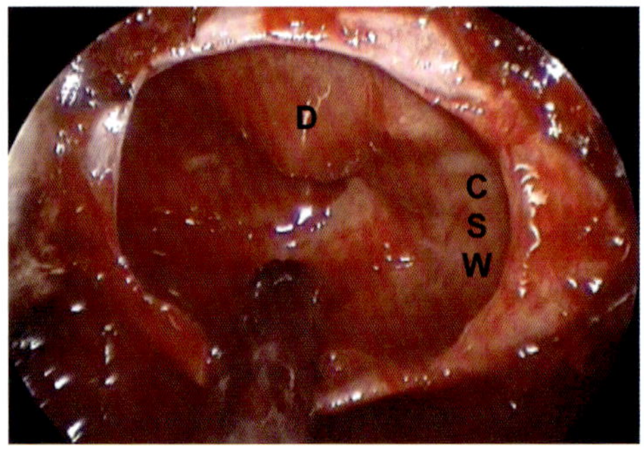

9

10
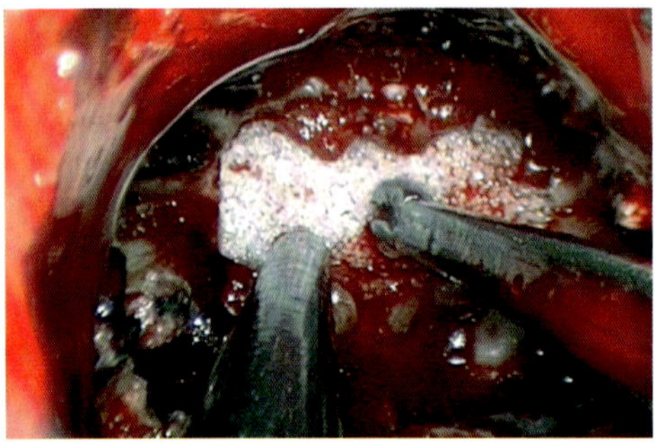

Fig. 4. Panoramic view afforded by the endoscope. Within the field can be visualized the sella (S), planum sphenoidale (Pl) and clival recess (C) as well as both optic (O) and carotid (C) protuberances and both opticocarotid recesses.

Fig. 5. Panoramic view afforded by the endoscope as seen from within the sella. Clearly visualized are the diaphragma sella (D), both cavernous sinus walls (CSW) as well as the tumor bed and sellar floor.

on the turbinate near its origin as this may result in fracture through the anterior cranial fossa. After lateralizing the middle turbinates, the superior turbinates should be clearly visible. With adequate lateralization, the sphenoid ostia should be visible at the inferior third of the superior turbinate. By identifying the anatomical landmarks early in the procedure, we hope to avoid the mistake of directing our dissection too far superiorly and thus arriving at the anterior cranial fossa as opposed to the rostrum of the sphenoid.

After identifying the sphenoid ostia, a suction cautery is used to coagulate and expose the bony rostrum of the sphenoid sinus. This exposure is carried across the midline septum to expose the contralateral bony rostrum and sphenoid ostia. The rostrum of the sphenoid sinus can then be removed with pituitary rongeurs or a high-speed drill, allowing early and definitive visualization of the sella, guiding the remainder of the exposure. The posterior septostomy is then advanced anteriorly using either a soft-tissue shaver or a back-biting thru-cut instrument. Care must be taken not to extend the septostomy too far anteriorly, using the anterior margin of the middle turbinates as the extreme anterior limit of the septostomy. An adequate septostomy will provide adequate working space for a bi-narial approach.

Sphenoidal Anatomy

The importance of performing a wide anterior sphenoidotomy cannot be overstated. Considering the additional working space occupied by the endoscope and the fact that larger tumors require instruments which may be angled, the wider the exposure the more likely a safe and successful resection. Intricate knowledge of sphenoid anatomy is essential in order to safely develop a wide enough exposure to perform this approach. The body of the sphenoid bone has numerous important arterial, venous and neural relationships which must be kept in mind while performing the sphenoidotomy. The cubical sphenoid body extends laterally and continues as two sets of wings. The lesser wings project superolaterally from the upper part of the body while the greater wings project from the lower part of the body. The sphenoid sinus is contained within the body. As it branches from the sphenoid body, the lesser wing forms the superior margin of the superior orbital fissure while the inferior and lateral

Fig. 6. Tumor (T)/gland (PG) interface as well as the diaphragma sella (D). The ability to manipulate the line-of-sight affords clear visualization during dissection.

Fig. 7. View from within the sella of the diaphragm (D) and right cavernous sinus wall (CSW) as seen with the 45° endoscope. Angled scopes allow for close inspection and the ability to 'see around corners'.

Fig. 8. View from within the sella of the diaphragm (D) and left cavernous sinus wall (CSW) as seen with the 45° endoscope.

Fig. 9. View of the sella including the diaphragm (D) and left cavernous sinus wall (CSW). One limitation of the endoscope is the two-dimensional view.

Fig. 10. Sellar reconstruction with a porex plate. The edges of the plate are tucked behind the lateral bony remnants of the anterior sella.

margins are formed by the greater wing. The optic strut is a bridge of bone which extends from the anterior clinoid process to the body of the sphenoid and separates the optic canal from the superior orbital fissure [17]. Clearly, the contents of both the optic canal and superior orbital fissure are at risk if the sphenoidotomy is too wide. This is one area where the wide field of view provided by the endoscope can yield a significant advantage by allowing for direct visualization of these structures so that the maximal exposure can be achieved with less risk.

Having already exposed the sphenoid sinus between the sphenoid ostia, various instruments including the suction cautery, Kerrison punches, high-speed drill, and soft-tissue shaver (micro debrider) are used to widen the sphenoidotomy in all directions. The inferior extent of the sphenoidotomy must be low enough to allow a suction to pass inferior to the sella. Removal of the superior aspect of the vomer bone is often accomplished with the high-speed diamond drill. Care must be taken during removal of bone from the inferolateral aspects of the sphenoid rostrum to avoid injury to the posterior nasal branch of the sphenopalatine artery, which can cause brisk expistaxis if injured. The superior extent of the exposure must allow for adequate visualization of the planum sphenoidale, the optic protuberances and the opticocarotid recess [9]. Upon entering the sphenoid sinus, it is common to encounter a bony septum in the sagittal plane, known as the intersphenoid sinus septum. This structure may be misleading as it is often mistaken as representing the anatomical midline. This is rarely the case and the true midline must be assessed by other means. The panoramic view afforded by the endoscope allows for use of other anatomic landmarks in the assessment of midline, including the vomer bone and the mid-point between opticocarotid recesses and the cavernous sinuses (once the anterior wall of the sella is removed). Rarely is it necessary to employ fluoroscopy in this effort.

Sellar/Cavernous Sinus Anatomy

While the nasal and anterior sphenoid portions of the approach are performed using a 'two-handed' technique and an 18-cm, 0° endoscope, the remainder of the operation utilizes a 30-cm endoscope which allows a third hand for operation of the camera. If the anterior wall of the sella is not already thinned by the pituitary tumor, the initial sellar opening is performed using either a high-speed drill or a small chisel to outline a square of bone in the posterior wall of the sphenoid sinus. Taking care not to disrupt the dura, this fragment of bone is then removed with a Kerrison punch. The sellar opening is then extended inferiorly to the sellar floor and laterally to the medial limits of the cavernous sinus. Extreme caution must be employed in widening the sellar opening due to the proximity of the carotids in their course through the cavernous sinus. Similarly, one must take care to avoid aggressive bony removal near the tuberculum as there is a significant risk for CSF leak.

After wide bony exposure is achieved, it is important to carefully inspect the dura. Of particular importance is recognition of the superior and inferior intercavernous sinuses which run horizontally between the two layers of dura. Care must be taken to avoid aggressive bipolar cauterization of the superior intercavernous sinus as CSF leak can easily occur due to its proximity to the suprasellar arachnoid. At this time it is also often possible to identify a small dural vessel which provides accurate localization of the anatomical midline.

The dura is then opened sharply using a #11 or #15 blade which is introduced through a nasal speculum to avoid injuring the nasal mucosa. The blade is used to make a window-type opening in the dura taking care not to interrupt the capsule of either the underlying pituitary gland or tumor. Keeping the pituitary capsule intact will facilitate development of an anatomical dissection plane and will allow for easier identification of the tumor in cases of microadenoma. If wider exposure is required, the corners of the dural window can be incised diagonally or the edges cauterized until sufficient visualization is possible.

Tumor Resection

Once identified, the tumor is then removed with a combination of techniques. A series of ringed curettes are useful in dissecting the tumor capsule away from surrounding structures. Dissection starts inferiorly, then laterally and finally superiorly. During this process, the dynamic view provided by the endoscope allows for direct visualization of vital structures to help prevent injury. This is particularly important while dissecting tumor away from the wall of the cavernous sinus and optic chiasm. Direct visualization allows for inspection of areas previously beyond the view of the microscope.

After a plane as been established and the tumor has been separated from the cavernous sinus wall, larger tumors may be entered sharply and internally debulked to allow descent of additional suprasellar components. Furthermore, the addition of angled scopes such as the 30° and 45° cameras allow for inspection of the suprasellar space and removal of tumor which extends there.

Suprasellar Anatomy

Suprasellar extension of pituitary macroadenomas is common and an intricate knowledge of the relevant anatomy is invaluable for safe resection of these tumors. Tumors in this region may often involve the circle of Willis, compress the floor of the third ventricle and even extend to involve the cerebral peduncles, mesial temporal lobes or anterior cranial fossa. The area involved by these tumors corresponds to the anterior incisural space located between the free edges of the tentorium and the front of the midbrain [17]. Inferiorly, it is bounded by the cerebral peduncles posteriorly and the uncus posterolaterally. Superiorly, it is bounded by the lamina terminalis posteriorly and the medial frontal lobes laterally. This space includes the interpeduncular cistern and the chiasmatic cistern which are separated by Liliequist's membrane. The optic chiasm lies at the anterior limit of the floor of the 3rd ventricle. Above the chiasm lie the anterior cerebral and communicating arteries, while the carotid arteries are found laterally. It is important to note that while in the majority of cases, the optic chiasm lies directly superior to the diaphragma sella it may be either prefixed (above the tuberculum) or postfixed (above the dorsum). Preoperative localization of the chiasm is essential to ensuring adequate exposure in cases where chiasmal decompression is required.

Repair and Closure Techniques

After tumor removal is complete, the cavity is again inspected using the 0° and often the 30° or 45° endoscopes to ensure that no tumor has been unintentionally left behind. Once meticulous hemostasis is achieved, we begin with our sellar reconstruction. The extent of reconstruction required depends almost entirely on whether an intraoperative CSF leak occurred. If no leak was observed, the sellar face is reconstructed with a small Porex plate, which can be cut to fit the size of the sellar opening. However, if a CSF leak did occur, we first close the sella with an autologous fat graft harvested from the periumbilical region, preferably a single, appropriately sized piece rather than multiple fragments. The size of the graft can be difficult to assess and extra fat is always harvested so a few options are available. Before insertion, the fat graft is prepared by soaking in chloramphenicol, dabbed in cotton fibers, and rolled in avitene. The graft should fit tightly enough to prevent CSF egress but should not be so large as to cause compression. Visualization of transmitted brain pulsations through the fat graft is used as an indicator that the sella has not been overpacked. After the fat graft is in place, the bony defect is repaired with a Porex plate which is tucked under the remaining rim of bone (fig. 10). Care must be taken while placing the plate to avoid injury to the cavernous sinus and carotid artery laterally. Finally, a layer of Dura-Seal is applied. Once the sellar repair is complete, the nasal cavity is irrigated and the middle turbinates are medialized. In cases of larger leaks in which the diaphragm is completely removed, we often also will place fat within the sphenoid sinus. In this circumstance, the sphenoid mucosa should be completely removed prior to fat insertion to avoid a postoperative mucocele. In these cases, the sphenoid fat graft is held in place by the medialized middle turbinates which are held in place with either nasal rockets or Naso-Pore placed lateral to the middle turbinates. We have found that absorbable materials placed lateral to the middle turbinates is preferable to nasal packing which patients generally do not tolerate as well. The stomach, esophagus and oropharynx are then suctioned to minimize digestion of blood which can contribute significantly to postoperative emesis. We do not routinely employ lumbar drainage even in the event of intra-operative CSF leak and do not administer postoperative antibiotics unless nasal rockets are used.

Patients usually are transferred from the recovery room to the neurosurgical floor and are discharged home on postoperative day two. They receive nasal decongestants for 2 days, and saline nasal sprays and nasal rinses for 6 weeks. Postoperative endocrine monitoring varies depending on the secretory characteristics of the tumor but always includes surveillance for diabetes insipidus and adrenal insufficiency. Consultation from the endocrinology service is routine.

Complications

Transsphenoidal surgery is considered one of the safest fields in modern neurosurgical practice with an overall mortality of less than 1% [18]. Mortality is usually a result of catastrophic vascular injury or meningitis. While the overall morbidity is generally low, there are several important complications which warrant discussion. Of these, postoperative CSF leakage can present a particular problem as it places patients at risk for meningitis and may be difficult to diagnose once the patient has left the hospital. Cappabianca et al. [6] reported an incidence of 2% which is similar to our experience. While these usually arise in the immediate postoperative period they can arise from days to weeks after the original surgery and usually present with headache and often copious clear nasal drainage. While clinical diagnosis remains paramount, confirmation of CSF rhinorrhea is accomplished by laboratory analysis of the fluid for beta-2-transferrin. Once CSF leak is confirmed, re-exploration and reclosure is the most effective technique to ensure adequate repair. While lumbar drainage has been attempted, it is our experience that its efficacy is inconsistent.

Injury to the anterior or posterior pituitary, infundibulum and hypothalamus are additional important complications that must be monitored. While these injuries usually occur from direct surgical insults, they can also arise from post-operative hemorrhage or ischemia. The most common of these is diabetes insipidus, with permanent loss occurring in 2–3% [9]. Frequent postoperative monitoring of fluid and electrolyte balance will allow for early recognition and treatment, if necessary, with DDAVP. Anterior pituitary loss can also be transient or permanent and measurement of post-operative cortisol is important to ensure continued function. Hypothalamic complications may present later and may include hyperphagia, poikilothermia and memory loss. Overall, the rate of endocrine complications has been found to be lower with endoscopic transsphenoidal surgery than with the traditional microscopic approach [6].

Visual loss can arise from direct surgical trauma including aggressive traction and cautery as well as from ischemia. This most commonly occurs while attempting to dissect tumor away from the optic chiasm and usually presents immediately post-operatively. As previously mentioned, the advantage of the endoscope is that it allows for this dissection to occur under direct visualization thus potentially decreasing the chance of injury. Delayed visual loss can also arise and is usually the result of compression from post-operative hematoma. Early recognition and evacuation are essential to preservation and recovery of normal visual function.

Additional complications include vascular injury, most commonly to the carotids which can be catastrophic and may require ICA sacrifice. While rare, this often can result in mortality and often be avoided by using only gentle traction when attempting to dissect tumor away from vascular structures. Endoscopic transsphenoidal pituitary surgery is also subject to the same variety of sinonasal complications as other endoscopic skull base techniques including sinusitis and epistaxis. A broader discussion of these complications is beyond the scope of this chapter.

Conclusions

The endoscopic endonasal transsphenoidal approach for resection of pituitary tumors is a safe and effective technique with low complication and high success rate. The advantages provided by the expanded field of view and maneuverability provide for enhanced visualization of previously hard to reach areas. This may be of particular importance when addressing macroadenomas and those with suprasellar and parasellar extension. As our experience grows and camera technology improves, our techniques and outcomes will continue to evolve.

References

1 Ezzat S, Asa SL, Couldwell WT, Barr CE, Dodge WE, Vance ML, McCutcheon IE: The prevalence of pituitary adenomas: a systematic review. Cancer 2004;101:613–619.

2 Vance ML, Thorner MO: Prolactinomas. Endocrinol Metab Clin North Am 1987;16:731–753.

3 Melmed S, Colao A, Barkan A, Molitch M, Grossman AB, Kleinberg D, Clemmons D, Chanson P, Laws E, Schlechte J, Vance ML, Ho K, Giustina A: Guidelines for acromegaly management: an update. Acromegaly Consensus Group. J Clin Endocrinol Metab 2009;94:1509–1517.

4 Shimon I, Cohen ZR, Ram Z, Hadani M: Transsphenoidal surgery for acromegaly: endocrinological follow-up of 98 patients. Neurosurgery 2001;48:1239–1243.

5 Barahona MJ, Sojo L, Wägner AM, Bartumeus F, Oliver B, Cano P, Webb SM: Determinants of neurosurgical outcome in pituitary tumors. J Endocrinol Invest 2005;28:787–794.

6 Cappabianca P, Cavallo LM, Colao A, Divitiis E: Surgical complications associated with the endoscopic endonasal transsphenoidal approach for pituitary adenomas. J Neurosurg 2002;97:293–298.

7 Young WF, Scheithauer BW, Kovacs KT, Horvath E, Davis DH, Randall RV: Gonadotroph adenoma of the pituitary gland: a clinicopathologic analysis of 100 cases. Mayo Clinic Proc 1996;71:649–656.

8 Arafah BM, Kailani S, Nekl KE, Gold RS, Selman WR: Immediate recovery of pituitary function after transphenoidal resection of pituitary macroadenomas. J Clin Endocrinol Metab 1994;79:348–354.

9 Fatemi N, Dusick JR, Mattozo C, McArthur DL, Cohan P, Boscardin J, Wang C, Swerdloff RS, Kelly DF: Pituitary hormonal loss and recovery after transsphenoidal adenoma removal. Neurosurgery 2008;63:709–718.
10 Jane Jr JA, Han J, Prevedello DM, Jagannathan J, Dumont AS, Laws ER: Perspectives on endoscopic transsphenoidal surgery. Neurosurg Focus 2005; 19:E2.
11 Hirsch O: Endonasal method of removal of hypophyseal tumors: with a report of two successful cases. JAMA 1910;5:772–774.
12 Halstead AE: Remarks on the operative treatment of tumors of the hypophysis: with the report of two cases operated on by an oronasal method. Trans Am Surg Assoc 1910;28;73–93.
13 Cohen-Gadol AA, Spencer DD: Pituitary Adenoma in the Legacy of Harvey Cushing: Profiles of Patient Care. Stuttgart, Thieme, 2007, pp 19–22.
14 Jho HD, Carrau RL: Endoscopic endonasal transsphenoidalsurgery: experience with 50 patients. J Neurosurg 1997;87:44–51.
15 Sharma K, Tyagi I, Banerjee D, et al: Rhinological complications of sublabial transseptal transsphenoidal surgery for sellar and suprasellar lesions: prevention and management. Neurosurg Rev 1996;19: 163–167.
16 Jane JA Jr, Thapar K, Kaptain GJ, et al: Pituitary surgery: transsphenoidal approach. Neurosurgery 2002;51:435–442.
17 Rhoton AL: The Sellar Region in Cranial Anatomy and Surgical Techniques. Philadelphia, Lippincott Williams & Wilkins, 2003, pp 363–393.
18 Ciric I, Ragin A, Baumgartner C, Pierce D: Complications of transsphenoidal surgery: results of a national survey, review of the literature, and personal experience Neurosurgery 1997;40:225–236.

John A. Jane Jr., MD
Department of Neurosurgery, University of Virginia Health System
PO Box 800212
Charlottesville, VA 22908–0711 (USA)
Tel. +1 434 243 5749, Fax +1 434 243 5204, E-Mail johnjanejr@virginia.edu

Kassam AB, Gardner PA (eds): Endoscopic Approaches to the Skull Base.
Prog Neurol Surg. Basel, Karger, 2012, vol 26, pp 76–86

Endoscopic Endonasal Approach for Olfactory Groove Meningiomas

Paul A. Gardner[a] · Allan Vescan[b] · John R. de Almeida[b] · Arif Janjua[b] · Amin B. Kassam[c] · Daniel M. Prevedello[d] · Ricardo L. Carrau[e] · Carl H. Snyderman[a,f]

[a]Department of Neurological Surgery, University of Pittsburgh, Pittsburgh, Pa., USA; [b]Department of Otolaryngology – Head and Neck Surgery, University of Toronto, Toronto, Ont., and [c]Department of Neurological Surgery, University of Ottawa, Ottawa, Ont., Canada; Departments of [d]Neurological Surgery and [e]Otolaryngology, Ohio State University, Columbus, Ohio, and [f]Department of Otolaryngology, University of Pittsburgh, Pittsburgh, Pa., USA

Abstract

Background: Endoscopic endonasal approaches (EEAs) have been applied for pathologies across the entire anterior skull base. Olfactory groove meningiomas are tumors of the anterior base that present significant challenges. **Objectives:** To evaluate the surgical techniques, challenges, advantages and disadvantages of EEA for olfactory groove meningiomas. **Methods:** We present our concepts of EEA for addressing these tumors by thoroughly discussing our surgical techniques, presenting the advantages of the approach such as early devascularization and complete lack of brain retraction, and reviewing outcomes, especially complications. **Conclusions:** Olfactory groove meningiomas can be addressed safely and effectively via EEA, with the conceptual advantage of accessing the tumor surface directly.

Evolution of Endoscopic Techniques

Advances over the last several decades have significantly improved treatment outcomes for skull base pathologies [1–4]. In 1941, Dandy [5] first described the removal of an orbital tumor involving the cranial base via a craniotomic approach. Smith et al. [6] later described the removal of a skull base tumor originating in the frontal sinus through a combined transfacial-transcranial approach. However, it wasn't until the 1960s that Ketchum described the first craniofacial resection using a bicoronal incision and craniotomy combined with facial incisions for removal of the inferior, intranasal, component of the tumor [7]. Over the ensuing decades, the landscape of skull base surgery changed very little. In 1997, Yuen et al. [8] described an endoscopic-assisted craniofacial resection applying the principles and instruments developed for inflammatory endoscopic sinus surgery to surgically address a malignant neoplasm. Stammberger et al. [9] described a completely endoscopic resection of an esthesioneuroblastoma in 1999. Since then, multiple case series have documented good results following endoscopic resection of esthesioneuroblastomas and other neoplasms of the skull base [9–12].

The goals of both endoscopic and open skull base resections remain the same—complete tumor extirpation for benign disease and with negative margins for oncologic cases [13]. The surgeon must take care to prevent or minimize associated morbidities such as neurological sequelae, visual dysfunction or resultant post-operative chronic sinus disease. Cosmesis, while not the primary goal, is an important concern to the patient especially when undergoing extensive open procedures. The use of advanced endoscopic technology has allowed for extensive resections to be performed without the need for facial or coronal incisions.

There are currently no systematic reviews comparing open techniques to endoscopic techniques for olfactory groove meningiomas. A recent systematic review did however compare endoscopic and open techniques for treatment of sinonasal inverting papillomas [14]. In patients treated endoscopically, the recurrence rate was significantly lower than those treated 'nonendoscopically' (12 vs. 20%). Casler et al. [15] compared endoscopic and open techniques for pituitary surgery in a cohort study and noted that patients undergoing trans-sphenoidal endoscopic resection of adenomas experienced less pain, less blood loss, fewer complications and shorter length of stay in the ICU and hospital. Additional benefits include superior visualization, lack of incisions, a reduction in swelling and decreased pain and bleeding [16–18]. However, indications for endoscopic and open approaches are not necessarily the same, and comparing these heterogeneous groups of patients may yield misleading conclusions.

Olfactory Groove Meningiomas

Olfactory groove meningiomas are a challenging group of tumors to treat with well described and effective craniotomic approaches for resection. These tumors are often associated with significant cerebral edema and usually do not directly contact the posterior frontal sinus wall, thus requiring some degree of frontal lobe retraction or manipulation for access. By definition, these tumors are based on the olfactory cribriform dura and, as such, are always in direct contact with the roof of the ethmoid sinuses. The endoscopic endonasal approach (EEA) takes advantage of this anatomic relationship to allow resection without any brain retraction.

There are several concerns about EEA for olfactory groove meningiomas including: adequate lateral access for complete resection, control of involved or associated cerebral vasculature, reconstruction with adequate separation of the cranial and sinonasal cavities, and prevention of postoperative CSF leak.

This chapter describes the surgical techniques developed for EEA for olfactory groove meningiomas. Outcomes will be briefly summarized from the early case series of olfactory groove meningiomas resected via EEA at the University of Pittsburgh Medical Center. The above concerns will be addressed in the context of the evolution of these techniques as well as recommendations for managing the learning curve associated with such cases.

Endoscopic Approaches

Endoscopic approaches allow for a concerted effort between Otolaryngologist and Neurosurgeon, whereby each step of the approach, resection and reconstruction is performed in tandem. At each stage after the initial exposure, one surgeon performs bimanual dissection via a binarial approach while the second surgeon provides dynamic movement of the endoscopic field of view and optimizes visualization while assisting with surgical decision making. This two-surgeon approach facilitates interdisciplinary collaboration and maximizes the therapeutic outcome by drawing on the distinct skills and experiences of both surgeons. In addition, this two-surgeon, four-hand technique can facilitate dealing with potentially catastrophic problems such as major vascular injury.

Sinonasal Approach

Initial exposure requires creating room for surgical manipulation and instrumentation. Opening the surgical corridor involves bilateral uncinectomies, complete ethmoidectomies and maxillary antrostomies. Either unilateral or bilateral middle turbinate resection(s) can be performed as needed. Bilateral sphenoidotomies are performed and joined via removal of the rostrum and the intersinus septum. This provides adequate visualization of the carotid arteries and optic nerves.

The frontal sinus ostia are identified and a modified endoscopic Lothrop procedure (Draf III) is then performed. This involves removal of the interfrontal sinus septum, the frontal sinus floor and the superior nasal septum [19–21]. A high-speed cutting drill is used to remove the nasofrontal 'beak' at the anterior aspect of the frontal sinus ostium on each side. During this dissection, care must be taken to avoid such structures as the anterior ethmoid arteries, which lie immediately posterior to the frontal sinus ostia at the level of the skull base. The superior nasal septum can be resected by outlining an inferior septal cut using suction cautery and extended from the anterior extent of the common enlarged frontal sinus opening to the rostrum of the sphenoid posteriorly.

Following wide opening of the frontal sinuses, it may be appropriate to ligate the anterior ethmoid arteries. This will aid in devascularizing the tumor bed and prevent any nuisance bleeding during the remainder of the neurosurgical dissection. The anterior ethmoid artery on each side courses posterolaterally to anteromedially from the orbit to the anterior cranial fossa. The artery can consistently be found one cell posterior to an opened frontal ostium between the second and third ethmoid lamellae. It is not uncommonly encased in a bony mesentery into which dura can extend [22]. Therefore, careful manipulation of this area is paramount to prevent unwanted CSF leaks. The artery may be exposed and ligated within the roof of the nasal cavity or alternatively, may be identified lateral to the lamina paprycea and ligated proximally. This lateral location is often a better position to ligate the anterior ethmoid vessels as the junction of the lamina papyracea and the skull base is routinely where the lateral osteotomes are made in anterior craniofacial resection. Exposure of the vessel in this location is achieved by breaching the lamina and removing it from inferior to superior. Gentle lateral retraction on the intact peri-orbita at the level of the skull base places the artery on stretch and allows for easy identification. The removal of the lamina may be continued posteriorly such that the posterior ethmoid artery, as well as additional accessory feeding vessels may be identified and ligated in a similar fashion. In each case the arteries may be ligated with bipolar cautery and/or surgical clips [23].

After achieving appropriate exposure anteriorly, posteriorly and laterally, the skull base osteotomies must be planned. These should be tailored to the extent of disease but are routinely located anteriorly at the junction of the posterior wall of the frontal sinus and cribiform plates, posteriorly within the planum sphenoidale and laterally within the fovea ethmoidalis at the junction of the medial orbital wall (lamina papyracea) with the skull base. These osteotomes are traditionally performed bimanually with a high-speed drill by the neurosurgeon while the endoscopic visualization is maintained by the otolaryngologist. The high-speed drill is used to thin the skull base and create a trough along the margins of the dissection in which the dura may be visualized. This sets the stage for the dural resection.

Neurosurgical Approach

Conceptually, approaching an olfactory groove meningioma via an EEA is similar to approaching a convexity meningioma. The dural and bony origin/involvement of the tumor presents to the surface following the initial exposure. Analogous to a convexity meningioma, bony removal and tumor devasularization are key early steps in the EEA, as they are with any meningioma. These steps are often difficult or impossible to achieve at the beginning of the resection of skull base meningiomas when approached via standard craniotomic avenues.

Bony Resection/Exposure

Olfactory groove meningiomas often involve the bone of the cribriform plate, either with direct tumor extension or hyperostosis. Either way, this bone may be thick and hypervascular. A high speed, hybrid/diamond drill bit can be helpful for controlling the bony

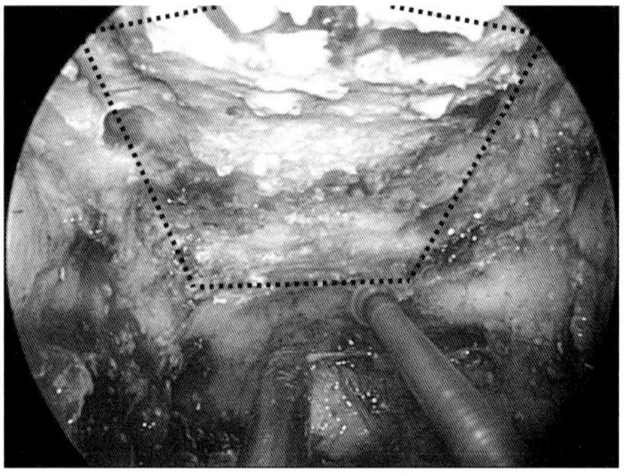

Fig. 1. Endoscopic endonasal view of the anterior skull base following the sinonasal portion of the approach. Dashed lines represent the osteotomies to be performed for dural access.

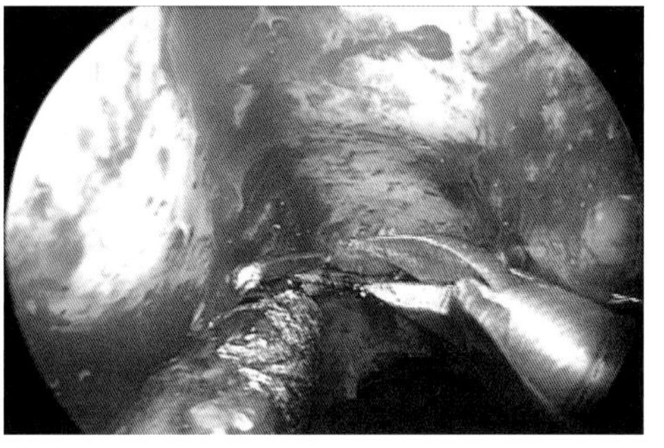

Fig. 2. Endoscopic endonasal view of the right posterior ethmoidal artery for bipolar coagulation and ligation.

bleeding associated with this aspect of the resection. Sometimes, however, this cannot be truly controlled until the bone is removed and the dura and tumor capsule coagulated.

The bone of the anterior base can be removed endonasally, usually in two pieces, separated in the center by the olfactory fimbrae. Osteotomies are made on either side, laterally next to the lamina papyracea in the fovea ethmoidalis (fig. 1). This lateral bony osteotomy can be extended over the orbital roof by removing the lamina papyracea and gently retracting the periorbita with a suction tip. The bony gutter is extended from the planum (as posterior as the optic canal) to the posterior wall of the frontal sinus as needed. As mentioned above, the ethmoidal arteries must be located and ligated when making these lateral osteotomies (see below, vascular control) (fig. 2).

Another osteotomy is made posteriorly across the planum sphenoidale. The exact location of this is variable depending upon tumor extent and can be determined using intraoperative image guidance. Sometimes, the planum itself must be removed separately, as a third bony piece. Occasionally, olfactory groove meningiomas will involve the tuberculum and optic chiasm directly. In this case, it is wise to leave the bone over the optic nerves and tuberculum until the rest of the tumor is resected. This portion of the skull base becomes the most posterior/caudal portion of the working area during an endonasal approach. As a result, this area may not always be well visualized during tumor resection, leaving the optic nerves susceptible to inadvertent injury when introducing instruments into the field. As a precaution, bone is left over these structures until the very end of the resection when attention and visualization can be directed only to this area.

The final osteotomies are made (again using a high speed drill) from the anterior aspect of the lateral osteotomy medially to the crista galli. This can be extended as far anteriorly as the posterior wall of the frontal sinus. This determination can be aided by image guidance and its visualization improved by ensuring an adequate frontal sinus opening (Draf). After this final disconnection, the anterior skull base has been divided into bilateral bony plates, separated in the midline by the cribriform plate. These bony plates can be dissected free from the dura with a dissector and removed, exposing the dura of the anterior skull base, underlying the tumor.

Vascular Control

When approaching an olfactory groove meningioma, regardless of approach, both the extra- and intradural arteries associated with the tumor must be controlled. The anterior and posterior ethmoidal arteries provide the major extradural blood supply to the tumor. These arteries are exposed during the EEA and easily bipolar coagulated and ligated (fig. 2) as described above. In addition, the dura underlying the tumor is exposed following bone removal and can be coagulated for further tumor devascularization.

There are often multiple fine falcine arterioles that provide additional blood supply to olfactory groove meningiomas. Following tumor debulking on either side of the falx, these arterioles can be carefully transected and coagulated during the resection of the falx to provide further tumor devascularization.

The anterior communicating and anterior cerebral arteries may be intricately associated or even enveloped by meningiomas in this region (fig. 3). This relationship should be fully understood preoperatively. The ability to control major arterial injury during an endoscopic endonasal approach has been questioned. In our experience, as long the surgical team has significant experience together, this situation can be controlled as easily and effectively endonasally as it can be via a craniotomic approach. Avoidance of such injury is preferred and it is important to apply careful microsurgical techniques of gentle counter-traction combined with sharp dissection. The use of two surgeons for tumor resection allows the dissecting surgeon to use both hands with appropriately designed endonasal instrumentation to dissect in the identical manner as he/she would if approaching the tumor via an open approach. In addition, if there is an arterial injury, having a skilled endoscopist is critical to maintain clear visualization while providing a dynamic view which allows such dissection and vascular control.

Tumor Resection

The basic principles of tumor resection via an EEA are identical to those of a standard, microsurgical approach. The tumor is sequentially internally debulked prior to careful extracapsular dissection using standard microsurgical techniques. There are some modifications of instrumentation required such as pistol-grip, angled microscissors

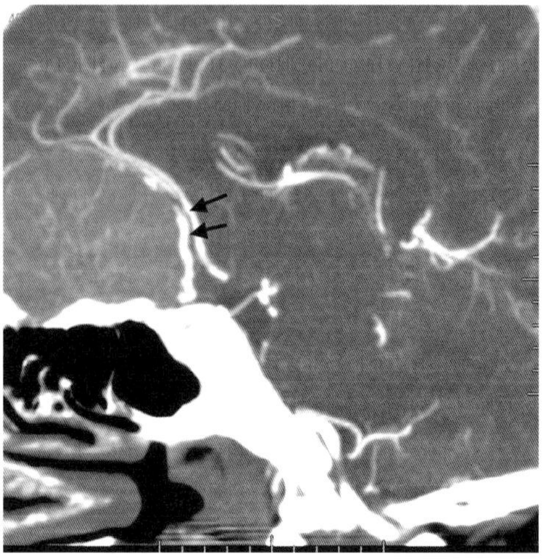

Fig. 3. Preoperative CT angiogram showing the close association of the tumor capsule of an olfactory groove meningioma with the anterior cerebral arteries (arrows).

and bipolars and extendable, nonbayonetted dissectors, but the techniques and concepts are identical.

Debulking begins by opening the dura and tumor capsule on either side of the falx and internally debulking the tumor up to the falx. The small, falcine arterioles that feed the tumor can be coagulated. Sacrificing these arteries early in the dissection provides further tumor devascularization. Once the falx is isolated from either side, it can be bipolar coagulated and carefully cut with scissors or micro through-cutting instruments at its most anterior aspect. This is done sequentially deeper and deeper into the tumor until the falx is completely transected, thereby creating a single tumor cavity and releasing the anterior attachment of the tumor. Care should be taken to ensure a frontopolar branch is not adherent to the surface of the tumor overlying the falx. The tumor should not be detached anteriorly before all of the internal debulking is complete, as frontal lobe descent can obscure visualization. The same obscuration can occur with excessive dural opening anteriorly.

Once the capsule is disconnected from the falx anteriorly, it can be sequentially dissected from the overlying cortex and associated structures (anterior cerebral arteries (ACAs) and optic apparatus). The tumor and capsule are debulked as they are dissected sequentially in an identical fashion to microsurgical approaches using a combination of blunt and sharp dissection (fig. 4). If there is significant involvement of the ACAs, then the capsule should be initially dissected posteriorly to provide proximal control.

Reconstruction

Prior to beginning the dissection, some consideration must be given to the reconstruction of the resultant defect. The nasoseptal flap can be raised in an anterior to posterior fashion pedicled on the posterior septal artery. This can then be stored in the nasopharynx until it is needed for subsequent reconstruction. Unlike in the

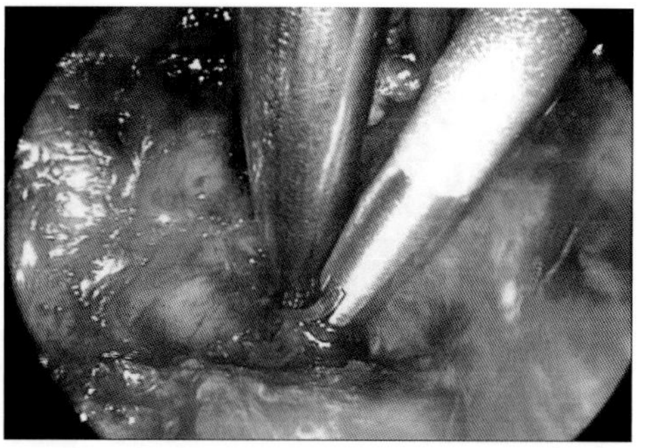

Fig. 4. Endoscopic view during extracapsular tumor dissection. Identical techniques (suction and microscissors) are applied during endonasal surgery as during open microsurgery to ensure similar results.

reconstruction of sinonasal tumors, the septal mucosa is not involved in olfactory meningiomas and, as such, the full extent of the septal flap can be utilized for reconstruction. If the planned resection extends as far anteriorly as the posterior wall of the frontal sinus, the nasoseptal flap may have insufficient length (or width, depending upon how it is turned) to seal to anterior margin of the skull base defect. In these setting, other options for reconstruction should be considered. Further reconstructive options are reviewed in the chapter by Zanation et al. [this vol.].

Case Series

Between 2003 and 2008, we performed EEA for 29 olfactory groove meningiomas. One early patient's surgery was aborted due to generalized bleeding secondary to obesity and associated venous congestion. All other patients had either complete resection or adequate resection for neural decompression depending upon the goals of surgery.

Complications consisted of one sterile Teflon granuloma that developed a superinfection, intracerebral hemorrhage following anterior cerebral artery (ACA) branch psuedoaneurysm and a CSF leak rate of 25% (7 of 28). This series was prior to the introduction of the vascularized nasoseptal flap which has dramatically decreased the risk of CSF leak following EEA [24]. Other than the pseudoaneurysm hemorrhage which resulted in an ACA infarct, no patient had neurological worsening following EEA. There were 4 thromboembolic events (DVT or PE) all treated with anticoagulation. One patient suffered a postoperative MI. One patient died 3 months following surgery of multiorgan system failure after she developed delayed renal failure.

Limitations of EEA for Olfactory Groove Meningiomas

The endoscopic endonasal approach is an approach to anterior skull base pathology from a medial, anterior and inferior trajectory. Therefore, the limitations are

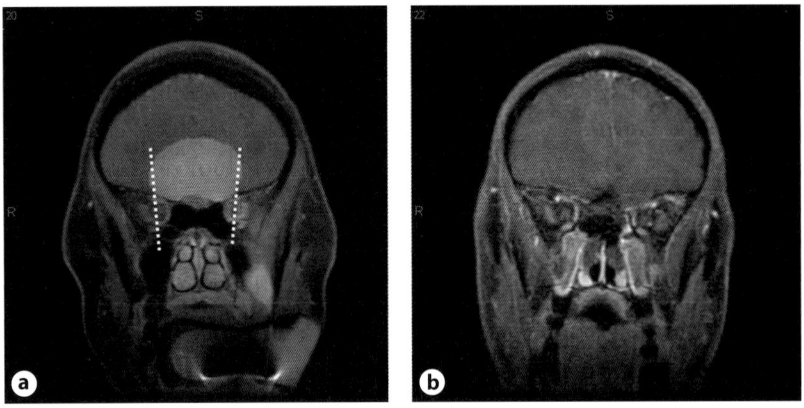

Fig. 5. **a** Coronal post-contrast T1-weighted MRI showing the lateral limit of resection at the midorbital vertical meridian (dotted line). **b** Postoperative post-contrast T1-weighted MRI showing complete resection out to midorbit via EEA.

potentially lateral, posterior and superior. In practice, these limitations can be minimized as long as safety and vascular control are maintained.

The lateral limit of resection for olfactory groove meningiomas is the midorbital vertical meridian (fig. 5). This limitation is created by, as we believe most limitations are, a nerve, in this case the optic nerve. Removal of the lamina papyracea allows gentle retraction of the periorbita and orbital contents to allow access to the orbital roof out to the midorbit.

The posterior limit for an EEA is essentially the same as for any anterior approach. Most olfactory groove meningiomas do not extend past the tuberculum sellae. They tend to displace the optic nerves and chiasm laterally and posteriorly and the anterior cerebral and communicating arteries superiorly and posteriorly. Therefore, unless there is significant tumor extending beyond these confines or wrapping around these structures, tumor is accessible via an EEA.

The same holds true for superior tumor extent with one caveat. Very tall tumors can be difficult to access and care must be taken not to remove too much of the inferior and anterior capsule before the apex of the tumor has been debulked. The frontal lobes can herniate into the field, obscuring view. Sometimes, very tall tumors need to be resected in stages, with a significant initial debulking allowing tumor descent over time prior to complete resection.

Image Guidance

Image guidance and navigation systems are critical for endoscopic skull base surgery. New image guidance systems help to localize pathology, enhance safety and reduce morbidity. They also have the potential benefit of enhancing confidence and safety in trainees. Better localization with image guidance can help delineate obscured tumor boundaries, aid in ensuring complete resection and to also identify inflammatory disease and adjacent vital structures. Identification and dissection around the internal carotid artery and multiple cranial nerves require optimal exposure and image guidance can assist in this regard [25]. The drawbacks for such systems include a necessary time delay in the order of 5–20 min for image registration [26].

Learning Curve

As with any EEA, the transcribriform approach for olfactory groove meningioma has a steep learning curve. We believe that these particular tumors, while often well suited for this approach, require an experienced team to be addressed safely. The extensive anatomic knowledge and intradural microdissection techniques necessary can only be acquired with time and exposure via other tumors. This full learning curve concept is better detailed in another chapter in this book, but we believe that olfactory groove meningiomas, as with other intradural tumors should not be approached until late in the learning curve of an endoscopic skull base team. It is critical to evaluate tumor involvement with the ACAs and their branches. If there is a cuff of cerebral cortex between the tumor and the ACAs, tumor resection is safer and simpler than if no such cuff exists, regardless of arachnoid and pial invasion. If the vessels are touched by the tumor, one will not know until the time of surgery how separable they are. The dissection and control of arteries during an EEA requires significant experience, both by the individual surgeon as well as the team together. Finally, if the vessels are enveloped by the tumor, there are many who believe that these tumors should not be approached endonasally as this dissection is perilous enough when using a microscope. At the very least, they should not be attempted until the endoscopic team has worked together on many such cases without vascular involvement.

Conclusions

The EEA for olfactory groove meningiomas represents the culmination of the approach via collaboration between otolaryngologists and neurosurgeons in an attempt to reach the ultimate goal of any skull base approach, maximal tumor resection with minimal or no neural or brain manipulation. Conceptually, the approach makes sense as it converts these tumors into 'convexity' meningiomas by approaching them from their surface of dural attachment and origin.

References

1 Arbit A, Shah JP: Combined craniofacial resection for anterior skull base tumors. Neurosurg Operative Atlas 1991;1:342–352.

2 Patel SG, Singh B, Polluri A, et al: Craniofacial surgery for malignant skull base tumors: report of an international collaboration study. Skull Base 2003; 13(suppl 1):7–8.

3 Lund V, Howard DJ, Wei WI, Cheesman AD: Craniofacial resection for tumors of the nasal cavity and paranasal sinuses-a 17-year experience. Head Neck 1998;20:97–105.

4 Har-El G, Casiano RR: Endoscopic management of anterior skull base tumors. Otolaryngol Clin N Am 2005;38:133–144.

5 Dandy WE: Orbital tumor: Results following the Transcranial Operative Attack. New York, Oskar Priest, 1941, pp 168–188.

6 Smith RR, Klopp CT, Williams JM: Surgical treatment of cancer of the frontal sinus and adjacent areas. Cancer 1954;7:991–994.

7 Ketcham AS, Wilkins RH, Van Buren JM, et al: A combined intracranial facial approach to the paranasal sinuses. Am J Surg 1963;106:698–703.

8 Yuen AP, Fung CF, Hung KN: Endoscopic cranionasal resection of anterior skull base tumor. Am J Otolaryngol 1997;18:431–433.

9 Stammberger H, Anderhuber W, Walch C, et al: Possibilities and limitations of endoscopic management of nasal and paranasal sinus malignancies. Acta Otorhinolaryngol Belg 1999;53:199–205.

10 Snyderman C, Carrau R, Kassam A, Zanation A, Prevedello D, Gardner P, Mintz A: Endoscopic skull base surgery: principles of endonasal oncological surgery. J Surg Onc 2008;97:658–664.

11 Casiano RR, Numa WA, Falquez AM: Endoscopic resection of esthesioneuroblastoma. Am J Rhinol 2001;15:271.

12 Castelnuovo PG, Delu G, Sberze F, et al: Esthesioneuroblastoma: endonasal endoscopic treatment. Skull Base 2006;16:25–30.

13 Kaplan MJ, Fischbein NJ, Harsh GR: Anterior skull base surgery. Otolaryngol Clin N Am 2005;38:107–131.

14 Busquets JM, Hwang PH: Endoscopic resection of sinonasal inverted papilloma: a meta-analysis. Otolaryng Head Neck Surg 2006;134:476–482.

15 Casler JD, Doolittle AM, Mair EA: Endoscopic surgery of the anterior skull base. Laryngoscope 2005,115:16–24.

16 Krouse JH: Endoscopic treatment of inverted papilloma: safety and efficacy. Am J Otolaryngol 2001;22: 87–99.

17 Baruah P, Deka RC: Endoscopic management of inverted papillomas of the nose and paranasal sinuses. Ear Nose Throat J 2003;82:317–320.

18 Kraft M, Simmen D, Kaufmann T, et al: Long-term results of endonasal sinus surgery in sinonasal papillomas. Laryngoscope 2003;113:1541–1547.

19 Dubin MG, Kuhn FA: Endoscopic modified Lothrop (Draf III) with frontal sinus Punches. Laryngoscope 2005;115:1702–1703.

20 Draf W: Endonasal micro-endoscopic frontal sinus surgery: the Fulda concept. Oper Tech Otolaryngol Head Neck Surg 1991;2:234–240.

21 Becker DG, Moore D, Lindsey WH, Gross WE, Gross CW: Modified transnasal endoscopic Lothrop procedure: further considerations. Laryngosocope 1995;105:1161–1166.

22 Floreani SR, Nair SB, Switajewski MC, Wormald PJ: Endoscopic anterior ethmoidal artery ligation: a cadaver study. Laryngoscope 2006;116:1263–1267.

23 Pletcher SD, Metson R: Endoscopic ligation of the anterior ethmoid artery. Laryngoscope 2007;117: 378–381.

24 Kassam AB, Thomas A, Carrau RL, Snyderman CH, Vescan A, Prevedello D, Mintz A, Gardner P: Endoscopic reconstruction of the cranial base using a pedicled nasoseptal flap. Neurosurgery 2008;63(1 suppl 1):ONS44–S52, discussion ONS52–S53.).

25 Carrau RL, Snyderman CH, Curtin HD, Janecka IP, Stechison M, Weissman JL: Computer-assisted intraoperative navigation during skull base surgery. Am J Otolaryngol 1996;17:95–101.

26 Petruzzelli GJ, Origitano TC, Stankiewicz, Anderson DE: Frameless stereotactic localization in cranial base surgery. Skull Base Surgery 2000;10:125–130.

Paul A. Gardner, MD
Department of Neurological Surgery
University of Pittsburgh School of Medicine
200 Lothrop Street, PUH, Suite B400
Pittsburgh, PA 15213–2582 (USA)
Tel. +1 412 647 3685, E-Mail gardpa@upmc.edu

Kassam AB, Gardner PA (eds): Endoscopic Approaches to the Skull Base.
Prog Neurol Surg. Basel, Karger, 2012, vol 26, pp 87–103

Endoscopic Anterior Skull Base Resection for Esthesioneuroblastoma

Adam M. Zanation[a] · Roy R. Casiano[b] · Ricardo L. Carrau[c] · Carl H. Snyderman[e,f] · Amin B. Kassam[g] · Paul A. Gardner[f] · Daniel M. Prevedello[d] · Candace A. Mitchell[a] · Arlan H. Mintz[e]

[a]Department of Otolaryngology, Head and Neck Surgery, Chapel Hill, N.C., [b]Department of Otolaryngology, Head and Neck Surgery, University of Miami Health System, Miami, Fla., Departments of [c]Otolaryngology, Head and Neck Surgery and [d]Neurological Surgery, The Ohio State University Medical Center, Columbus, Ohio, and Departments of [e]Otolaryngology, Head and Neck Surgery, and [f]Neurological Surgery, University of Pittsburgh Medical Center, Pittsburgh, Pa., USA; [g]Division of Neurological Surgery, University of Ottawa, The Ottawa Hospital Civic Campus, Ottawa, Ont., Canada

Abstract

Esthesioneuroblastomas (ENB) are relatively rare neoplasms accounting for less than 5% of malignant sinus tumors. The presentation, preoperative evaluation, imaging, and staging are described. The roles of endoscopic endonasal resection and the traditional transcranial subfrontal approach are compared. The endoscopic surgical technique is emphasized including postoperative repair. The early outcomes of patients who have undergone this approach as well as the role of adjunctive treatment including radiation therapy are described. Potential complications from CSF leak to infectious to vascular are reviewed.

Esthesioneuroblastomas (ENB) are relatively uncommon accounting for approximately 3–5% of primary malignant sinus tumors [1, 2]. Berger et al. [3] first described ENB in 1924, initiating significant controversies as to the cell of origin, staging and management. Its management has been studied and advanced for more than 80 years; however, throughout this period, surgical resection has been the keystone of treatment. The most recent surgical advancement is the use of endoscopic endonasal approaches (EEA) for the resection of ENBs that originate or involve the anterior skull base. In appropriately selected patients, EEA offers excellent visualization that facilitates a complete resection while avoiding external incisions and frontal lobe retraction. The purpose of this review is to outline the current management of ENB including endoscopic surgical techniques and their complications, adjunctive treatments, management of the neck, and treatment outcomes.

The exact cell of origin of ENB is controversial. Proposed sources include the vomeronasal organ, the sphenopalatine ganglion, autonomic ganglia in the nasal mucosa, and the olfactory epithelium. It has also been proposed that ENB is a variant of Ewing's sarcoma or neuroblastoma; however, ENB lack the (11:22) trans-location that is characteristic of Ewing's sarcoma [4, 5] and are genetically distinct from conventional neuroblastoma [6, 7]. Currently, ENBs are presumed to arise from the olfactory epithelium, which would account for their intimate relationship with the cribiform plate, the midline superior nasal structures and the anterior skull base.

Presentation

ENB presents within a wide age range with a bimodal peak: one in the second and third decades of life, and again in the sixth and seventh decades [3]. Twenty percent of all ENBs present in patients under the age of 20, with the youngest reported case being 3 years of age [1].

ENB presents with a multitude of nonspecific symptoms, the most common being nasal obstruction (70%). Other presenting symptoms include epistaxis, anosmia, and less frequently cranial neuropathy, headache, vision changes, mental status changes, proptosis and diplopia. These symptoms and signs, although not specific for a histological diagnosis, do reflect the location of the tumor and may be predictive of the extent of involvement of adjacent anatomic structures. Nonetheless, the clinical presentation of the tumor may be identical to that of inflammatory sinus disease and a delay in diagnosis is not uncommon. Diplopia may be associated with invasion of orbital structures. Intracranial extension with significant involvement of the frontal lobes may occur without any specific symptom. Owing to this 'silent' area of the brain, the first indication of invasion of the brain may be symptoms associated with elevated intracranial pressure, such as headache. On further questioning (especially in patients with extensive intracranial disease), one may be able to detect short-term memory deficits and personality changes with disinhibition and inappropriate responses.

Because of the internal location of these tumors, the external clinical examination may not detect any manifestations until the tumor reaches an advanced stage. Widening of the nasal dorsum and pseudotelecanthus may be seen with slow-growing anterior tumors. Lateral extension into the orbit may result in chemosis, periorbital swelling, proptosis or restriction of extraocular movements and/or diplopia. Visual loss is a late occurrence and is seen more often with tumors that originate close to the optic chiasm or orbital apex. Intracranial extension may be associated with signs of elevated intracranial pressure, such as papilledema.

Intranasal examination may be difficult due to the mass effect of the tumor, deviation of the nasal septum, edema, or obstructing nasal polyps. The examination is greatly facilitated with the use of flexible fiberoptic or rigid rod lens endoscopes. A tumor that originates from the nasal vault, medial to the attachment of the middle turbinate in the olfactory sulcus, suggests an ENB. Extension of a neoplasm into the maxillary sinus or into the orbit from the anterior cranial base may be evident. Posteriorly, involvement of the Eustachian tube or nasopharynx may be detected, indicating that involvement of the internal carotid artery is a possibility and that appropriate imaging is necessary.

Preoperative Evaluation, Imaging and Staging

Some aspects of the physical examination have been addressed above. Endoscopic visualization of the nasal cavity and nasopharynx is considered a routine part of the examination. This may provide useful information regarding the origin, extent, and vascularity of the tumor. Additional preoperative testing may include assessments of olfactory function using 'scratch-and-sniff' panels; however, this testing will not change the management. A neuro-ophthalmologic examination including visual acuity and visual field testing is warranted because of the potential for subtle changes given the location of the tumor and also to have a baseline examination for any potential post-operative vision changes. Biopsies are most commonly obtained in the operating room setting owing to concerns of bleeding and possible communication with cerebrospinal fluid (CSF). However, large fungating tumors that are easily visualized in the anterior nasal cavity may be biopsied with minor risk in the office setting. Debulking of the tumor before imaging is not recommended as it may alter the magnetic resonance imaging (MRI) characteristics of the tumor and it may even cause difficulty with the visualization of the intraoperative margins.

Imaging is an essential part of the evaluation of these patients. Involvement of the orbit and intracranial extension may not be clinically apparent. A paranasal sinus computed tomography (CT) scan with contrast is the preferred initial examination (fig. 1a–c). Images through the skull base are obtained at intervals of 1 mm or less in order to achieve maximum resolution. The CT scan provides excellent bone detail and is superior to MRI in detecting bony erosion of the anterior cranial base and paranasal sinuses. A contrast agent provides an assessment of the overall vascularity of the tumor as well as its relationship with intracranial vasculature. Coronal and sagittal images of the anterior cranial base are superior to axial images in demonstrating intracranial extension and the skull base bone anatomy (fig. 1a–c). MRI provides much greater detail of soft tissue structures and complements CT scanning in most patients. Bone detail is poorly visualized with MRI. MRI is particularly valuable for demonstrating dural involvement and invasion of the brain. MRI is also superior for demonstrating perineural extension of tumor. When a sinus is opacified, a CT scan may not be able to differentiate tumor from retained secretions. MRI with T_1- and T_2-weighted images allows differentiation of tumor and secretions.

Angiography is usually not necessary for ENB unless there is neoplastic involvement of the cavernous sinus or extensive extracranial involvement with extension of

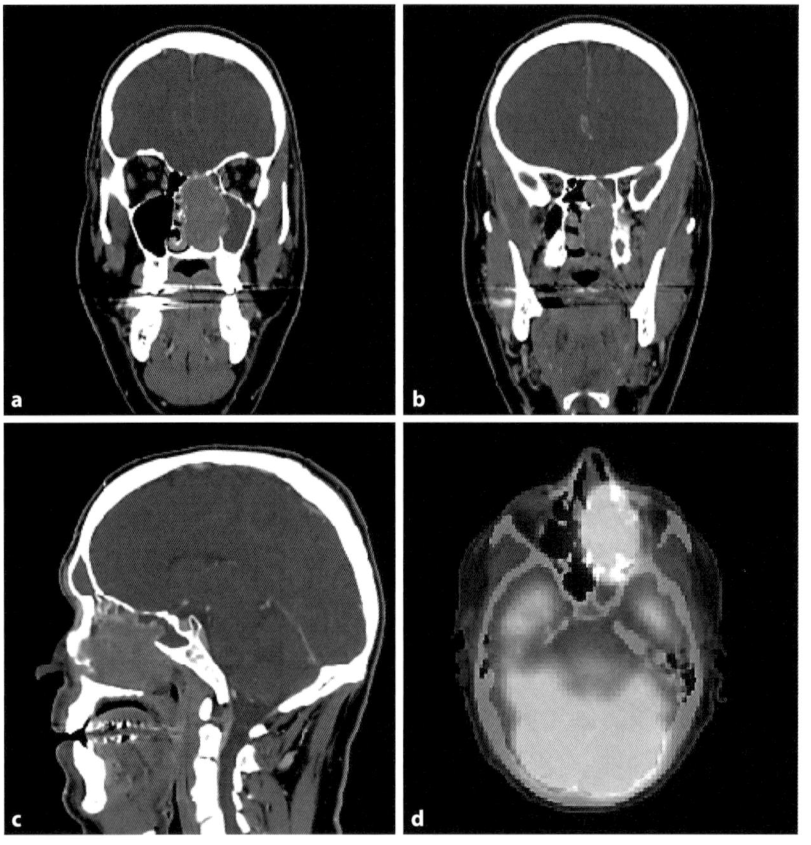

Fig. 1. **a** Coronal CT of patient 'X' with a left Kadish C ENB. **b** Coronal CT patient 'X' with a left Kadish C ENB with sphenoid involvement but no orbital apex involvement. **c** Sagittal CT of patient 'X'. **d** PET/CT of patient 'X'.

tumor to the infratemporal skull base. CT or MR angiography is usually adequate to establish the status of the vasculature in these areas and for potential carotid involvement. PET or PET/CT scanning is useful for staging of potential distant and regional metastasis (fig. 1d).

There are several staging systems for ENB. The most common was described by Kadish [8] in 1976 (see below). More recently, a staging system based upon a TMN type classification system was proposed (see below) to include a more specific description of regional and distant metastasis into the staging system [9].

Modified Kadish Staging System

Stage A: Tumor confined to the nasal cavity.
Stage B: Tumor confined to the nasal cavity and paranasal sinuses.

Stage C: Tumor confined beyond the nasal cavity and paranasal sinuses, including involvement of the cribriform plate, base of the skull, orbit or intracranial cavity.
Stage D: Tumor with metastasis to cervical lymph nodes or distant sites.

TMN Esthesioneuroblastoma Staging System
T1: Tumor involving the nasal cavity and/or paranasal sinuses (excluding sphenoid), sparing the most superior ethmoidal cells.
T2: Tumor involving the nasal cavity and/or paranasal sinuses (including the sphenoid) with extension to or erosion of the cribriform plate.
T3: Tumor extending into the orbit or protruding into the anterior cranial fossa, without dural invasion.
T4: Tumor involving the brain.
N0: No cervical lymph-node metastasis.
N1: Any form of cervical lymph-node metastasis.
M0: No metastases.
M1: Distant metastasis.

Traditional Open Craniofacial Technique

Open anterior craniofacial resection most often consists of two approaches combined; one transfacial and the other a subfrontal craniotomy. The transfacial approach can be accomplished via a lateral rhinotomy, facial degloving, or Weber-Ferguson incision with or without orbital exenteration. Once the transfacial exposure is accomplished, the septum is transected as the inferior margin, the ethmoid arteries are controlled and the lamina papyraceae are removed as the lateral margins (periorbita and orbital contents can be removed if needed to clear the margins). The sphenoid is then entered and exposed so the planum sphenoidale or optic chiasm can be seen as the posterior margin. The neurosurgical team approaches from above after a bifrontal craniotomy and supraorbital osteotomies via a bicoronal incision. The frontal lobes are retracted from the anterior base to visualize the median anterior skull base and dural margins. A partial frontal lobectomy can also be performed to remove gross tumor or clear margins (Kadish C tumors). Using both the transcranial and transfacial routes, the median anterior skull base is removed from lamina papyracea to lamina papyracea and from the posterior wall of the frontal sinus to the planum sphenoidale. The dura adjacent to this area, the olfactory bulbs and tracts are also removed. The resection comprises the entire ethmoid sinuses bloc, superior septum, lamina papyraceae, anterior skull base and dura. Margins of resection are analyzed intraoperatively to ensure complete removal of the tumor. Once margins are clear, the pericranial flap raised and placed under the frontal lobes and over the anterior skull base to cover the entire defect. The cranial and supraorbital bone grafts are then fixated in their original anatomical position using adaptation plates. Any transfacial incisions are closed meticulously. Nasal packing is rarely necessary, although we commonly use hemostatic agents such as absorbable gelatin sponges. An anterior craniofacial resection provides direct visualization and the ability to take wide dural and intracranial margins (especially lateral over the orbital roof). It also allows an excellent skull base reconstruction with vascularized tissue. Disadvantages include the cosmetic facial deformity, frontal lobe retraction, illumination limited by external light sources and magnification limited by the extent of the surgeon's loupes. Even in experienced hands, it is associated with a very high frequency of complications ranging from 30 to 60%.

Combined Endoscopic and Open Techniques

This technique combines a transnasal endoscopic resection of tumor with a traditional transcranial-subfrontal exposure. It requires a bicoronal incision but involves no facial or oral incisions and it allows for reconstruction using a pericranial or galeo-pericranial flap. This technique has the advantage of sparing the facial cosmesis while offering excellent intranasal visualization provided by the superior illumination and magnification of the endoscope; however, it does not eliminate the morbidity of a craniotomy and the need for frontal lobe retraction.

Expanded Endoscopic Endonasal Anterior Craniofacial Resection

We have described several endoscopic 'modules' based on the exposure and control of key skull base and neurovascular structures. Although this chapter addresses the resection of the anterior skull base for the specific indication of ENB, we consider this approach as a part of an encompassing modular system that provides endoscopic exposure of the entire anatomy of the sinonasal tract and the anterior skull base and clival regions [10–15].

Patients are positioned supine on the operating table with the head in neutral position and fixed by a three-pin head holder with the neck slightly rotated to the right side. Exposure of the frontal sinus (endoscopic Lothrop or Draf III) is required for the resection of most ENBs, and its exposure is enhanced by a mild extension of the neck. The video monitor is placed at the left side of the patient. If two video-monitors are available, they are positioned directly in front of each surgeon.

The nasal cavity is decongested with cottonoids soaked in oxymetazoline 0.05% and then examined with 0° and 45° endoscopes (fig. 2a). Lidocaine 1% with 1:100,000 epinephrine solution may be infiltrated in the lateral nasal wall, anterior attachment of the middle turbinates, anterior nasal septum and rostrum of the sphenoid sinus for additional hemostasis. Infiltration of vasoconstrictors must be avoided in areas involving the vascular pedicle for a nasoseptal flap if one is to be harvested

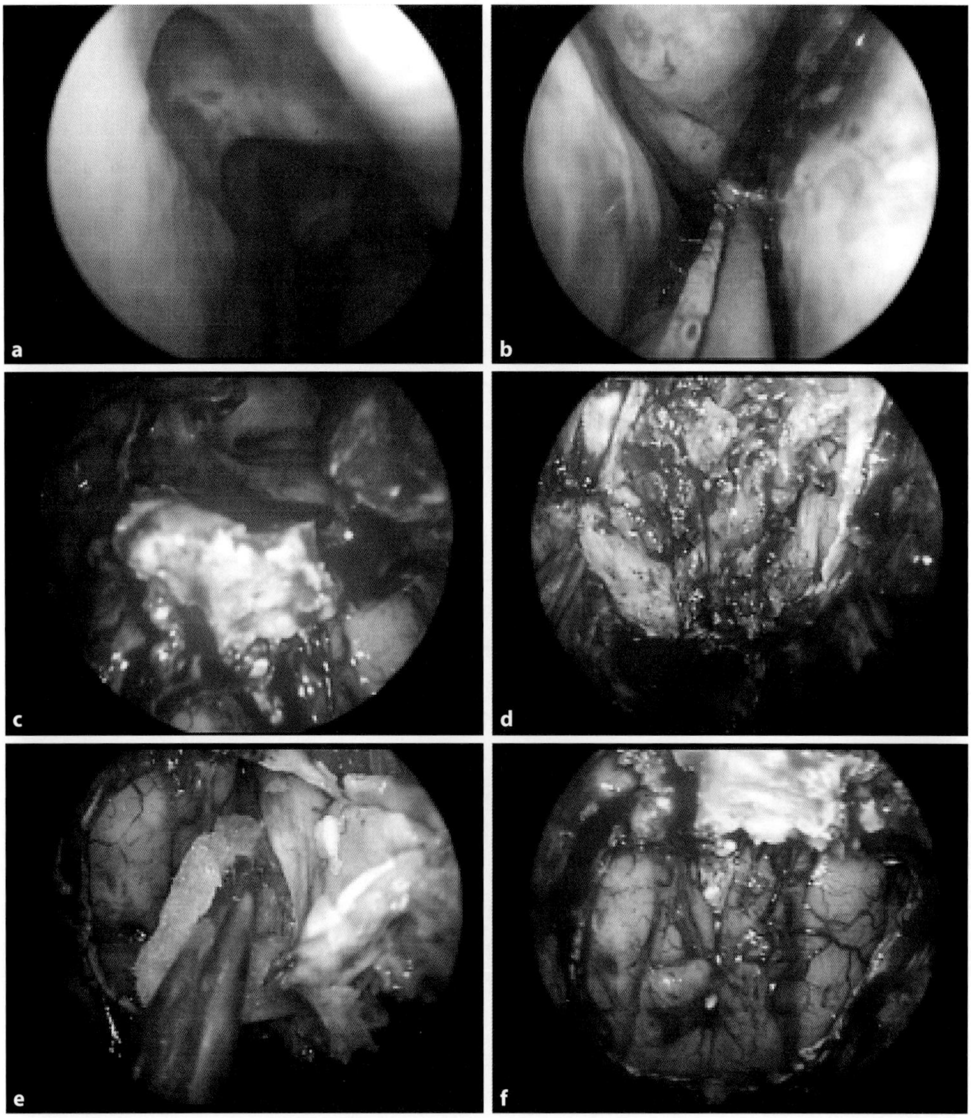

Fig. 2. **a** Intraoperative zero degree endoscopic view of patient 'X' after preoperative chemoradiation with persistent left sided disease. **b** Intraoperative zero degree endoscopic view of HB flap elevated on right side while a superior frozen section margin is taken. **c** Intraoperative 45 degree endoscopic view of the Draf III sinusotomy. **d** Intraoperative zero degree endoscopic view of lateral dural cuts with the olfactory groove intact in the midline. **e** Intraoperative zero degree endoscopic view of the removal of the anterior skull base dura. **f** Intraoperative zero degree endoscopic view of the entire skull base defect.

(see below). The operation begins with the debulking of the tumor and resection of the middle turbinate(s). Using a microdebrider, the tumor is debulked to increase exposure of the tumor site of origin, skull base and nasal margins. Resection of the middle turbinate further enhances the visualization of these areas. Dissection of the paranasal sinuses follows a technique similar to that one used for the management of inflammatory disease. The dissection can be unilateral or bilateral depending on the extent of the tumor. An uncinectomy is followed by the identification and widening of the natural ostium of the maxillary sinus in a posterior and inferior direction. A wide middle meatal antrostomy helps to define the inferior and medial walls of the orbits and exposes the posterior wall of the antrum, thus facilitating control of the sphenopalatine and posterior nasal arteries. Completion of anterior and posterior ethmoidectomies and exposure of the nasofrontal recess will define and expose the paramedian anterior skull base including the fovea ethmoidalis, the vertical and horizontal lamellae of the cribiform plate and its olfactory filae, and the anterior and posterior ethmoidal artery canals. A Draf III or endoscopic Lothrop procedure exposes the posterior wall of the frontal sinus and enhances the exposure of the anterior margin of the tumor (fig. 2c).

At this point, a vascularized nasoseptal flap is harvested for reconstruction, provided that does not interfere with the oncologic resection (fig. 2b). Until recently, the options for endoscopic reconstruction of the skull base were limited to the use of nonvascularized tissue. This yielded CSF leak rates of 12–20% (anterior skull base resection of sinonasal tumors) and became a major obstacle for the widespread acceptance of these techniques. Recently, the Haddad-Bassagaisteguy flap (HBF) or nasoseptal flap has proven to be a versatile, robust vascularized flap for the reconstruction of endonasal dural defects [16]. Since its adoption we have seen our CSF leak rates drop to numbers comparable to those of traditional techniques (5%). The advantage of this flap as a reconstructive option is that a second approach or incision is not necessary and the flap can be harvested endoscopically. The major drawback of the HBF is that its need must be anticipated prior to the resection as the vascular pedicle of this flap is frequently compromised during the sphenoidotomy and posterior septectomy. In addition, if a revision procedure is necessary, the flap may have been used previously or the pedicle previously damaged. In patients with ENB the septum may be involved by tumor; therefore the HBF will not be available.

The flap should be designed based on the anticipated size of the defect. This is counterintuitive to most reconstructive surgeons, as the flap is harvested before the resultant defect is created; thus, one can be left with a flap that is inadequate. Due to this potential flaw, we tend to harvest the largest possible flap. The most critical incision involves the use of needle electrocautery along the free edge of the choana from the lateral nasal wall toward the nasal septum. This incision is exceedingly difficult to perform once the flap has been elevated; thus, extra time and patience is warranted to ensure a full incision carried down to the level of the bone of the sphenoid floor. Two longitudinal incisions are then created from posterior to anterior. The most inferior incision is placed along the maxillary crest; however, it can be extended inferiorly and laterally to harvest the mucoperiosteum of the nasal floor. The superior incision is created 1–1.5cm inferior to the cribiform plate in order to preserve olfactory epithelium. Occasionally this incision must be moved inferiorly due to tumor involvement; if this is the case, the margin should be analyzed histologically to ensure that the flap is free of tumor (fig. 2b). The superior incision crosses the rostrum of the sphenoid at the level of the sphenoid sinus os. This leaves a pedicle across the anterior face of the sphenoid that is approximately 1–2 cm wide. Both of these incisions are joined anteriorly with a vertical incision at the most rostral end of the septal mucoperichondrium, just posterior to the columella. Once all of the incisions are completed, the flap is elevated from anterior to posterior in a subperichondrial and subperiosteal plane back to the origin of its vascular pedicle at the sphenopalatine foramen. The flap can then be 'stored' for the duration of the resection, in the nasopharynx or inside the antrum through a wide maxillary antrostomy.

In the event that a flap cannot be harvested due to involvement with tumor or because of a compromised blood supply, the nasal septum is separated from the sphenoid rostrum using a transfixion incision with a Cottle elevator. A similar vertical transfixion incision is performed at a level just posterior to the nasofrontal recess (this may be modified to include the anterior extent of the tumor). A third septal transfixion incision, horizontal and parallel to the floor of the nose, connects these two vertical transfixion incisions and leaves the bony nasal septum attached to the cribiform plate. These steps are part of the tumor resection even if the HBF is harvested. Bilateral wide sphenoidotomies, which remove the entire rostrum, help define the posterior limit of the tumor (planum sphenoidale) and further delineate the position of the skull base. At this point of the surgery, the skull base from orbit to orbit and from frontal sinus to sella turcica, as well as the base of the tumor, are completely exposed and resection is ready to proceed (fig. 3a). The lamina papyracea may be removed as a lateral margin or as part of an endoscopic medial maxillectomy (unilaterally or bilaterally according to the necessary resection), taking care to preserve the periorbita while identifying the anterior and posterior ethmoidal arteries at their entry into their respective bony canals. Gentle curettage or drilling removes the bone over the canal, exposing the arteries, which can then be dissected and controlled using clips or bipolar electrocautery.

Using a high-speed drill with a 3- or 4-mm coarse diamond (hybrid) burr, a horizontal osteotomy is made at the planum sphenoidale, parallel and anterior to the sphenoid rostrum. Another horizontal osteotomy is made just posterior to the frontal sinus posterior wall. These osteotomies are then connected by bilateral osteotomies performed lateral to the cribiform plate and running parallel to the superomedial wall of the orbits, thereby forming a rectangle which surrounds the tumor and adjacent structures such as the nasal septum, the entire cribiform plate and the planum sphenoidale. The resection then proceeds in an anterior to posterior direction. The olfactory nerves are identified and transected after bipolar

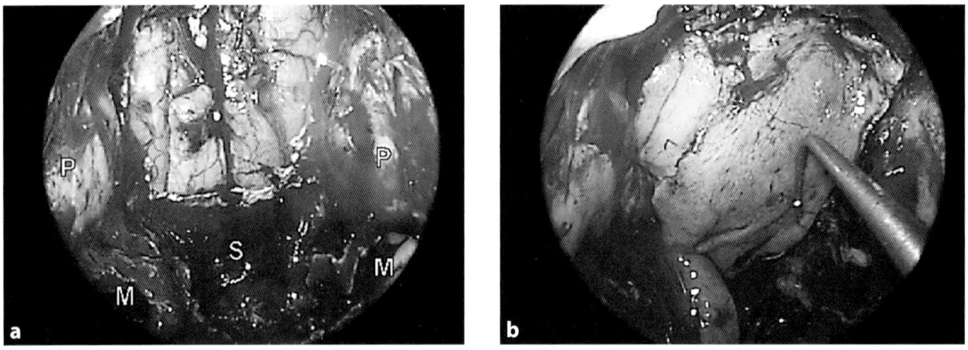

Fig. 3. **a** Intraoperative endoscopic view of the ACF from patient 'X' with free margins (P = periorbita; M = maxillary sinus; S = sphenoid sinus) prior to reconstruction. **b** Placement of the HB flap over the ACF defect.

cauterization. An alternative – and most often safer – technique is to remove the median anterior skull base in layers. First, the mucosa and olfactory epithelium are removed, then the bone, then the dura (fig. 2d–f). The dural surface can be coagulated using a bipolar cautery and is then incised. It is critical to establish the completeness of the resection with the use of intraoperative frozen section analysis. Any positive margin mandates additional resection. Resection of the olfactory bulbs and tracts is based on the intraoperative frozen section analysis, but should be performed at least unilaterally.

The crista galli is most often disconnected from the rest of the skull base. It must be removed, nonetheless, to improve visualization and to facilitate the reconstruction. It should be noted that the crista galli can extend for a variable depth into the intracranial cavity; thus, its removal involves drilling internally until it becomes thin so it can be fractured. Meticulous hemostasis completes the anterior cranial base resection. As previously stated, the resection can be unilateral, preserving the contralateral turbinates and possibly the olfactory fibers, but only in cases where tumor involvement allows it.

Endoscopic Anterior Skull Base Reconstruction

We have dedicated a chapter to endoscopic skull base reconstruction; however, a brief description follows. A collagen matrix dural substitute is placed as an inlay graft under (superior to) the dural and bone margins. The septal flap is then rotated over the defect with the mucosal surface facing the nasal cavity (fig. 3b, 4a, b). The entire defect is covered and oxidized cellulose cut to 1 by 1.5 cm sizes are used to 'picture frame' the external edge to fix the HBF flap in place. Duraseal (Confuent Surgical Inc., Waltham, Mass., USA) is then sprayed over the HBF. Absorbable gelatin sponges are

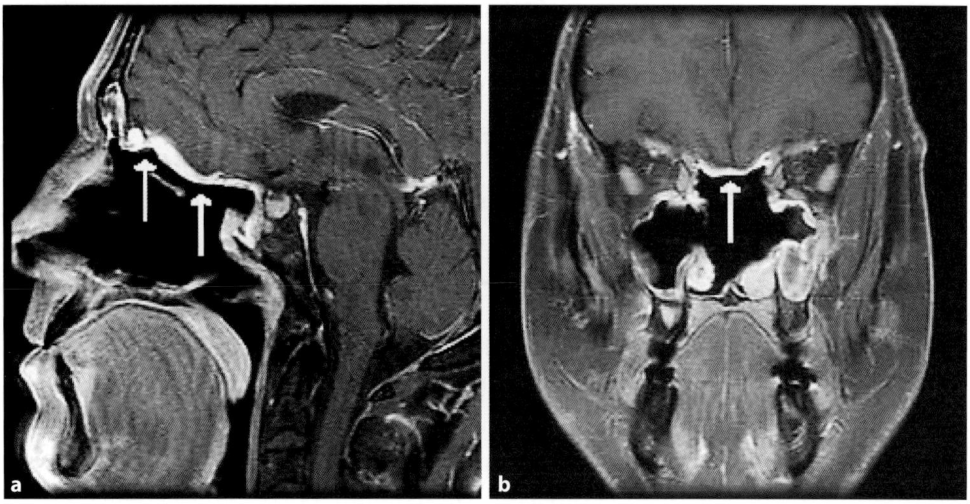

Fig. 4. Postoperative sagittal (**a**) and coronal (**b**) T1 with contrast MRI of patient 'X' showing no evidence of disease and excellent HB flap reconstruction (arrows)

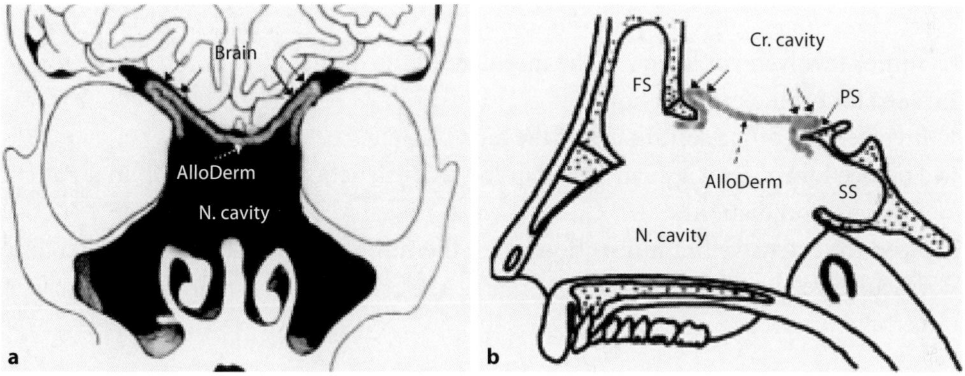

Fig. 5. Artistic representation in coronal (**a**) and sagittal (**b**) planes of an alloplastic graft reconstruction technique for anterior skull base defects.

then applied and an expandable sponge packing or a Foley catheter balloon is placed to hold press the flap against the defect. If the optic nerves or chiasm are exposed during the operation, the use of a Foley catheter balloon is relatively contraindicated.

An alloplastic graft technique reconstructive option is also available. It is the reconstructive option of choice at the University of Miami (Dr. Casiano) and is also utilized at the University of Pittsburgh in situations where an HBF is not available. This option for repairing large anterior skull base defects involves the use of Alloderm (AlloDerm, Life Cell Corp. Woodlands, Tex., USA) or lyophilized dura, as an onlay graft [22] (fig. 5 a, b). Large defects are repaired using a technique in which the graft material is positioned intracranially, to overly the bony margins of the defect circumferentially over the medial orbital roof, planum sphenoidale, and posterior wall of the frontal sinus (fig. 5). The graft is 'rolled' onto itself and extended intranasally over the de-epithelialized superomedial orbital wall, postero-inferior frontal sinus, and common sphenoid sinus cavity roof. The intracranial pocket created by this rolling of the graft is filled with gelfoam pledgets (Gelfoam; Pharmacia and Upjohn, Kalamazoo, Mich., USA). Merocel tampons (usually 2) are placed inferior to the grafted defect to provide counterpressure against the weight of the brain. The merocel is removed on postoperative day seven. The gelfoam is left undisturbed to fall off on its own. The reconstructed area will go through approximately a 6-month period of mild crusting, eschar formation, and healing by secondary intention that should be left undisturbed. During this time, the graft is replaced with a thick band of re-epithelialized granulation tissue and fibrosis. Patients can still undergo radiation therapy within a month of reconstruction. In a few patients, prolonged crusting (greater than 6 months) may ensue. These patients are treated with topical wound care including culture-directed topical antibiotics.

Relative Contraindications to Endoscopic Anterior Skull Base Resection

1. Tumor involvement lateral to the meridian of the orbits.
2. Need for orbital exenteration.
3. Involvement of the soft tissues of the face.
4. The need for microvascular free flap for reconstruction (absent HBF in a patient after chemoradiation).
5. Need for extensive brain resection when the tumor involves the anterior cerebral vasculature.

Outcomes

In a recent meta-analysis of ENB, the overall and disease-free survival at 5 years averaged 45 and 41% [9]. This rate is considerably lower than the 60–70% range that some of the larger ENB series report; however, these studies are often the result of controlled treatment protocols and patients often received aggressive multi-modality treatment and excellent follow-up. In this meta-analysis, histological grading according to the Hyams classification and cervical metastases emerged as prognostic factors. Survival rates in patients Hyams' grades I–II was 56% compared with 25% for patients with grades III–IV (odds ratio 6.2). In patients with N+ disease at initial presentation (approximately 5% of the total number of patients) survival was 29%, compared to 64% for patients with N0 disease (OR 5.1). Survival rates according to treatment modalities were 65% for surgery plus radiotherapy, 51% for radiotherapy and chemotherapy, 48% for surgery alone, 47% for surgery plus radiotherapy and chemotherapy, and 37% for radiotherapy alone. A combination of surgery and radiotherapy seems to be the best treatment; in this study no endoscopic resection trials were analyzed. The role of chemotherapy as adjunctive treatment with surgery and radiation is still unclear.

In a large combined series of endoscopic resection for cure of ENB, the University of Pittsburgh Medical Center and the University of Miami reviewed their outcomes in 23 patients. Of the 23 patients, 19 were treated for primary disease while 4 were treated for recurrent tumors. The most common stage at presentation was stage B (58.9%), then C (26.3%), A (10.5%), and D (5.3%). One patient required conversion to an endoscopic assisted approach, complementing the endoscopic approach with a transcranial approach, to clear a positive margin along the supraorbital dura. Only one patient had a positive margin at the orbital apex at the conclusion of the procedure. Post-operative radiation therapy was administered to 16 patients. The mean length of follow-up for the study group was 37 months (3–144 months). All of the patients who presented for primary surgery showed no evidence of disease (NED) at their last follow-up visit. Of the 4 patients who had recurrent disease at presentation, 3 were NED at their last follow-up. Complication rates were reasonable: there were no cases of tension pneumocephalus, 8 cases exhibiting chronic nasal crusting, 4 CSF leaks, 2 cases of dacryocystitis, 1 case of epistaxis, and 1 case of osteomyelitis of the bone flap. In this series, endoscopic resection with clear margins and post-operative radiation therapy provided excellent disease control.

Castelnuovo et al. [17] reported on their series of 10 patients with ENB treated with endoscopic techniques. Eight of the 10 patients were Kadish A (n = 3) or B (n = 5). The mean follow-up was 38 months and they had no patients with recurrent disease. Again, this series supports endoscopic resection as an effective technique for disease control.

Adjunctive Treatment

Standard radiotherapeutic techniques include daily radiation treatment for 6–7 weeks. The dose ranges from 5,500 to 7,000 cGy and in most cases is above 6,000 cGy. Protection of the optic chiasm and optic nerves is given considerable planning to deliver the highest radiation exposure to the tumor site while minimizing potential vision problems. Possible roles of proton beam radiotherapy and IMRT are currently being studied.

Neoadjuvant chemotherapy has been advocated by many groups for patients with advanced disease. At the University of Virginia, patients with Kadish stage C disease are first treated with two cycles of chemotherapy followed by full course radiotherapy, which is then followed by planned open craniofacial resection [18]. With this regimen the 5-year actuarial survival was 72% and that at 10 years 60%. The extent to which chemotherapy contributed to these cure rates is unclear. At Harvard, adjunctive chemotherapy followed by proton radiation was studied in nine patients. They did not have a planned surgical treatment modality in their protocol. They reported excellent results with complete responses in 8 of 9 patients; these data are promising but their number of patients is small and the follow-up is short [19]. There is significant data to support surgical therapy as a part of multimodal treatment in ENB patients and protocols without a planned resection should be done as a clinical trial only.

Treatment of the Neck

Management of the neck in cases of ENB is controversial. There is substantial evidence that this disease is associated with a rate of cervical metastases as high as 25%, most of which may not become apparent until after 2 years. In a review by David and Weissler, patients with Kadish C disease (24/55) had 44% overall rate of neck metastasis compared with an overall rate of 18.8% (39/207) and 10% (15/152) in patients with Kadish A and B disease [20]. In the estimated 5% of patients who present initially with neck metastases, treatment should proceed with a neck dissection and radiotherapy [21]. Another 15–20% of these patients present with late cervical metastasis after treatment at the primary site; these patients are then candidates for salvage treatment [21]. Additional staging with PET/CT for distant metastasis is warranted in these patients at the time of new cervical disease.

Complications

Metabolic

The fluid and electrolyte balance of patients undergoing skull base surgery should be monitored closely. Postoperative hyponatremia is usually the result of inappropriate fluid balance in the operating room, but patients with cerebral edema or contusion may develop the syndrome of inappropriate antidiuretic hormone (SIADH) or cerebral salt wasting. In SIADH, excessive antidiuretic hormone (ADH) secretion leads to water retention with a serum sodium usually less than 130 mg/dl. SIADH is usually self-limited and may be treated with fluid restriction of less than 1000 ml/day, whereas patients with cerebral salt wasting should be hydrated with saline solutions. If the patient shows signs of disorientation, seizures, or muscle irritability, 3% saline solution is slowly administered intravenously in the ICU setting.

On the contrary, ischemia or trauma to the hypothalamus may lead to insufficient production of ADH, resulting in diabetes insipidus. During diabetes insipidus, the patient loses the ability to concentrate urine, leading to increased free water loss and hypovolemic hypernatremia. Serum sodium is usually higher than 145 mg/dl, and urine specific gravity is less than 1.005. Careful replacement of fluids is necessary, since urine output can be more than 2 liters every hour. Aqueous ADH (2.5 units intramuscularly every 4 h) or DDAVP (0.5 μg i.v. or i.m. every 12 h) may be replaced initially. Iatrogenic SIADH, through overuse of parenteral ADH, should be avoided.

Hyperglycemia is very common in patients receiving steroids and should be ruled out in any patient with increased diuresis and hypernatremia. It is treated by a sliding scale of regular insulin titrated to glycemia. Other electrolyte disorders such as hypomagnesemia (<1.8 mg/dl), hypophosphatemia (<2 mg/dl), and hypocalcemia (<8.0 mg/dl) are common in patients after skull base surgery. This is especially true if the patient requires replacement of a significant blood loss (>5 units of packed red blood cells). These disorders can add to postoperative delirium and diminished mental state.

Vascular

DVTs are prevented using sequential compression stockings and ambulation if possible. Heparin is contraindicated initially because of the risk of postoperative intracranial bleeding. Coagulopathies may be induced by rapid bleeding and blood replacement, which may temporarily exhaust the coagulation factors. This deficit is treated by replacing coagulation factors in the form of fresh frozen plasma.

Central Nervous System/Skull Base

Seizures owing to frontal lobe trauma are rare. Nevertheless, in the presence of significant brain contusion or when parenchymal resection is necessary, seizure prophylaxis in the form of phenytoin (Dilantin) is recommended. The treatment for a grand mal type seizure is diazepam (Valium) 10 mg intravenous and ventilatory support, followed by phenytoin 15 mg/kg loading dose and 5 mg/kg/day maintenance dose. It is essential to rule out electrolyte or acid-base imbalances as well as an intracranial space occupying lesion or inflammation as a cause for the seizures.

CSF leaks that present in the immediate postoperative period are managed with an immediate endoscopic repair. Some high-flow leaks also require addition of a lumbar spinal drain. The drain bag is kept at shoulder level and 50–80 ml are drained every 8 hours. This approximates the physiologic production of CSF in 24 h. Overdrainage may lead to pneumocephalus. Repair of the leak usually involves repair of the CSF fistula by moving or bolstering the flap repair to separate the leak from the upper aerodigestive tract. Patients who develop hydrocephalus require a ventriculoperitoneal shunt. Since introducing the pedicled nasoseptal flap, CSF leak rates are around 5% [19].

A small amount of pneumocephalus is frequently seen in the early postoperative period. This usually resolves spontaneously over about 1 week. Persistent or large amounts of pneumocephalus imply a CSF leak but may be managed conservatively. Tension pneumocephalus, which is the accumulation of intracranial air under pressure, may compress cerebral tissue and cause impairment of the sensorium or focal neurologic deficits. This is treated by needle aspiration when there are neurologic changes or evidence of increasing pressure. Tension pneumocephalus requires repair of the dura. A tracheotomy may be used in order to bypass positive pressure mask ventilation.

Wound infection and meningitis are rare complications of anterior cranial base surgery. Antibiotic therapy is directed by Gram stain or culture and the ability to achieve adequate CSF penetration. It is essential to achieve separation of the cranial cavity from the upper aerodigestive tract.

Encephalocele and pulsatile exophthalmos rarely present as late postoperative complications. They are corrected by reoperation and reconstruction of the dural and bone defects. Loss of medial orbital support and imprecise realignment of the medial canthus may result in ocular asymmetry and a disconjugate gaze. Whenever possible, large orbital defects should be reconstructed.

Conclusions

ENB is a tumor whose anatomic location makes treatment complex with significant risk to CNS and optic structures. Surgical treatment combined with radiation provides long-term disease control of 45–70% at 5 years. The latest advance in the treatment of this disease is endoscopic anterior craniofacial resection (ACF) of the tumor. This involves resection of the same anatomic structures and ability to clear margins as open ACF while avoiding external incisions, offering excellent visualization and magnification, avoiding frontal lobe retraction, and allowing for endoscopic vascularized tissue reconstruction. Disease control in 23 ENB patients who underwent endoscopic ACF was excellent (22/23), with complication rates comparable to open resections. Endoscopic ACF is an acceptable treatment option for cure of ENB in the hands of appropriately trained endoscopic skull base tumor surgeons.

References

1 Broich G, Pagliari A, Ottaviani F: Esthesioneuroblastoma: a general review of the cases published since the discovery of the tumor in 1924. Anticancer Res 1997;17:2683–2706.

2 Bradley PJ, Jones NS, Robertson I: Diagnosis and management of esthesioneuroblastoma. Curr Opin Otolaryngol Head Neck Surg 2003;11:112–118.

3 Berger L, Luc R, Richard D: L'esthesioneuroepitheliome olfactif. Bull Assoc Fr Etude Cancer 1924;13:410–421.

4 Kumar S, Perlman E, Pack S, et al: Absence of EWS/FLI1 fusion in olfactory neuroblastomas indicates these tumors do not belong to the Ewing's sarcoma family. Hum Pathol 1999;30:1356–1360.

5 Mezzelani A,Tornielli S,Minoletti F, Pierotti MA, Sozzi G, Pilotti S: Esthesioneuroblastoma is not a member of the primitive peripheral neuroectodermal tumour Ewing 's group. Br J Cancer 1999;81: 586–591.

6 Riazimand SH, Brieger J, Jacob R, Welkoborsky H-J, Mann WJ: Analysis of cytogenetic aberrations in esthesioneuroblastomas by comparative genomic hybridization. Cancer Genet Cytogenet 2002;136: 53–57.

7 Bockmuhl U, You X, Pacyna-Gengel-bach M, Arps H, Draf W, Petersen I: CGH pattern of esthesioneuroblastoma and their metastases. Brain Pathol 2004; 14:158–163.

8 Kadish S, Goodman M, Wang CC: Olfactory neuroblastoma: a clinical analysis of 17 cases. Cancer 1976;37:1571–1576.
9 Dulguerov P, Allal AS, Calcaterra TC: Esthesioneuroblastoma: a meta-analysis and review. Lancet Oncol 2001;2:683–690.
10 Kassam A, Snyderman CH, Mintz A, Gardner P, Carrau RL: Expanded endonasal approach: the rostrocaudal axis. Part II. Posterior clinoids to foramen magnum. Neurosurg Focus 2005;19:E4.
11 Kassam A, Snyderman CH, Mintz A, Gardner P, Carrau RL: Expanded endonasal approach: the rostrocaudal axis. I. Crista galli to the sella turcica. Neurosurg Focus 2005;19:E3.
12 Kassam A, Carrau RL, Snyderman CH, Gardner P, Mintz A: Evolution of reconstructive techniques following endoscopic expanded endonasal approaches. Neurosurg Focus 2005;19:E8.
13 Cavallo LM, Messina A, Cappabianca P, et al: Endoscopic endonasal surgery of the midline skull base: anatomical study and clinical considerations. Neurosurg Focus 2005;19:E2.
14 Snyderman CH, Kassam AB, Carrau R, Mintz A: Endoscopic reconstruction of cranial base defects following endonasal skull base surgery. Skull Base 2007;17:73–78.
15 Carrau RL, Kassam AB, Snyderman CH, Duvvuri U, Mintz A, Gardner P: Endoscopic transnasal anterior skull base resection for the management of sinonasal malignancies. Oper Tech Otolaryngol Head Neck Surg 2006;17:102–110.
16 Hadad G, Bassagasteguy L, Carrau RL, et al: A novel reconstructive technique after endoscopic expanded endonasal approaches: vascular pedicle nasoseptal flap. Laryngoscope 2006;116:1882–1886.
17 Castelnuovo PG, Delu G, Sberze F, Pistochini A, Cambria C, Battaglia P, Bignami M: Esthesioneuroblastoma: endonasal endoscopic treatment. Skull Base 2006;16:25–30.
18 Eden BV, Debo RF, Larner JM, et al: Esthesioneuroblastoma: long-term outcome and patterns of failure – the University of Virginia experience. Cancer 1994;73:2556–2562.
19 Bhattacharyya N, Thornton AF, Joseph MP, et al: Successful treatment of esthesioneuroblastoma and neuroendocrine carcinoma with combined chemotherapy and proton radiation: results in 9 cases. Arch Otolaryngol Head Neck Surg 1997;123:34–40.
20 Davis RE, Weissler MC: Esthesioneuroblastoma and neck metastasis. Head Neck 1992;14:477–482.
21 Ferlito A, Rinaldo A, Rhys-Evans, PH: Contemporary clinical commentary: esthesioneuroblastoma: an update on management of the neck. Laryngoscope 2003;113:1935–1938.
22 Casiano RR, Germani RM, Vivero R, Herzallah IR: Endoscopic reconstruction of large anterior skull base defects using acellular dermal allograft. Am J Rhinol 2007;21:615–618.

Prof. Ricardo L. Carrau
Director of the Comprehensive Skull Base Surgery Center
Department of Otolaryngology-Head and Neck Surgery, The Ohio State University Medical Center
915 Olentangy River Road, Suite 4000
Columbus, OH 43212 (USA)
Tel. +1 614 293 8074, E-Mail carraurl@gmail.com

Kassam AB, Gardner PA (eds): Endoscopic Approaches to the Skull Base.
Prog Neurol Surg. Basel, Karger, 2012, vol 26, pp 104–118

Endoscopic Approaches to the Skull Base: The Coronal Plane

Daniel M. Prevedello[a] · Amin B. Kassam[c] · Bradley A. Otto[b] · Leo F.S. Ditzel Filho[a] · Danielle de Lara[a] · Ricardo L. Carrau[b]

Departments of [a]Neurological Surgery and [b]Otolaryngology, Head and Neck Surgery, The Ohio State University, Columbus, Ohio, USA; [c]Department of Neurological Surgery, University of Ottawa, Ottawa, Ont., Canada

Abstract

Background: Endoscopic endonasal skull base surgery has become an important part of the arsenal of contemporary skull base surgery. The coronal or paramedian plane is defined as the region lateral to the internal carotid artery (ICA) as it courses along the ventral skull base. The endoscopic approaches performed in the coronal plane for paramedian pathology are the most complex of the expanded extrasellar procedures. **Method:** We reviewed our experience with over 1,000 patients who underwent fully endoscopic expanded endonasal skull base surgery. In this report, we describe a modular system organized around the course of the ICA oriented in the anterior, middle, and posterior coronal planes. **Results:** The anterior coronal plane has an intimate relation with the anterior fossa and orbit, the mid-coronal plane with the middle fossa and temporal lobe and the posterior coronal plane with the posterior fossa and jugular foramen. The middle and posterior paramedian approaches are further divided in 7 modular zones based on the anatomy of the ICAs. **Conclusion:** The standardization of anatomic modular approaches to the skull base in the coronal plane simplifies the complexity of accessing paramedian lesions through a midline endonasal corridor optimizing the surgical strategy and, consequently, outcomes. The standardization of modular approaches herein provides for a systematic way of approaching segments via individual or combined endoscopic endonasal corridors.

The paramedian skull base is a complex anatomical region, harboring critical arteries and cranial nerves housed in the cavernous sinus. Accordingly, lesions in this region are challenging to manage. To date, most procedural descriptions related to paramedian pathology have focused on progressive skull base approaches requiring craniotomy that gain incremental access to the ventral skull base while minimizing manipulation of central neurovascular structures. However, the lateral to medial trajectory of such approaches requires mobilization of peripheral neurovascular structures, leading to considerable morbidity.

Transsphenoidal approaches to the midline skull base have been performed for a century. Initially, such procedures were restricted to the pituitary fossa. More recently, the endoscope and advanced computer assisted stereotactic navigation systems have allowed surgeons to expand this approach to incorporate lesions located in more anatomically complex regions, such as the paramedian plane. Dissection in the paramedian plane requires manipulation of the internal carotid artery (ICA) and carries the risk of vascular compromise. While carotid artery complications are rare, they are frequently devastating when they do occur. Accordingly, surgeons must master not only the ICA anatomy to reduce risk of inadvertent damage, but also the techniques used to control large vessel rupture endoscopically.

Internal Carotid Artery

The ICA is divided into the following segments at the ventral skull base: the parapharyngeal ascending segment, the horizontal petrous segment, the lacerum segment (second genu), the paraclival segment (proximal posterior vertical segment of cavernous ICA), carotid siphon (cavernous ICA), and the paraclinoid segment. Distal to the paraclinoid segment the ICA enters the subarachnoid space. This caudal to rostral progression of the ICA helps define the coronal plane as the region lateral to these successive segments. The coronal plane approaches described herein allow access to this region.

Mastery of the ICA anatomy within the ventral skull base is an essential prerequisite to dissection in the coronal plane. This is even more important in situations where the carotid canal is dehiscent or the ICA course is distorted. Image guidance systems (IGS) can be used as an adjunct to help confirm vital structures; however, such devices should never replace the clinical judgment and mastery of relevant anatomy.

Coronal Planes

The coronal plane approaches described in this chapter are divided into three sagittal segments. The anterior coronal plane comprises the anterior cranial fossa and orbits, the mid-coronal plane the middle fossa and temporal lobes and the posterior coronal plane the posterior cranial fossa. The mid and posterior paramedian modules are divided based on the course of the ICAs. The vidian nerve is a key landmark for mid- and posterior coronal plane expanded approaches as the vidian canal represents a reliable landmark to identify the petrous ICA.

Modular Approaches

Anterior Coronal Plane

The anterior coronal plane approaches are utilized for extra- and intraconal orbital pathology located medial to the optic nerve. Examples of extraconal procedures, where the periorbita is generally preserved, include medial orbital decompression and optic nerve decompression. Supraorbital pathology is addressed through this approach as well. Intraconal procedures, where dissection transgresses the periorbita, allow for the removal of lesions medial to the optic nerve. Usually, the corridor between the inferior and medial rectus muscles is utilized. It is important to isolate these muscles to prevent inadvertent damage. Transconjunctival isolation of the muscles as they insert in the globe allows for distraction and mobilization of the recti, easing endonasal dissection. Furthermore, this approach can also amplify the endonasal approach, allowing for improved access to the anterior orbital compartment. Together, these approaches allow for full access of the medial orbit, from the anterior limit through the apex.

Mid-Coronal and Posterior Coronal Planes

The mid-coronal and posterior coronal planes are divided into 7 anatomic zones based on the relationship to the ICA. The 'infrapetrous' and 'suprapetrous' planes referred to in this discussion pertain to the plane to the petrous ICA, not necessarily the petrous bone. The 7 anatomic zones are as follows:

Zone 1 represents the anterior petrous apex.

Zone 2 represents the mid-body of the petrous bone below the level of the horizontal segment of the petrous carotid.

Zone 3 represents the suprapetrous region consisting of the quadrangular space. The quadrangular space is defined medially by the paraclival ICA, inferiorly by the horizontal segment of the petrous ICA, laterally by the second division of the trigeminal nerve, and superiorly by the course of the sixth cranial nerve within the cavernous sinus. Through this approach Meckel's cave and the gasserian ganglion can be reached.

Zone 4 represents the superior lateral cavernous sinus, representing the region through which the oculomotor (III), trochlear (IV), first division of the trigeminal nerve, and abducens (VI) nerves traverse.

Zone 5 represents the transpterygoid /infratemporal space with direct access to the middle fossa.

Zone 6 represents the region of the condyle. It is the paramedian area located immediately lateral to the inferior third of the clivus and foramen magnum. It is antero-laterally bounded by the eustachian tube and fossa of Rosenmuller that mark the parapharyngeal ICA laterally. Superiorly, it has its limit on the petroclival synchondrosis. Lesions in this region can involve the hypoglossal canal.

Zone 7 represents the region lateral to the parapharyngeal ICA. The approach for this region extends along the floor of the maxillary sinus and contains the lateral pterygoid plate and attached soft tissue. Most importantly, this region contains the jugular foramen posteriorly.

For the subsequent portion of the chapter, these zones will be referred to as above and the corridors used will be described accordingly.

Surgical Technique

Preparation. Preoperative imaging consists of computed tomographic angiography and fine cut magnetic resonance imaging. These are used for frameless stereotactic image guidance during the procedure (Stryker-Leibinger Corp., Kalamazoo, Mich., USA). Following orotracheal intubation the patient is placed in Mayfield pins with the head turned to the right side and tilted to the left. The nose is topically decongested with 0.05% oxymetazoline soaked ½ × 3 inches neuro patties. The nasal skin and vestibule are prepped and sterilized in standard fashion. The periumbilical region is also prepped and sterilized, in the event that an autologous fat graft is necessary for reconstruction.

Exposure. The exposure is initiated using a zero degree Karl Storz endoscope (Culver City, Calif., USA). The middle turbinate is resected on the side ipsilateral to the lesion. Hemostasis is then achieved along the insertion of the middle turbinate with selective cauterization. Lateralization or resection of the contralateral middle turbinate is then undertaken and out fracture of the inferior turbinates is performed to increase space for binarial, bimanual surgery. Next, a Hadad-Bassagasteguy (H-B) nasoseptal flap is created, usually on the side contralateral to the lesion [1]. The nasoseptal flap is raised and placed either in the nasopharynx or in a wide maxillary antrostomy for storage and to avoid inadvertent trauma during dissection.

Generally, a posterior nasal septectomy in addition to a wide bilateral sphenoidotomies and posterior ethmoidectomies is then performed. The posterior ethmoidectomy provides space for endoscope placement during instrumentation of the skull base. For certain approaches, such as the transorbital approach, anterior ethmoidectomy may be necessary as well. Following the posterior septectomy, the contralateral septal mucosa is draped around the posterior margin of the remaining septum (reverse flap) and secured anteriorly to the cartilage exposed from creation of the H-B flap. Absorbable sutures are placed to secure this mucosa.

Anterior Coronal Plane (Anterior fossa)

Transorbital Approach

The transorbital approach [2] is defined by the removal of the lamina papyracea, the medial optic canal or the orbital roof. This module requires a total (anterior and posterior) ethmoidectomy in order to expose the lateral wall of the sinonasal cavity. It can be performed unilaterally or bilaterally as dictated by the pathology. The lamina papyracea and orbital apex are the lateral limits of resection of the ethmoid cells. The most important structures related to this module are the optic nerves, the anterior and posterior ethmoidal arteries and the ophthalmic artery with its central retina artery branch.

An extraconal transorbital approach is indicated for resection of sinonasal lesions that are invading the medial wall of the orbit, such as sinonasal malignances, to

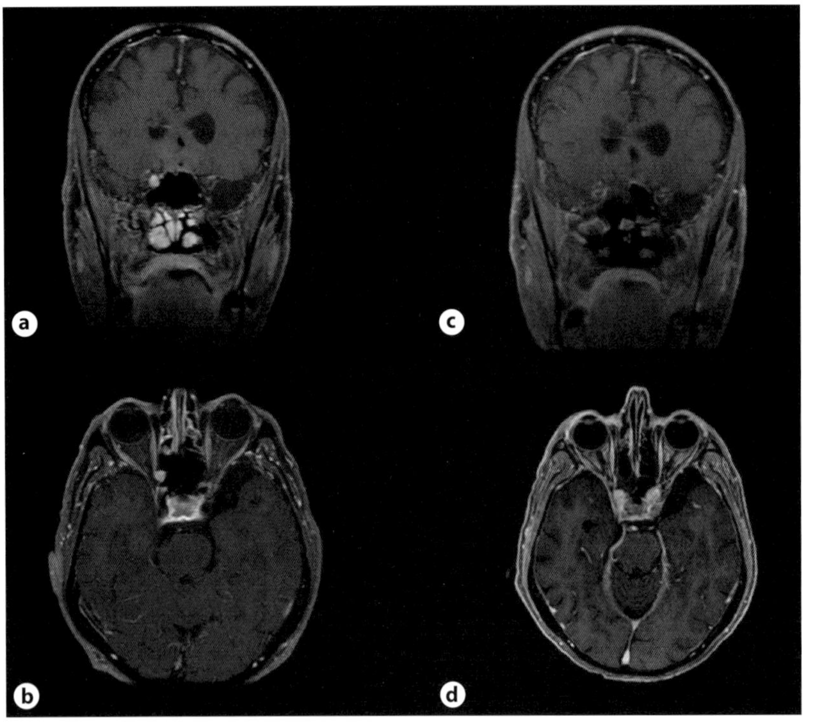

Fig. 1. Preoperative T_1-weighted MRI coronal (**a**) and axial (**b**) views of a small orbital apex schwannoma in a 72-year-old male patient. This lesion was removed through an anterior coronal plane intraconal approach. Postoperative coronal (**c**) and axial (**d**) MRI views confirm the total resection of the tumor.

decompress the optic nerves in the presence of unresectable intraconal pathology, such as optic sheath meningiomas and optic gliomas, or to access the lateral extension of intradural anterior cranial fossa disease such as the dural tail of olfactory groove meningiomas.

Alternatively, intraconal transorbital approaches are designed for the resection of intraconal lesions located medial to the optic nerve (fig. 1). Characteristic lesions include orbital schwannomas, cavernomas and meningiomas.

Mid-Coronal and Posterior Coronal Planes

Transpterygoid Approach

All of the modules in the mid-coronal and posterior coronal plane require a transpterygoid approach [3] as a common initial corridor. A transpterygoid approach is performed on the side ipsilateral to the pathology of interest. Initially, a maxillary antrostomy is performed, exposing the posterior wall of the maxillary sinus. The sphenopalatine artery (SPA) is identified and its branches are coagulated and ligated. The posterior wall of the maxillary sinus is removed and the contents of the pterygopalatine fossa are retracted laterally. This allows for subsequent identification of the pterygoid base and access to the medial temporal fossa through the lateral recess of the sphenoid sinus. At this point the vidian nerve and artery bundle (if present) can be seen clearly at the vidian canal (pterygoid canal) along the base of the pterygoid process. Image guidance can be used to confirm the depth and location of the vidian canal [4]. The floor of the sphenoid sinus is then drilled flush with the clival recess using a 3- or 4-mm hybrid cutting/diamond burr.

Theoretically, a letter 'H' is anatomic formed at the skull base, which is extremely helpful for surgical orientation. The superior vertical limb represents the paraclival ascending carotid and the descending vertical limb is represents the medial pterygoid plate. The horizontal bar of the 'H' is represented by the sphenoid sinus floor. The vidian complex is encountered at the confluence of the vertical and horizontal segments of the 'H'. The vidian canal is an important landmark to the identification and dissection of the carotid artery. As previously described, the bone around the vidian canal is drilled along its inferior half (from 3 o'clock to 9 o'clock) until the carotid artery is identified at the lacerum segment [4].

Mid-Coronal Plane (Middle Fossa)

The suprapetrous approach (zone 3) is also called the quadrangular space. This module is indicated to access lesions located in the Meckel's cave (fig. 2, 3) [5].

Once the lacerum segment of the internal carotid artery is identified, the middle fossa bone is drilled. Depending on the disease to be approached, the exposure includes the petrous horizontal ICA under V2 as well as the paraclival carotid (vertical cavernous segment). The dura is then opened within the quadrangular space bounded by the ICA medially, V2 laterally, and the horizontal petrous ICA inferiorly. The abducens nerve will be located running obliquely and superiorly and it marks the superior limit of the quadrangular space. Neurophysiology is crucial during this procedures and the dura should be stimulated before being incised with attention to VI cranial nerve responses. III and IV cranial nerve should also be monitored any time the tumor approached is located lateral to the ICA in the middle fossa.

For lesions that infiltrate the Gasserian ganglion, as sinonasal malignancies, the trigeminal nerve is not respected and the resection of the tumor is accomplished along with the trigeminal segments that are involved. Intraoperative pathology consultation is frequently necessary in order to determine clear margins in cases a total resection is planned. For benign lesions occupying the medial inferior compartment of the Meckel's cave, the trigeminal nerve is kept intact at the superolateral position against the middle fossa dura. Occasionally, the anteromedial (between V1 and V2) and anterolateral (between V2 and V3) middle fossa triangles can be utilized to reach the lateral aspect of Meckel's cave, particularly when the trigeminal nerve is pushed medially by a laterally located disease. At these levels, the meningeal dural layer can

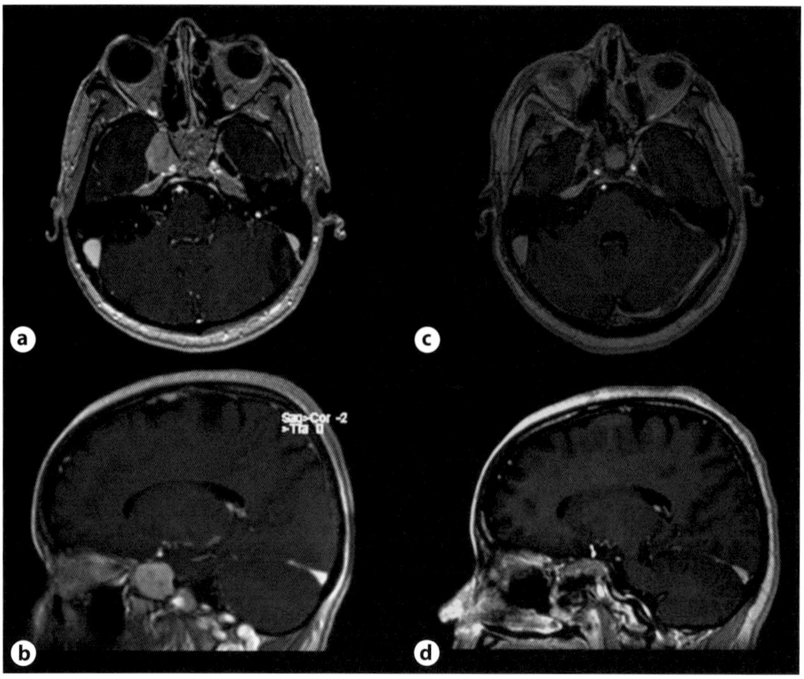

Fig. 2. Preoperative T_1-weighted MRI axial (**a**) and sagittal (**b**) views of an adenoid cystic carcinoma invading Meckel's cave. After a suprapetrous approach to the quadrangular space the lesion was thoroughly removed, as seen in the postoperative axial (**c**) and sagittal (**d**) T_1 MRI views. The maxillary pain with which the patient presented initially resolved after surgery.

be opened lateral to Meckel's cave in order to expose the anterior temporal fossa subarachnoid space, if dictated by the pathology.

Pathologies commonly encountered in this region are invasive adenoid cystic carcinomas, meningiomas, schwannomas and invasive pituitary adenomas. The important structures related to this module are exactly the boundaries: ICA, VIth cranial nerve and trigeminal nerve.

Cavernous Sinus Approach (Zone 4) [3]

It is anatomically defined by the area lateral to the sella turcica where the cavernous ICA is located. The cavernous sinus is approached laterally to the ICA siphon. It is rarely indicated since it is a compact area where the cranial nerves (III, IV, VI) are passing lateral to the ICA. In general, we prefer to either observe slow benign intracavernous residual tumors or radiate them when they demonstrate tendency of growth.

The ICA exposure and bone resection is undertaken as described in the quadrangular (zone 3) module. The dural opening, however, is made above the quadrangular space. In the majority of cases, the tumor has already thrombosed the sinus and little

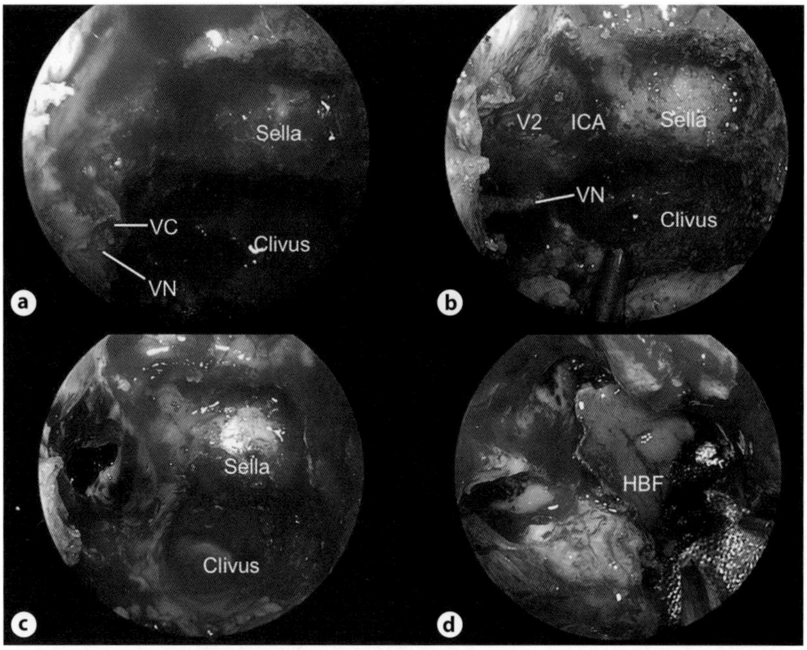

Fig. 3. Stepwise approach and resection of the lesion seen in figure 2. **a** Exposure of the anterior opening of the vidian canal (VC) at the pterygopalatine fossa. **b** Opening of the VC and exposure of the vidian nerve (VN). **c** Final image after resection of the lesion through the quadrangular space. **d** Reconstruction with the H-B flap (HBF). V2 = Maxillary nerve.

venous bleeding is encountered during the initial opening. It is often advisable to open the sella turcica and identify the medial margin of the ICA in the sella. Once the ICA is identified medially, it can be protected with a dissector during the lateral opening.

The structures at risk for this approach are the III, IV, V, VI cranial nerves and the ICA with its sympathetic fibers.

Infratemporal Approach (Zone 5) [3]

Tumors often create a corridor through the pterygomaxillary fissure, extending rostrally to the middle cranial fossa, laterally to the infratemporal fossa (fig. 4) and often medially to the pterygopalatine fossa. The foramen rotundum and the lacerum ICA are identified as previously described. During the lateral dissection, the internal maxillary artery and its branches must be systematically isolated and ligated. The dissection can be pursued laterally until the lateral pterygoid plate (LPP) is identified. The LPP can be drilled rostrally until it is flush with the middle cranial fossa and foramen ovale. Pathologies encountered in this region are invasive carcinomas, CSF leaks, encephaloceles, and skull base meningiomas. It is common to encounter profuse venous bleeding from the pterygopalatine venous plexus which is controlled with

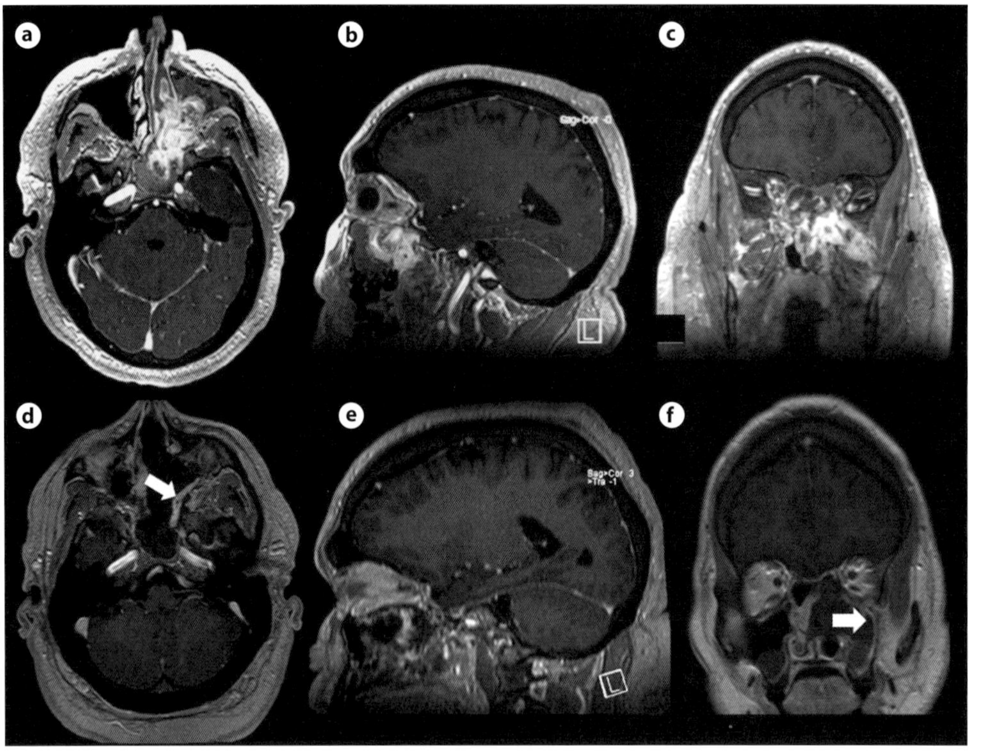

Fig. 4. Preoperative axial (**a**), sagittal (**b**) and coronal (**c**) T_1-weighted MRI views of an extensive juvenile angiofibroma that invades the infratemporal fossa. The lesion was resected through a coronal plane zone 5 approach and reconstruction was based on an H-B flap (white arrow). Postoperative axial (**d**), sagittal (**e**) and coronal (**f**) scans demonstrate the gross total resection of the tumor.

packing. The anatomy in this space can be difficult to navigate because the osseous landmarks (MPP and LPP) are often destroyed by the tumor thus making image guidance imperative.

The relevant structures in this module are the internal maxillary artery with its branches, the vidian nerve, the trigeminal nerve (V2 and V3) with branches and the superior orbital fissure superiorly.

Posterior Coronal Plane (Posterior Fossa)

Petrous Apex (Zone 1) [3]

It is basically a lateral extension of a transclival approach in its middle third. After identifying and exposing the lacerum ICA, the artery is mobilized laterally so that the underlying petrous apex can be accessed directly. Drilling the portion of the clivus at its junction with the petrous apex further facilitates this medial-to-lateral access. This

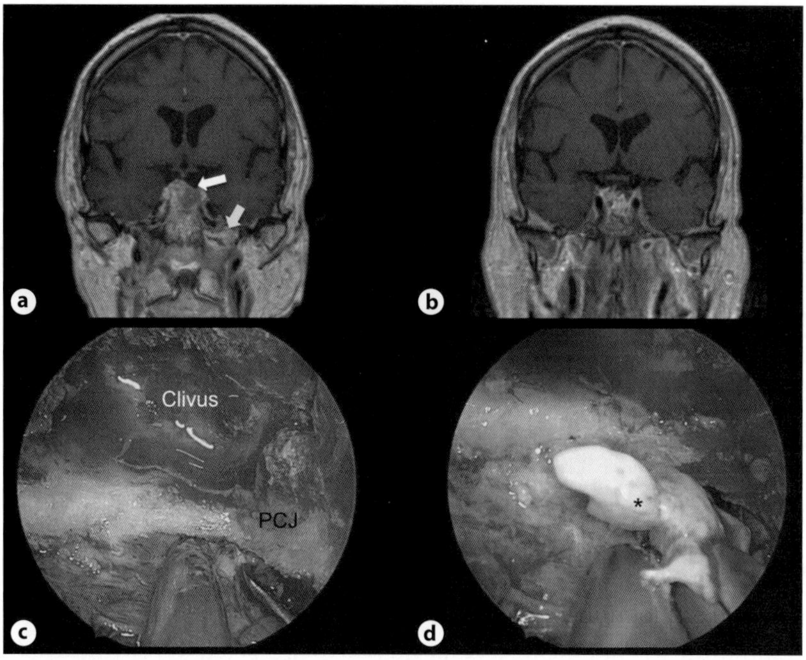

Fig. 5. Preoperative (**a**) and postoperative (**b**) coronal T_1-weighted MRI scans of a patient with a synchronous recurrent pituitary tumor (white arrow) and an expansive process on the left petroclival junction region (white arrow). This patient had been previously operated on elsewhere for a nonfunctioning pituitary macroadenoma. The recurrent tumor was addressed using a transsellar approach; the petroclival junction lesion (star) was removed through a coronal plane zone 2 approach with anterior exposure of the foramen lacerum (**c**, **d**). Pathology showed that this mass was indeed a *Pseudomonas* granuloma.

approach provides access as far as the medial anterior margin of the internal auditory canal. If the posterior dura is incised, it opens to the posterior fossa. Chondrosarcomas and cholesterol granulomas are typical pathologies at this location. The most relevant structures are the ICAs and the VIth cranial nerve at the Dorello's canal immediately above the petrous bone.

Infrapetrous Approach (Zone 2) [3]

This is defined by resections at the petroclival junction (fig. 5). An initial transclival exposure provides access to more caudally oriented regions. After identifying and isolating the lacerum ICA, the bone over the petrous segment (horizontal), lacerum and paraclival (cavernous) ICA is removed using a high-speed, extended drill and fine Kerrison rongeurs. The lateral clivus at the petroclival junction is drilled laterally beneath the horizontal (petrous) ICA. The petrous bone under the ICA in its petrous segment can be removed until underlying dura of the posterior fossa and venous plexus is identified. The middle fossa represents the superolateral boundary.

Chondrosarcomas are the commonest pathology in this region. If required, the dura mater posterior to the drilled petrous bone can be opened to provide access to the paramedian portion of the pre-pontine cistern as to improve the corridor to approach petroclival meningiomas for instance. The vital structures related to this module are the inner ear with VIIth and VIIIth nerves laterally, the petrous ICA superiorly and the XIIth cranial nerve inferolaterally in the occipital condyle.

Occipital Condyle/Hypoglossal Canal Approach (Zone 6) [3]
The Eustachian tube is an important landmark to safely determine the position of the internal carotid artery in its ascending parapharyngeal segment at the point it penetrates the carotid canal in the petrous bone. The Rosenmüller fossa is followed laterally. The medial aspect of the occipital chondyle is encountered lateral to the foramen magnum and followed laterally. The hypoglossal canal is localized rostro-lateral to the condyle and should be navigated carefully.

Following binarial general exposure, the basal nasopharyngeal mucosa is resected, exposing the midline musculature (longus capitis and rectus capitis anterior). This exposes the midline component of the foramen magnum. The posterior margin of the Eustachian tube at the level of the torus tubarius can be resected to provide direct access to the underlying parapharyngeal carotid prior to its entrance into the skull base. This provides the lateral margin of the module. Superiorly, the vidian nerve and artery is exposed to provide the superior and medial margins.

In order to address the paramedian extension, the parapharyngeal ICA can be further mobilized laterally allowing for exposure of the superior articular facet of C1 and its articulation with the occipital condyle. Approximately 20% of the occipital condyle, at the medial aspect, can be drilled away providing for direct access to the hypoglossal canal and vertebral artery proximal control. Care should be taken when drilling away the medial occipital condyle to stay along its most medial margin as the hypoglossal canal will be incorporated within the occipital condyle obliquely orienting from medial to lateral. If the foramen magnum is considered as a clock, the hypoglossal canal is located in the 2 and 10 o'clock positions. The hypoglossal nerve is exposed free of the canal distally and laterally and therefore drilling medially and proximally will prevent injury to this. In addition, care should be taken while drilling the medial condyle to not disrupt the synovial joint. A supra-articular drilling is preferable.

The approach to zone 6 can be divided into two areas: a transcondylar approach, where the occipital condyle is drilled as explained above, and the supracondylar approach, where the condyle is preserved and only the supracondylar bone is drilled up to the petroclival synchondrosis. When a supracondylar approach is performed, the jugular tubercle (from an intracranial perspective) is removed.

Pathologies encountered in this region are invasive carcinomas, paragangliomas, schwannomas and skull base meningiomas. The relevant structures in this region are the internal maxillary artery, the ICA (parapharyngeal lateral and petrous segment above), and the XIIth cranial nerve exiting the hypoglossal canal inferiorly.

Jugular Foramen Approach (Zone 7)
Zone 7 is lateral to zone 6. Once the parapharyngeal ICA is localized, any dissection performed laterally occurs at zone 7. The jugular foramen is located immediately lateral. The cranial nerves IX, X and XI are located in between the jugular vein and the ICA.

This requires proximal control of the parapharyngeal ICA prior to entering the carotid canal. Having established the distal control at the level of the vidian, proximal control can be established at the level of the Eustachian tube in the parapharyngeal space. Therefore, in order to get lateral to the parapharyngeal ICA, the initial maxillary antrostomy is converted to a complete maxillectomy providing even greater access to the pterygomaxillary fissure, the entire pterygopalatine fossa, and infratemporal fossa. The medial and lateral pterygoid plates are resected along with the medial and lateral pterygoid muscle attachments in these regions. At this point, the contents of the infratemporal fossa were isolated. The foramen ovale and the mandibular branch (V3) need to be identified.

Next, to gain proximal control of the parapharyngeal carotid, the Eustachian tube is identified and transected. As described in zone 6, the torus tuberus of the Eustachian tube is then resected providing direct visualization of the parapharyngeal free segment of the carotid just lateral to it. This is then followed into the carotid canal providing the lateral margin of the exposure and proximal control.

The mobile parapharyngeal component is mobilized first medially, and any tumor lateral to the parapharyngeal carotid extending towards the jugular fossa can be resected and planes prepared between the carotid and jugular sheath. The jugular vein is identified lateral to the ICA lower in the field allowing for proximal control. The jugular foramen is then directly accessed.

Pathologies encountered in this region are invasive carcinomas, paragangliomas, schwannomas and skull base meningiomas. The relevant structures in this region are the internal maxillary artery, the ICA (pharyngeal and petrous segments), the trigeminal nerve, the jugular foramen with jugular vein and lower cranial nerves (IX, X, XI), and the XII cranial nerve exiting the hypoglossal canal inferiorly.

Discussion

The expanded endonasal approach represents an additional tool that is of value when medial-to-lateral approaches are required to gain access to lesions in which the critical neurovascular structures are located along the perimeter. This trajectory has the potential of providing a direct route into the lesion, minimizing the need to manipulate structures located circumferentially along the perimeter.

The primary contraindication to the approach is encountered when the critical neurovascular structures are located medial or ventral to the tumor, requiring manipulation before entering the lesion. For example, if a lesion is located lateral to the optic nerve inside the orbit, the endonasal approach is totally contraindicated. It would be completely against the principles of neurovascular protection to approach such a lesion intensively manipulating the optic nerve. We have not found tumor size, vascularity, fibrosity or calcification to represent contraindications.

Using the expanded endonasal approach we have been able to resect large tumors as well as significantly calcified lesions, such as chondrosarcomas. In this report we have restricted the discussion to the technical anatomic considerations associated with approaches. Despite all else, an important contraindication to the expanded endonasal approaches is the surgeon's experience. We consider endoscopic endonasal approaches to paramedian lesions of the skull base as the most complex and risky procedure of this nature. It requires a team formed by an otolaryngologist experienced in endoscopy and skull base procedures and a neurosurgeon experienced in endoscopy, cranial base, and cerebrovascular surgery.

Because of the enhanced and panoramic view that is offered by the endoscope, lesions beyond the sella can be accessed. Several cadaveric anatomical dissections have evaluated the accessibility of the cranial base from crista galli to the odontoid process. Cappabianca and his group reviewed the access to various corridors of the skull base from the olfactory groove to the lower clivus [6, 7]. They identified many clear advantages to this approach including decreased retraction on the brain, minimizing manipulation of the optic apparatus, early identification of the pituitary gland and greater likelihood of preserving neuroendocrine function and concluded that the endoscopic endonasal approach to the skull base has great potential benefit [3].

The use of the endoscopic endonasal approaches to treat paramedian lesions can offer minimal morbidity and a short postoperative hospital stay. Obviously, long-term data will be required to determine if the low morbidity and mortality is sustainable and if resection is durable. Similarly, the modular approach to lesions of the skull base provides a method of systematically defining and approaching lesions based on various zones and modules.

We fully understand that on occasion large lesions lateral to the carotid such as those located in the infratemporal fossa and the pterygopalatine fossa can be tempting for an endonasal approach as they may have provided a corridor into the midline via the sphenoid or maxillary sinus. However, we would like to emphasize that many of these lesions can engulf or be circumferentially bound by the ICA, internal maxillary artery and the pterygopalatine venous plexus, all of which can represent sources of arterial and/or venous hemorrhage.

We consider all procedures in which manipulation or exposure of the ICA is necessary as the most complex and risky of the expanded endonasal approaches [3, 8]. Trying to access paramedian lesions without first isolating these ICA segments can prove dangerous. Particularly in the case of malignancies where tumors may be adherent to or invade these structures, lack of proximal control at the terminal portion of the dissection in the absence of proximal and distal ICA control can lead to life-threatening hemorrhage [9].

In a more caudal direction, the space between the ICAs and the parapharyngeal space (the region between the Eustachian tubes) is difficult to be navigated because the dissection proceeds through the soft tissue (pterygoid muscles, Eustachian tubes, venus plexus). These dissections can be disorienting because of the lack of normal bony anatomy, venous bleeding, and the need to use angled endoscopes. In summary, despite the temptation to pursue lesions located in the paramedian space, mainly when they have a midline extension, we consider these procedures remarkably complex, therefore, should be reserved for experienced endoscopic surgeons.

Conclusions

In this chapter we detail an anatomical classification that provides a practical guide for access to the paramedian region via a fully endoscopic, completely transnasal approach. The key anatomical landmarks are provided for each modular approach. These modules can be used in isolation or in combination, based on the extent of the lesion.

There are two key features to be considered for the application of EEA for paramedian lesions:

1 The critical neurovascular structures must be located along the perimeter of the lesion.

2 The surgical team must have developed progressive and incremental experience with fully endoscopic endonasal approaches. The management of the carotid and regional anatomy is imperative for success. This can only be achieved by pursuing a progressive and systematic approach to gain experience.

It is our strong belief that when surgeons consider a tumor for endoscopic endonasal resection, that same team must be comfortable in offering a conventional external approach to the patient. The surgical team must be able to tailor the approach based on the anatomy of each case. Only surgeons comfortably performing conventional skull base procedures and with proper experience in performing endonasal skull base surgery are able to offer patients the best option of surgical treatment.

Disclosure Statement

A.B.K. is a paid consultant for Karl Storz-Endoscopy and Stryker and holds an equity stake in NICO Corporation.

References

1 Hadad G, Bassagasteguy L, Carrau RL, et al: A novel reconstructive technique after endoscopic expanded endonasal approaches: vascular pedicle nasoseptal flap. Laryngoscope 2006;116:1882–1886.

2 Snyderman CH, Pant H, Carrau RL, Prevedello D, Gardner P, Kassam AB: What are the limits of endoscopic sinus surgery? The expanded endonasal approach to the skull base. Keio J Med 2009;58:152–160.

3 Kassam AB, Gardner P, Snyderman C, Mintz A, Carrau R: Expanded endonasal approach: fully endoscopic, completely transnasal approach to the middle third of the clivus, petrous bone, middle cranial fossa, and infratemporal fossa. Neurosurg Focus 2005;19:E6.

4 Kassam AB, Vescan AD, Carrau RL, et al: Expanded endonasal approach: vidian canal as a landmark to the petrous internal carotid artery. Journal of Neurosurgery 2008;108:177–183.

5 Kassam AB, Prevedello DM, Carrau RL, et al: The front door to meckel's cave: an anteromedial corridor via expanded endoscopic endonasal approach-technical considerations and clinical series. Neurosurgery 2009;64(3 suppl):71–82; discussion 82–73.

6 Cappabianca P, Frank G, Pasquini E, de Divitiis E, Calbucci F: Extended endoscopic endonasal transsphenoidal approaches to the suprasellar region, planum sphenoidale and clivus; in de Divitis E, Cappabianca P (eds): Endoscopic Endonasal Transsphenoidal Sugery. Wien, Springer, 2003, pp 176–187.

7 Cavallo LM, Messina A, Cappabianca P, et al: Endoscopic endonasal surgery of the midline skull base: anatomical study and clinical considerations. Neurosurg Focus 2005;19:E2.

8 Cavallo LM, Messina A, Gardner P, et al: Extended endoscopic endonasal approach to the pterygopalatine fossa: anatomical study and clinical considerations. Neurosurg Focus 2005;19:E5.

9 Snyderman C, Kassam A, Carrau R, Mintz A, Gardner P, Prevedello DM: Acquisition of surgical skills for endonasal skull base surgery: a training program. Laryngoscope 2007;117:699–705.

Daniel M. Prevedello, MD
The Ohio State University
Department of Neurosurgery, N-1011 Doan Hall
410 W. 10th Avenue, Columbus, OH 43210 (USA)
Tel. +1 614 293 7190, E-Mail dprevedello@gmail.com

Kassam AB, Gardner PA (eds): Endoscopic Approaches to the Skull Base.
Prog Neurol Surg. Basel, Karger, 2012, vol 26, pp 119–139

Cavernous Sinus: Endoscopic Endonasal Approaches

Giorgio Frank[a] · Ernesto Pasquini[b]

[a]Center of Surgery for Pituitary Tumors, Department of Neuroscience, Bellaria Hospital, and
[b]Center of Endoscopic ENT Surgery, ENT Department Sant'Orsola-Malpighi Hospital, Bologna, Italy

Abstract

The endoscopic transsphenoidal extended approach to the cavernous sinus is a recent but still evolving technique which may contribute to the management of cavernous sinus pathologies. As with other transsphenoidal extended approaches, it is direct and extracerebral having the advantage of being rapid and well-tolerated. Many variants exist (midline transsphenoidal endoscopic approach, ethmoid-pterygoid-sphenoidal endoscopic approach, trans-maxillo-pterygoid endoscopic approach) which should be tailored according to tumor extension in order to allow the best access to the compartments involved by the tumor. **Clinical Material:** Since 1998, we have performed 793 endoscopic transsphenoidal procedures, 141 (18%) of them for pathologies involving the cavernous sinus. In this chapter, we consider pituitary adenomas, chordomas and chondrosarcomas the most frequent groups (132 procedures). Pituitary adenomas invading the cavernous sinus (103 patients, 107 procedures) were the most representative group involving the superior portion of the cavernous sinus. Chordomas and chondrosarcomas (19 patients, 25 procedures) were the second group of tumors invading the cavernous sinus and affected mainly the inferior portion of the cavernous sinus. **Results:** The median hospital stay was 4 days for adenomas and 5 days for chordomas and chondrosarcomas. Radical tumor removal, according to postoperative MRI, was obtained in 53% of pituitary adenomas and in 44% of chordomas/chondrosarcomas. The biological cure of secreting adenomas, according to the modern remission-criteria, was obtained in 27% of the patients. A clinical improvement was observed in the great majority of patients; neurological symptoms (trigeminal neuralgia and ophthalmoplegia) responded to the release of tumoral compression. Major complications included 1 case of adjunctive oculomotor nerve palsy, 4 cases of delayed CSF leak, 1 case of hemorrhagic infarction of the residual tumor and one case of carotid artery injury. There was no perioperative mortality. **Conclusion:** Due to the different biological and morphological characteristics of tumors involving the cavernous sinus, a single surgical procedure of choice does not exist. Endoscopic endonasal surgery represents an adjunctive technique in the armamentarium of skull base surgeons. It is indicated in selected cases (intracavernous, soft tumors not invading the vessels and/or the nerves) and represents the most balanced technique as regards safety, tolerability and efficacy. Surgery still plays a central role in the treatment of cavernous sinus tumors; sometimes surgery alone is sufficient but, more frequently, multimodal therapy is required in which medical and radiation therapy contribute to controlling neoplastic disease.

Cavernous sinus (CS) surgery represents a surgical challenge due to the anatomical complexity and high functional value of the structures contained in this 'jewelry box'. Since the 1960s, surgical interest in this region has increased as has the anatomical knowledge of this region. Before then, it had been considered to be a large, intradural, trabeculated venous cavern, similar to other dural sinuses. This belief is due to Claudius Galen who dissected animals with parasellar carotid retia bathed in venous blood and then transposed his findings to human anatomy. Winslow [1] christened this structure the 'cavernous sinus', presumably thinking that it resembled the corpus cavernosum of the penis. When it was first entered deliberately in a case of long-standing arteriovenous fistula, the engorged and thickened arterialized veins were noted to be neither cavernous nor dural sinus but a plexus of veins [2]. Multiple surgical explorations, gross dissections and microscopic views led to the present belief: the lateral sellar compartment is extradural and the venous structures contained within consist of a variable plexus of thin-walled veins. This compartment continues along the clivus and basiocciput with the extradural space of the spine. Anteriorly, the compartment is continuous through the superior orbital fissure with a similar arrangement in the orbit. 'Lateral sellar compartment' is the name proposed to replace the old term 'cavernous sinus' which is inappropriate [3]. However, since all scientific texts today continue to call this compartment and the veins within it exclusively the cavernous sinus, we will continue to use this nomenclature due to its general acceptance, even if it is incorrect and misleading.

Pioneers of cavernous sinus surgery [2, 4, 5] used a craniotomic approach to penetrate the cavernous sinus through the narrow windows existing between the nerves on its superior and lateral walls; the main advantage of the transcranial approach is the safety given by the proximal and distal control of the internal carotid artery. After an enthusiastic phase with this type of surgery which lasted 20 years, its use has been steadily decreasing, partly due to the appearance of alternative non-surgical therapies such as radiosurgery and partly due to its high morbidity. In the 1980s, one of the most famous skull base neurosurgeons wrote about cavernous sinus surgery that the 'very early enthusiasm will undoubtedly be tempered in time by the poor results and complications that will be encountered in some patients' [5]. At present, the strategy for the management of cavernous sinus tumors is changing; the aim is to control the mass effect and not necessarily radically remove the tumor, achieving improvement of neuropathies and avoiding the risk of increasing neural damage [6]. Therefore, a multidisciplinary strategy is preferred in which surgery, radiation therapy and pharmacological therapy all contribute to obtaining the final result. The transcranial approach still remains the main surgical procedure for meningiomas, vascular malformations, or tumors with a major intradural component.

Currently, there is increasing interest in anterior extracranial approaches to the cavernous sinus for tumors growing within the cavernous sinus or those extending to it but having an extradural extracranial location.

The first anterior extracranial approach to the cavernous sinus was described by Laws et al. [7] in 1979 for the treatment of a carotid-cavernous fistula using a contralateral ethmoid-sphenoidal approach. Subsequently, several microscopic anterior approaches were proposed for the treatment of cavernous sinus pathologies: transsphenoethmoidal [8], transmaxillosphenoidal [9], transmaxillary [10] transmaxillary-transnasal [11] and, recently, an extended transsphenoidal approach with submucosal posterior ethmoidectomy [12]. The aim of these approaches is to overcome the strictly median exposure and the reduced peripheral vision characteristic of the transsphenoidal approach, creating a wider surgical channel in order to allow adequate exposure of the surgical field.

The emergence of the endoscope on the neurosurgical landscape [13] has introduced the possibility of wide peripheral and endocavitary vision through a limited surgical channel.

Detailed anatomical studies [14, 15] have shown the feasibility and the advantages of the endoscope in approaching the cavernous sinus. Three types of approaches, paraseptal, middle turbinectomy and middle meatal, have been described which are tailored according to the mediolateral extension of the tumor.

Regarding the endoscopic approach to the CS, the Bologna group has suggested a 'far lateral' approach, the etmoido-pterygo-sphenoidal approach, which is appropriate for tumors which also invade the lateral compartment of the cavernous sinus [16]. A further extreme lateral approach may be suggested, the transmaxillo-pterygoid approach, which is of value in tumors extending from the cavernous sinus through the foramen rotundum to the pterygo-maxillary fossa, or vice versa. Therefore, multiple endoscopic endonasal approaches are currently available and they should be selected according to the CS compartments which are involved by tumor.

Anatomical Remarks

The following paragraph is not intended to describe the anatomy of the cavernous sinus but simply to make some observations useful in understanding surgical strategy.

The cavernous sinuses are located near the center of the head on each side of the sella and body of the sphenoid bone. The cavernous sinuses have an oblique converging direction extending from the lower surface of the anterior clinoid process and from the posterior edge of the superior orbital fissure to the posterior clinoid process above the junction of the petrous apex with the body of the sphenoid bone. A cavernous sinus has four walls: lateral, medial, roof, posterior. The roof faces the basal cisterns, the lateral wall faces the temporal lobe, the medial wall faces the sella turcica, the pituitary gland and the sphenoid bone, and the posterior wall faces the posterior cranial fossa. The medial and lateral walls join inferiorly in a 'keel-like' formation at the level of the superior margin of the maxillary nerve. The medial wall may be divided into a superior part (sellar part) and into an inferior part (sphenoidal part or inferior wall) [17]. The cavernous sinus walls envelop the cavernous carotid segment and its branches: the sympathetic plexus, the IIIrd, IVth and VIth cranial nerves, the first trigeminal division and multiple venous structures.

The walls of the CS are composed of two layers: the external meningeal layer and the internal endosteal layer. Only the medial wall, in the sellar part and in the sphenoidal part or inferior wall, is formed by one layer. This layer is formed by the meningeal layer in the sellar part and by the endosteal layer in the sphenoidal part or inferior wall [17]. The intercavernous sinuses, connecting the two cavernous sinuses, are found between the two layers covering the anterior, posterior and inferior surfaces of the sella. The IIIrd, IVth and ophthalmic branch of the Vth cranial nerve are embedded in the reticularis membrane that forms the lateral wall of the CS [18]. The abducens nerve and the sympathetic plexus around the intracavernous carotid artery are the only nerves which have a real intracavernous course. The abducens nerve penetrates the CS by passing through Dorello's canal and courses inside the lateral venous space lateral and inferior to the horizontal segment of the intracavernous carotid artery and medial to the ophthalmic nerve to reach the superior orbital fissure.

The intracavernous carotid artery begins where the petrous segment of the internal carotid artery passes between the cartilaginous foramen lacerum below and the petrolingual ligament above to become intracavernous and ends when it leaves the cavernous sinus by piercing the dura medially from the upper surface of the anterior clinoid process. Alfieri and Jho [14] proposed a classification of the ICA suitable for the anterior endoscopic perspective. The ICA can be recognized on the posterior wall of the sphenoidal sinus by its bony protuberance: caudally, the paraclival protuberance and cranially, the parasellar protuberance. The paraclival segment of the ICA includes: (1) a caudal part, the lacerum segment of the artery corresponding to the extracavernous portion of the vessel, and (2) a rostral part, the trigeminal, intracavernous portion of the artery, so-called because the Gasserian ganglion is posterior to it and the trigeminal divisions are lateral to it. A landmark of the lacerum segment is the vidian canal which is located inferomedial to the foramen lacerum [19]. The parasellar carotid protuberance is a C-shaped bone protuberance with the convexity of the C facing anterolaterally. It covers four segments of the ICA: (1) the hidden segment; (2) the inferior horizontal segment; (3) the anterior vertical segment, and (4) the superior horizontal segment. The hidden segment is located at the level of the posterior sellar floor and includes the posterior bend of the ICA. The inferior horizontal segment appears short due to the perspective view, but is the longest segment of the intracavernous ICA. It courses along the sellar floor. The anterior vertical segment corresponds to the convexity of the C-shaped parasellar protuberance. The superior horizontal segment includes the clinoidal segment which courses medially to the optic strut, is anchored by the proximal and distal dural ring and continues in the subarachnoid portion of the vessel. Two main branches may be described in the intracavernous portion of the ICA: the meningohypophyseal trunk arising medially from the posterior bend and the inferolateral trunk arising from the middle or lateral surface of the inferior horizontal segment.

The intracavernous course of the carotid artery allows the cavernous venous spaces to be divided into four virtual compartments: medial, lateral, posterosuperior, and anteroinferior [20] (fig 1).

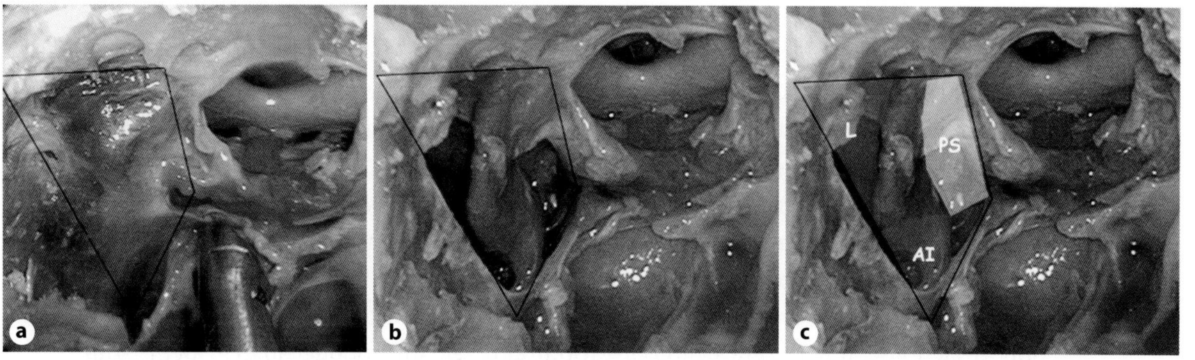

Fig. 1. Right cavernous sinus dissection. The quadrilateral delimits the right cavernous sinus area. **a** Before periosteal layer removal. **b** After periosteal layer removal. **c** Cavernous sinus compartments. L = Lateral; AI = antero-inferior; PS = posterosuperior compartment of the cavernous sinus (the medial is a virtual space in continuity with the AI and PS).

The medial and lateral compartments are located between the ICA and the medial wall and the lateral walls respectively. The posterosuperior compartment is confined between the internal carotid artery and the roof of the cavernous sinus. The anteroinferior space is situated in the concavity below the posterior bend of the cavernous carotid artery. Medial and posterosuperior compartments are in strict continuity and do not contain nerves, representing a surgical corridor without risk of neural damage. The anteroinferior and lateral compartments contain the abducens nerve and, as surgical corridors, they are exposed to the risk of injury to the VIth nerve.

Indications for Endoscopic Endonasal Cavernous Sinus Surgery

In agreement with many authors [3, 21], we believe that the cavernous sinus is an extradural vascular venous structure in continuity with other similar structures along the craniospinal axis. Following the general surgical rule of removing extradural tumors by an extradural approach, we believe that endoscopic endonasal cavernous sinus surgery should be used in cavernous sinus tumors having an extradural location (more frequently adenomas, chordomas and chondrosarcomas). The advantages of an extradural approach are multiple: it is extracerebral, avoiding any brain manipulation, the CS is penetrated through the medial wall in its sellar or sphenoidal part which is devoid of any cranial nerves, and the operation proceeds through surgical corridors with no (medial and postero-superior compartments) or low risk (antero-inferior or lateral compartments) of cranial nerve damage. If there is an intradural growth, a craniotomic approach or a combined or multistaged craniotomic and endoscopic approach is preferred.

It is of paramount importance to have adequate instrumentation and to plan the approach according to the CS compartments involved by the tumor.

Instrumentation

The instrumentation used in the endoscopic technique is a xenon 300-watt cold light fountain source, an endoscopic video camera and a video recorder. The endoscopes are 0, 30 and 45° Hopkins® telescopes, 4 mm in diameter and 18 mm long. A cleaning system with pedal control is used to reduce the necessity of extracting the telescope from the nose every time vision becomes unclear. At the end of the approach phase and during the tumor removal phase, we use a mechanical holder for the endoscope to allow the surgeon to work with both hands. The camera zoom allows better definition of anatomical features and the positioning of the endoscope further away from the surgical field, reducing the possibility of contamination of the tip of the telescope by blood.

Technical Adjuncts

Computer-assisted navigation and micro-Doppler help to precisely localize the internal carotid artery before the incision of the cavernous sinus wall and during tumor debulking. Modern navigation systems using a magnetic field to localize the pointer are especially suitable for endoscopy. They allow more continuous navigation, avoiding interruptions due to the body of the surgeon and/or the endoscope itself coming between the pointer and the optic system.

Intraoperative MRI or CT scans may be extremely useful. We believe that they are technologically advanced and should be additional and not substitutive to the navigation system and the Doppler.

Surgical Technique

The surgical technique is described using the pituitary adenoma, the most frequently treated tumor, as a model.

Surgery is carried out under general anesthesia using orotracheal intubation. The patient is placed in a half-sitting position with his head turned towards the surgeon and resting freely in a horseshoe head holder. The oropharynx is packed with moist gauze to prevent blood and secretions from reaching the stomach from the operative site. The nose and face are cleaned with soap and aqueous solutions. The nasal mucous membranes are decongested with Xilocaine® 5%. The periumbilical abdomen is routinely prepared for the eventual harvest of a free fat graft.

Different surgical approaches can be used for tumors involving the cavernous sinus: the midline transsphenoidal endoscopic approach (MTea), the ethmoid-pterygoid-sphenoidal endoscopic approach (EPSea) and only occasionally the trans-maxillo-pterygoid endoscopic approach (TMPea).

The approach is selected according to the compartments involved by the tumor. An MTea is adequate when the invasion is confined to the medial and posterosuperior compartments. When the tumor invades the anteroinferior and lateral compartments of the cavernous sinus or invades the entire CS, the EPSea is required. In the rare circumstance of a tumor extending from the lateral compartment through the foramen rotundum to the pterygo-maxillary fossa we have used the TMPea.

At the beginning of our experience, surgery was usually performed through only one nostril which was the one with the larger cavity in MTea and ipsilateral to the cavernous sinus involved in EPSea. At present, we gain access to the operative field through both nasal fossae by using a simple posterior septostomy and, therefore, the selection of the nostril is less important.

Midline Transsphenoidal Endoscopic Approach

The surgical procedure can be divided into 3 stages: approach phase, tumor removal and closure.

Stage I: Approach Phase

The lateral dislocation of the middle and upper turbinate allows localization of the sphenoethmoidal recess and the natural ostium of the sphenoid sinus.

The opening of the sphenoidal sinus starts with the enlargement of the natural ostium, using a Kerrison rongeur or a Stammberger punch. A semilunar incision is made in the vomer to separate the mucoperiostium from the bone and the natural ostium. In cases of difficult visualization of the sphenoidal ostium, it is possible to enter the sphenoid sinus by a direct perforation of the anterior wall at the junction of the keel of the sphenoid bone and the posterior nasal septum, approximately one centimeter above the rim of the choana and close to the septum.

The anterior sphenoidotomy should be wide, extending from the roof to the floor of the sphenoid sinus vertically and exceeding the sphenoidal ostia laterally.

To gain access to the surgical field from both nostrils, 1 cm of the posterior end of the nasal septum has to be removed using a back-biting forceps.

All the sphenoidal septa have to be removed. The sphenoidal mucosa may be preserved because the wide opening of the natural ostia avoids the risk of postoperative mucocele; preserving the mucosa permits a faster postoperative stabilization of the sphenoid cavity with a decreased incidence of sphenoidal inflammatory sequels.

The opening of the sellar floor is performed using a drill and is enlarged using the Kerrison rongeur; it should be wide, from the superior to the inferior intercavernous sinus and from one cavernous sinus to the other. The bone overlying the invaded cavernous sinus must be carefully removed from the optic-carotid recess to the paraclival carotid protuberance vertically and 1 cm laterally to the sella, exposing the main bulge of the parasellar carotid artery. This bone removal later increases the capacity of inspection of the cavernous sinus content by gently displacing the anterior membranous cavernous sinus wall laterally.

Stage II: Tumor Removal Phase

The dural opening starts in the sellar area. The sellar component of the tumor is removed first. Subsequently, the medial compartment of the cavernous sinus is entered, either enlarging the opening of the medial wall created by the tumor itself or (more rarely) making an incision in to the medial wall in a safe area (normally located in the posterior 2/3 of the medial wall of the cavernous sinus). Recognition of this 'safe' area requires identification of the bulging of the tumor and an accurate mapping of the internal carotid artery course (using direct vision, micro-Doppler and neuronavigation). The removal of the tumor inside the medial and posterosuperior compartments of the cavernous sinus is performed under direct view and has no risk of neural damage due to the absence of cranial nerves in this location. Usually, a 0° endoscope is adequate for the procedure. A gentle lateral displacement of the residual anterior medial wall of the CS sometimes helps to increase the vision of the contents of these compartments.

Stage III: Final Exploration and Closure of the Surgical Field

Hemostasis is obtained by packing with cottonoid. At the end of the removal phase, free-hand exploration into the surgical field using angled 30° and 45° optic scopes is recommended.

In the absence of a CSF leak, the surgical cavity is simply packed with Gelfoam®. If a CSF leak is detected or suspected, a multilayer repair is performed by applying autologous fat in the cavity, a piece of bone or cartilage (if available) extradurally and a mucoperiosteal flap overlay (from the middle turbinate or from the septum). It is important to remember that to have a viable graft it is necessary to remove the mucosa and to apply the graft directly over the bleeding surface.

The sphenoid sinus is packed with Gelfoam and, finally, the middle turbinate is medially displaced to its original position. Nasal packing is not routinely required. Lumbar drainage is not used.

Ethmoido-Pterygo-Sphenoidal Endoscopic Approach (EPSea)

EPSea is used for tumors invading the anteroinferior and/or the lateral compartments of the cavernous sinus or for tumors invading the entire CS. This procedure is the most versatile allowing the total exposition of the cavernous sinus with the possibility of simultaneous direct control of all compartments of the cavernous sinus (fig. 1, 2). The procedure can be schematically divided into 3 stages.

Stage I: Approach Phase

It is performed holding the endoscope freehand. Normally, a 0° endoscope is sufficient; a 30° endoscope is seldom required. The middle turbinate is resected through the ipsilateral nasal fossa, gaining a wide peripheral view and improving the maneuverability of the surgical instruments. An ethmoidal route is used and a complete sphenoethmoidectomy with a wide meatotomy is performed. The medial portion of the posterior wall of the maxillary sinus is resected to expose the posterior wall of the maxillary antrum

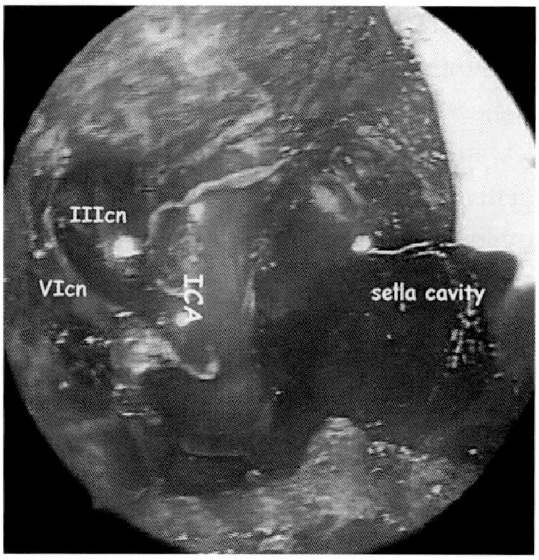

Fig. 2. Intraoperative EPSea right cavernous sinus vision.

and the vertical process of the palatine bone. After ligation of the sphenopalatine artery, the medial pterygoid process is drilled out. The resection of the medial pterygoid process permits the exposition of the inferolateral portion of the cavernous sinus. A partial resection of the pterygoid process is carried out taking into account the degree of pneumatization of the lateral recess of the sphenoid and the need for visualization of the lateral and inferior walls of the sphenoid sinus. The sphenoid sinus is exposed and its septa are removed. As in the MTea, contralateral access to the surgical field may be gained by removing 1 cm of the posterior end of the nasal septum with a back-biting forceps.

Stage II: Opening of the Cavernous Sinus and Removal of the Tumor

We divide the opening phase into two steps: (1) removal of the bone in front of the cavernous sinus, and (2) opening the dura of the cavernous sinus.

(1) Removal of the bone. To expose the anterior cavernous sinus, it is necessary to remove part of the bone of the posterolateral wall of the sphenoid sinus. The bone to be removed is a quadrilateral-shaped structure located between the optic-carotid recess and the paraclival carotid protuberance medially and the orbital apex and the trigeminal nerve protuberance laterally. The vidian canal on the floor of the sphenoidal sinus is a useful landmark because it indicates the junction of the horizontal, petrosal part of the carotid artery with the ascending paraclival segment of the vessel and, therefore, is a guide to the inferior portion of the cavernous sinus [19].

(2) Opening of the dura of the cavernous sinus. This step is performed using the endoscope fixed on its holder. The precise site of the opening of the inferior cavernous sinus wall (or sphenoidal part of the medial wall) depends on the displacement which the tumor produces along the course of the carotid artery and is to be performed in a safe area away from the carotid artery. The tumor may displace the ICA medially or laterally when its main bulk is in the lateral or medial compartments of the cavernous

sinus, respectively, and, therefore, the incision of the wall is to be performed lateral or medial to the vessel respectively. Moreover, besides the displacement of the ICA in the coronal plane, the displacement in the sagittal plane is also important. In cases of lesions involving the anteroinferior compartment of the cavernous sinus, the ICA is generally displaced posteriorly; in this case, the lesion covers the vessel making the opening of the dura less dangerous. Conversely, in cases of lesions involving the posterosuperior compartment, the ICA is displaced forward and is in strict contact with the anterior wall of the cavernous sinus. In the latter circumstance, before any dura incision, it is mandatory to locate the exact position of the ICA with the combined use of neuronavigation and micro-Doppler.

With the exception of a tumor exclusively located in the lateral compartment of the cavernous sinus, the dural opening is made in the sellar region and progressively enlarged following the tumor from its medial to its lateral and inferior portion. As pointed out earlier, maximal care is required during the sectioning of the dura in front of the carotid artery to avoid injury to the vessel, but also to avoid injury to the abducens nerve which, in the inferior portion of the cavernous sinus, runs close to the dura in an inferolateral direction toward the superior orbital fissure (fig. 2).

After dural incision, the tumor is mobilized by means of curettes and fragments are removed using an aspirator and forceps. The tumor is removed piece by piece, gradually gaining an increasing working area and obtaining good visual control of the contents of the cavernous sinus.

Stage III: Final Exploration and Closure of the Surgical Defect

Venous bleeding is usually not noteworthy. It may be more evident after tumor removal and is well controlled with Gelfoam or Floseal and cotton packing.

At the end of the tumor resection, inspection of the surgical field with 30° and 45° angled endoscopes permits the detection and removal of remnants.

Nasal packing with a single Merocel® is usually kept in place for 2 days.

Pterygo-Maxillary Endoscopic Approach (PMea)

This procedure is indicated when there are rare tumors extending through the foramen rotundum from the CS to the pterygomaxillary fossa (mainly neuromas and meningiomas) [22]. This approach is the combination of an EPSea and an endoscopic medial maxillectomy.

The procedure starts with a sphenoethmoidotomy ipsilateral to the cavernous sinus involved. Then, the inferior turbinate is resected, the vertical portion of the maxillary bone is drilled out and the medial wall of the maxillary sinus is removed. In this way, wide exposition of the lateral and posterior wall of the maxillary sinus is achieved. The nasolacrimal duct is transected immediately below the lacrimal sac in order to maintain its patency. The next step is characterized by the identification of the vidian canal after the resection of both the vertical process of the palatine bone and the medial pterygoid process. The posterior bone of the maxillary sinus is removed up to

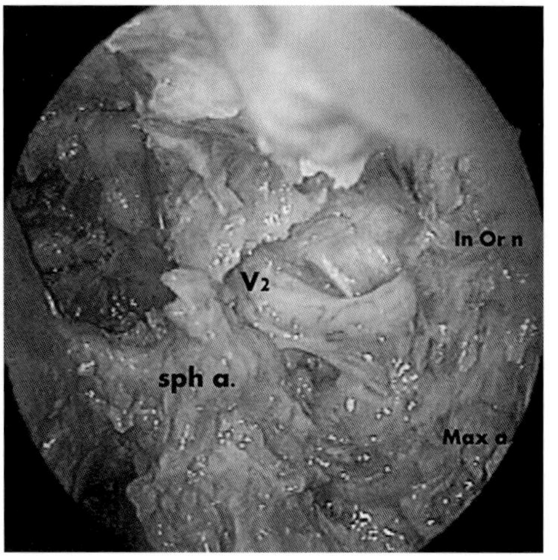

Fig. 3. Right pterygomaxillary fossa after fat removal. V_2 = Second branch of trigeminal nerve; sph a. = sphenopalatine artery; In Or n = infraorbital nerve; Max a = maxillary artery.

the course of the infraorbital nerve, and the periostium of the pterygomaxillary fossa is exposed. The exposure is tailored to tumor extension into the pterygomaxillary fossa. The landmarks are: medially, the vidian canal with the vidian nerve to localize the paraclival portion of the ICA; laterally and inferiorly, the maxillary artery and the pterygoid muscles, and superiorly, the infraorbital nerve and V2 following which, by passing through the foramen rotundum, makes it possible to arrive in the inferolateral compartment of the CS (fig. 3).

Material and Methods

Between May 1998 and December 2007 at the Neurosurgical Department of 'Bellaria' Hospital in Bologna, Italy, 793 patients underwent transnasal transsphenoidal endoscopic surgery for tumors involving the sella and parasellar regions. We performed an intraoperative evaluation of cavernous sinus invasion in each case [16]. Invasion of the cavernous sinus was detected in 141 cases. In this study, we reported our experience on 103 patients (107 procedures) with pituitary adenomas and 19 cases (25 procedures) with chordomas and chondrosarcomas (table 1). All other sporadic tumors with cavernous sinus invasion were excluded from this report.

The type of surgical approach is summarized in table 2.

The results are given using three parameters: (1) the degree of tumor removal, according to a 3-month MRI follow-up; (2) the remission of clinical symptoms, according to a 3-month postoperative examination; (3) a comprehensive evaluation which summarizes MRI, clinical and biochemical data after no less than a 6-month follow-up (table 3).

The degree of tumor removal was judged according to MRI imaging: (1) radical: no evidence of residual tumor; (2) subtotal: residual tumor less than 20%; (3) partial: residual tumor less than 50%; (4) insufficient: residual tumor more than 50%.

Clinical symptoms due to tumor mass effect (hemianopia, ophthalmoplegia and trigeminal neuralgia) are described as remission or persistence according to the physical and instrumental examination (visual field, Hess screen test) performed at a three month follow-up.

Table 1. Incidence of cavernous sinus invasion

Type of tumor	Number of procedures	CS invasion	%
Adenomas			
GH	154	27	16.8
PRL	91	15	16.4
ACTH	97	7	7.2
TSH	10	2	20
NF	328	56	17.3
Total	680	107	15.7
Chordomas	27	21	77.7
Chondrosarcomas	4	4	100
Total	31	25	80.6

Table 2. Patient population and surgical approaches

Type of approaches	Histopathology						Intraoperative CSF leak	
	adenoma, n	%	chordoma, n	%	chondrosarcoma, n	%	n	%
MTes	63	59	5	24			19	28
EPSea	43	40	13	62	3	75	14	24
PMAea	1	1	3	14	1	25	1	20
Total	107		21		4		34	25

Table 3. Parameters used for surgical outcome analysis

	MRI evaluation	Clinical evaluation	Comprehensive evaluation
1	Radical Radical removal No residue	Remission Resolution of symptoms	Cured (no residual tumor; no symptoms; endocrinological remission)
2	Subtotal Remnant <20%	Persistence Partial or no resolution	Controlled (residual tumor without symptoms or no residual tumor; mild symptoms)
3	Partial Remnant <50%		
4	Insufficient Remnant >50%	–	Not cured (residual tumor with symptoms not controlled with other therapy)

Finally, the comprehensive evaluation was defined as: (1) cured: radical removal, clinical and biohumoral cure (according to strict modern remission-criteria [16]); (2) controlled: subtotal removal with symptom resolution or radical removal with persistence of symptoms and/or biohumoral oversecretion; (3) not cured: residual tumor with persistent clinical and/or biohumoral symptoms.

Our postoperative protocol consists of an endocrinological evaluation on the third day and, for pituitary adenomas, at 1, 3 and 6 months. MRI follow-up is performed within 72 h, 3 months postoperatively, and then yearly. An endoscopic rhinologic evaluation is carried out after 1 month postoperatively to evaluate the normalization of the nasal and sphenoid cavities. A neuro-ophthalmological check-up is performed 3 months postoperatively only in the case of preoperative dysfunctions or postoperative referred visual disturbances.

Results

Adenomas

The median surgical time was 90 (60> to <180) min. In no case was a blood transfusion required. An intraoperative CSF leak was observed in 26 (24%) procedures and a plastic repair of the sella was performed intraoperatively. In general, in case of thin diaphragma sellae (with augmented postoperative risk of rupture), minimal CSF oozing or small dural defect with leak, we pack the surgical cavity through abdominal fat and the subsequent repositioning on the top of this of the previously undermined sphenoid mucosa is generally the repair of choice. In larger defects, a multilayer reconstruction through fat and mucoperiosteum is generally accomplished. Finally, in case of very large defects, we opt for a multilayer reconstruction with fascia lata, mucoperiostium and less often with pedicled nasal septal flap. CSF leaks appeared after 3 (3 cases) and 4 (1 case) days, and required endoscopic transsphenoidal repair. In 1 case, we had an increase of visual disturbance related to an overpacking of the sella which was only partially corrected by early surgical revision. One patient, who underwent partial removal of his tumor, was re-operated on using a transcranial approach due to hemorrhagic infarction of residual tumor in the temporal lobe.

One case of adjunctive cranial nerve palsy was observed: a third cranial nerve palsy occurred in a TSH adenoma. It was related to a blind curettage during a median approach. No intraoperative and perioperative deaths were observed.

One hundred and three patients, who underwent 107 procedures, had 3-month MRI follow-up to evaluate the degree of tumor removal (fig. 4, 5). The overall results showed no residual tumor in 59% of cases, subtotal removal in 32%, partial removal in 9% and insufficient removal in 1% (table 4). Compressive symptoms due to the mass effect (trigeminal neuralgia, ophthalmoplegia, hemianopia) disappeared in 86% and persisted in 14% (table 5).

A comprehensive evaluation was performed only in patients with not less than a 6-month follow-up. Eighty-nine patients with a median follow-up of 32 months (6–102 months) were analyzed (table 6).

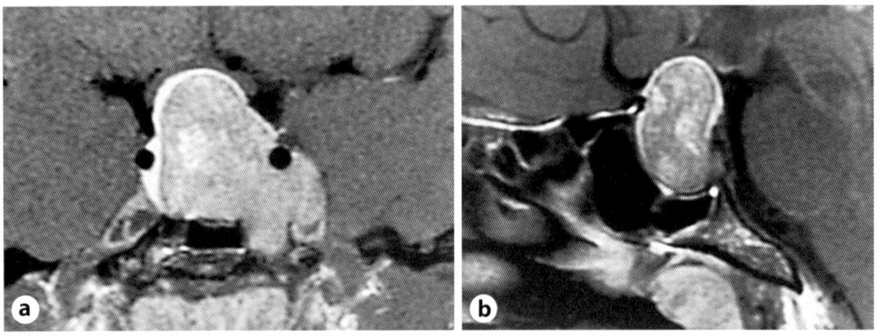

Fig. 4. GH-secreting adenoma invading the left cavernous sinus. Preoperative MRI view. **a** Coronal view. **b** Sagittal view.

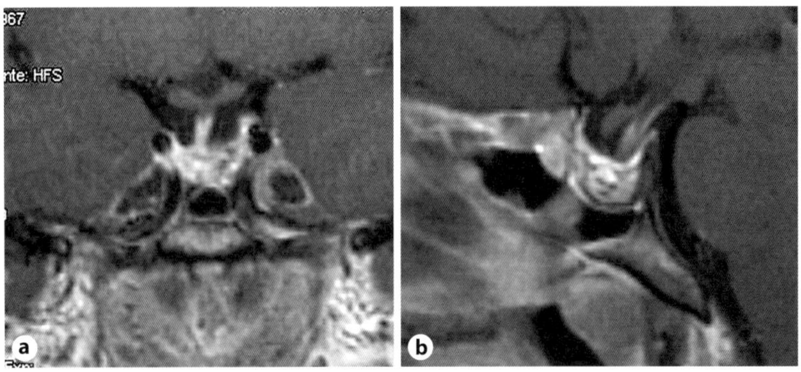

Fig. 5. GH-secreting adenoma invading the left cavernous sinus. Postoperative 3-month MRI confirms tumor removal in the sella and in the left cavernous sinus. **a** Coronal view. **b** Sagittal view.

The patients were considered cured in 43% of the cases, controlled in 50.5% and not controlled in 6.5% of the cases.

Four patients died after surgery due to tumoral progression: 3 months, 1 year, 5 years, and 6 years after surgery, respectively. In all cases, multiple brain metastases were discovered on MRI or at autopsy.

Chordomas and Chondrosarcomas

The median surgical time was 120 (60> to <260) min. In no case was a blood transfusion required. Intraoperative CSF leaks occurred in 7 procedures (28%) and a plastic repair of the sella was performed immediately. No postoperative CSF leaks appeared. No adjunctive cranial nerve palsy was observed. A tear of the ICA occurred during dissection so the surgical cavity was packed, and the tumoral resection was interrupted. This patient did not have any postoperative neurological deficit, and an endovascular procedure was carried out one week later to occlude a pseudoaneurysm of the injured ICA.

Table 4. Evaluation of tumor removal at 3-month MRI follow-up

Type of tumor	3-Month MRI follow-up				
	patients, n	1	2	3	4
GH	26	16	8	2	
PRL	15	7	7	1	
ACTH	7	3	3	1	
TSH	1		1		
NF	54	35	13	5	1
Total	103	61 (59%)	32 (31%)	9 (9%)	1 (1%)
Chordoma	21	7	10	2	2
Chondrosarcoma	4	4			
Total	25	11 (44%)	10 (40%)	2 (8%)	2 (8%)

Table 5. Pre- and postoperative neurological symptoms

Symptoms	Adenomas		Chordoma/chondrosarcoma	
	preop.	postop.	preop.	postop.
Ophthalmoplegia	13	2	17	2
Visual deficit	40	5	1	1
Visual neuralgia	4	1	6	0
Other cranial nerve palsy			2	1
Total	57	8	26	4

Table 6. Comprehensive evaluation referring to patients with more than a 6-month follow-up

Type of tumor	Cured	Controlled	Not controlled
Adenomas			
GH	8	15	1
PRL	3	9	1
ACTH		1	2
TSH		1	
NF	27	19	2
Total	38 (43%)	45 (50.5%)	6 (6.5%)
Chordomas	5	3	7
Chondrosarcomas	4	0	0
Total	9 (47%)	3 (16%)	7 (37%)

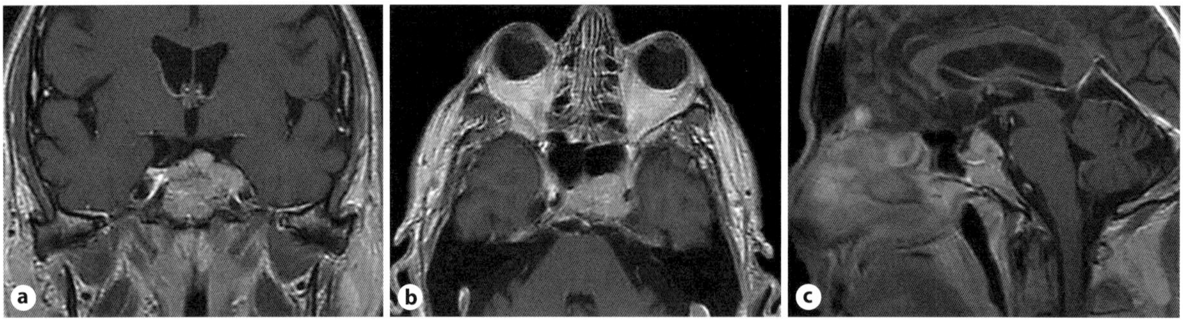

Fig. 6. Clivus chordoma invading the left cavernous sinus. Preoperative MRI. **a** Coronal view. **b** Axial view. **c** Sagittal view.

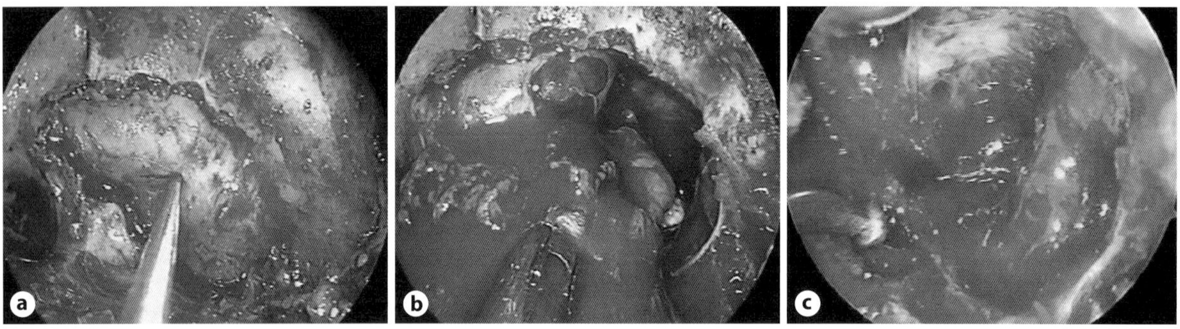

Fig. 7. Clivus chordoma invading the left cavernous sinus. Intraoperative view. **a** Incision of the inferior wall of the left cavernous sinus. **b** Tumoral dissection from the paraclival and parasellar segment of the left internal carotid artery. **c** Final view of the surgical cavity after the tumor removal.

The median follow-up was 37 months (11–112 months).

MRI was used to determine the extent of tumor removal (fig. 6–9); it was radical in 44% of cases, subtotal in 40%, partial in 8%, and insufficient in 8% (table 4). Visual and neurological disturbances regressed in 85% of the cases (table 5). A comprehensive evaluation was performed only in those patients with no less than a 6-month follow-up: 47% of patients were cured, 16% were controlled, and 37% were not controlled. Four patients died due to tumoral progression at 16, 23, 25 and 80 months after surgery, respectively (table 6).

Discussion

Surgery of the CS began in the 1960s. Since that time, some neurosurgeons [2, 4, 5] pioneered surgery in this region which had previously been considered a 'no

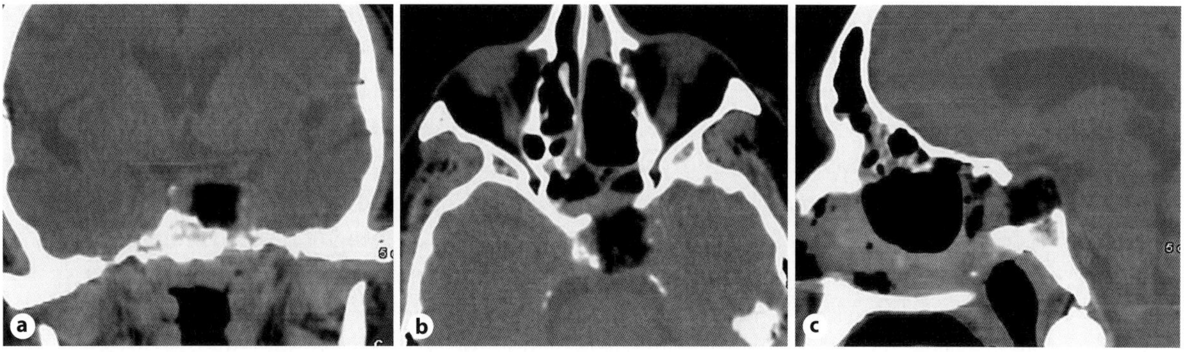

Fig. 8. Clivus chordoma invading the left cavernous sinus. One day postoperative CT scan. It is well visible the surgical trajectory through the ethmoidal region and the drilling out of the bone of the medial portion of the pterygoid process. The posterior and the left wall of the sphenoid sinus are removed. **a** Coronal view. **b** Axial view. **c** Sagittal view.

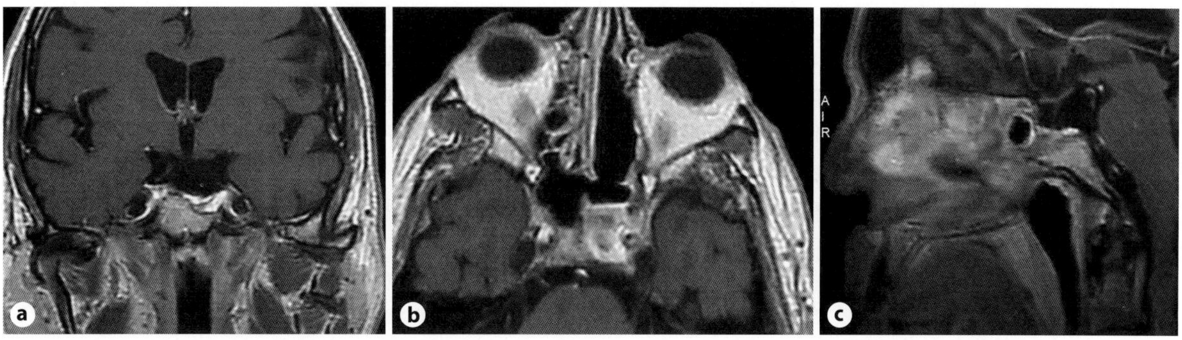

Fig. 9. Clivus chordoma invading the left cavernous sinus. Postoperative MRI no remnant tumor is visible. **a** Coronal view. **b** Axial view. **c** Sagittal view.

man's land'. With the advent of surgical interest, the anatomy of the structure was also re-evaluated [3, 17, 18, 20, 21]. Currently, even the name 'cavernous sinus' is being debated because this space is considered to be an extradural venous compartment in continuity with other similar venous extradural compartments of the orbit, i.e. the basiocciput and the spine [3, 21]. However, we continue to use this old term because 250 years of using the term 'cavernous sinus' makes it universally accepted in identifying this anatomical space. Moreover, the proposed new name 'lateral compartment' is currently being used to identify one of the compartments of the CS.

At present, different surgical approaches to the CS are available, including intra- and extradural craniotomic approaches and extended transsphenoidal approaches. A gold standard does not exist. The approach must be selected on the basis of many factors: extension of the tumor, biology of the tumor, and experience and confidence of the surgeon with the different techniques.

We believe that extended transsphenoidal approaches to the CS are options for tumors having an extradural location; they are represented mainly by pituitary adenomas and chordomas or chondrosarcomas [16, 23].

The extended transsphenoidal approaches consist of direct and extracerebral access which avoids brain manipulation and allows the opening of the CS through the medial wall which is devoid of any cranial nerves. Working within the venous compartments, the risk of damaging nerves depends on the compartments with tumor involvement. The median and posterosuperior compartments do not contain nerves; therefore, this localization does not expose the patient to the risk of nerve damage. The lateral and antero-inferior compartments contain the sixth cranial nerve which runs free inferiorly and laterally to the carotid artery directed towards the superior orbital fissure. Normally, the tumor displaces the nerve to its periphery, and great caution is required at the boundaries of the tumor to avoid or respect the nerve. Other nerves, IIIrd, IVth and V1, pass through the lateral wall of the CS, embedded and protected between the endosteal and meningeal layers composing the lateral wall, and may be injured only by the transection of this wall.

Extended transsphenoidal approaches to the cavernous sinus were first performed using the microsurgical technique [6–12]. The emergence of the endoscope in the neurosurgical landscape introduced the possibility of wide peripheral and endocavitary vision through a limited surgical channel, avoiding the need for wide access and the use of the speculum, which may be per se injurious and may also reduce surgical trajectories [13]. Anatomical studies demonstrating the feasibility of endoscopic endonasal cavernous surgery [14, 15] have been followed by clinical reports [16]. Unfortunately, until now, few series of microscopic extended transsphenoidal approaches to the CS have been reported. However, a recent study carried out using a microsurgical extended transsphenoidal approach for pituitary adenomas invading the cavernous sinus reported by Kitano et al. [24] shows excellent results confirming our experience. However, there are some discrepancies; even if we obtained an overall higher percentage of total and subtotal removal (92%) in GH adenomas, we verified a lower percentage of cure (32%). Furthermore, we did not have the problem of bleeding that Kitano et al. [24] describe; we experienced only 1 case of 3rd cranial nerve palsy with respect to the more frequent occurrence of ophthalmoplegia, even if transient, referred to by the same authors. The main limitation of all extended approaches consists of the difficulty in controlling the carotid artery in case of bleeding. We experienced one case of ICA injury in a patient affected by a chordoma: even though the bleeding was dramatic, the hemorrhage was controlled by packing the cavernous sinus endoscopically. Subsequent angiography showed a pseudoaneurysm and endovascular occlusion of the carotid artery was performed; finally, after 53 days, she was reoperated and the chordoma was removed.

Table 7. Complications referring to the procedures

	Adenomas (n = 107)		Chordomas (n = 25)	
Surgical complications				
Postoperative CSF leak	4	3.7%	1	4%
Epistaxis	1	0.9%	1	4%
Hematoma	2	1.8%	0	–
IIIrd cranial nerve palsy (no EPS)	1	0.9%	0	–
Overpacking	1	0.9%	0	–
Carotid injury		–	1	4%
Endocrine complications				
Adrenocortical insufficiency	2	1.8%	0	–
Transient DI	1	0.9%	0	–
Permanent DI	2	1.8%	0	–

Recent technical and instrumental advances may be helpful: perfected bipolar forceps are available which permit attempting the repair of a small hole in the carotid wall [25] and pistol clip appliers may allow putting a temporary or definitive clip on the bleeding carotid artery [24]. However, the main thing is to prevent such dramatic circumstances either by selecting patients without major involvement of the wall of the vessel or by using devices which localize the artery course. We avoid using an endoscopic technique to operate on tumors invading the wall of the vessel (meningiomas stenosing the carotid artery, carcinomas). During the procedure, we repeatedly perform precise mapping of the course of the carotid artery using neuronavigation and Doppler.

In addition to surgical treatment, radiation and pharmacological treatment have also made great strides. Radiosurgery has demonstrated that it is capable of controlling the growth of many tumors (meningiomas, adenomas) with low complication rates [26]. In functioning adenomas, medical therapy has been proven to be able to reduce and control the majority of prolactin-secreting adenomas [27] and control GH-oversecretion in a high percentage of GH-secreting adenomas [28]. Therefore, at present, surgery is not indicated for prolactin-secreting adenomas in which medical therapy is well-tolerated and effective. In GH adenomas invading the cavernous sinus, we were able to cure 33% of the patients, but an additional 62.5% were controlled using medical therapy [29, 30]. All these advances make it necessary to view the present role of surgery in the treatment of CS tumors in the correct perspective. The current strategy consists of controlling the mass effect and not necessarily radical removal, thereby achieving improvement of the neuropathies and minimizing deficits [6]. Neuropathies were responsive to surgical debulking and we obtained the regression of 85.5% (table 5) of neuropathies. Therefore, the preferred strategy should be multidisciplinary; surgery, radiation therapy and pharmacological therapy all contribute to the final result. However, it must be remembered that surgery still plays a central role in the complex treatment of CS tumors. It contributes to the diagnosis, confirming true cavernous sinus invasion by means of surgical inspection and furnishing material for pathologic analysis. It reduces the mass of the tumor, improving compressive symptoms and increasing the safety and efficacy of radiation [26] and medical therapy [29, 30]. Finally, in many cases, surgery alone permits the patients to be cured [16, 24].

Conclusions

In our experience, the endoscopic endonasal approach allows safe and effective management of tumors invading the cavernous sinus due to increased visualization, thus avoiding blind curettage. MTea is adequate for invasion limited to the medial or posterosuperior compartments. We have used the EPSea for major lateral or anteroinferior involvement of the CS.

The actual low complication rates and important benefits that can be obtained with endoscopic endonasal cavernous sinus surgery confirm the central role of surgery in the multidisciplinary treatment of tumors invading the cavernous sinus, particularly pituitary adenomas. It allows definition of true cavernous sinus invasion, histopathological diagnosis and, when cure is not feasible, tumor volume reduction which may be an important factor in the response to adjuvant therapy.

References

1 Winslow JB: Exposition Anatomique de la Structure du Corps Humain. London, N. Prevast, 1734, vol II, p 29.
2 Parkinson D: A surgical approach to the cavernous portion of the carotid artery: anatomical studies and case report. J Neurosurg 1965 23:474–483.
3 Parkinson D: Lateral sellar compartment OT (cavernous sinus): history, anatomy, terminology. Anat Rec 1998;251:486–490.
4 Dolenc VV: General approach to the cavernous sinus; in Dolenc VV (ed): Anatomy and Surgery of the Cavernous Sinus. New York, Springer, 1989, pp 139–169.
5 Sekhar LN, Goel A, Sen CN: Cavernous sinus tumors; in Apuzzo MLJ (ed): Brain Surgery: Complication Avoidance and Management. Churchill-Livingstone, New York, 1993, pp 2197–2218.
6 Couldwell WT, Weiss MH, Rabb C, Liu JK, Apfelbaum RI, Fukushima T: Variations on the standard transsphenoidal approach to the sellar region, with emphasis on the extended approaches and parasellar approaches: surgical experience in 105 cases. Neurosurgery 2004;55:539–547.
7 Laws ER Jr, Onofrio BM, Pearson BW, McDonald TJ, Dirrenberger RA: Successful management of bilateral carotid-cavernous fistulae with a transsphenoidal approach. Neurosurgery 1979;4:162–167.
8 Lalwani AK, Kaplan MJ, Gutin PH: The transsphenoethmoid approach to the sphenoid sinus and clivus. Neurosurgery 1992;31:1008–1014.
9 Fraioli B, Esposito V, Santoro A, Iannetti G, Giuffre R, Cantore G: Transmaxillosphenoidal approach to tumors invading the medial compartment of the cavernous sinus. J Neurosurg 1995;82:63–69.
10 Sabit I, Schaefer SD, Couldwell WT: Extradural extranasal combined transmaxillary transsphenoidal approach to the cavernous sinus: a minimally invasive microsurgical model. Laryngoscope 2000;110:286–291.

11 Rabadan A, Conesa H: Transmaxillary-transnasal approach to the anterior clivus: a microsurgical anatomical model. Neurosurgery 1992;30:473–481; discussion 482.
12 Kitano M, Taneda M: Extended transsphenoidal approach with submucosal posterior ethmoidectomy for parasellar tumors: technical note. J Neurosurg 2001;94:999–1004.
13 Jho HD, Carrau RL: Endoscopic endonasal transsphenoidal surgery: experience with 50 patients. J Neurosurg 1997;87:44–51.
14 Alfieri A, Jho HD: Endoscopic endonasal approaches to the cavernous sinus: surgical approaches. Neurosurgery 2001;49:354–360.
15 Cavallo LM, Cappabianca P, Galzio R, Iaconetta G, de Divitiis E, Tschabitscher M: Endoscopic transnasal approach to the cavernous sinus versus transcranial route: anatomic study. Neurosurgery 2005;56(2 suppl):379–389.
16 Frank G., Pasquini E: Endoscopic endonasal cavernous sinus surgery, with special reference to pituitary adenomas. Front Horm Res 2006;34:64–82.
17 Yasuda A, Campero A, Martins C, Rhoton AL Jr, Ribas GC: The medial wall of the cavernous sinus: microsurgical anatomy. Neurosurgery 2004;55:179–189; discussion 189–190.
18 Umansky F, Nathan H: The lateral wall of the cavernous sinus – with special reference to the nerves related to it. J Neurosurg 1982;56:228–234.
19 Kassam AB, Vescan AD, Carrau RL, Prevedello DM, Gardner P, Mintz AH, Snyderman CH, Rhoton AL: Expanded endonasal approach: vidian canal as a landmark to the petrous internal carotid artery. J Neurosurg 2008;108:177–183.
20 Harris FS, Rhoton A: Anatomy of the cavernous sinus: a microsurgical study. J Neurosurg 1976;45: 169–180.
21 Taptas JN: The parasellar osteo-dural chamber and the vascular and neural elements that traverse it: an anatomical concept that would replace the cavernous sinus of classical anatomy. Neurochirurgie 1990; 36:201–208.
22 Pasquini E, Sciarretta V, Farneti G, Ippolito A, Mazzatenta D, Frank G: Endoscopic endonasal approach for the treatment of benign schwannoma of the sinonasal tract and pterygopalatine fossa. Am J Rhinol 2002;16:113–118.
23 Frank G, Sciarretta V, Calbucci F, Farneti G, Mazzatenta D, Pasquini E: The endoscopic transnasal transsphenoidal approach for the treatment of cranial base chordomas and chondrosarcomas. Neurosurgery 2006;59(1 suppl 1):ONS50–57.
24 Kitano M, Taneda M, Shimono T, Nakao Y: Extended transsphenoidal approach for surgical management of pituitary adenomas invading the cavernous sinus. J Neurosurg 2008;108:26–36.
25 Kassam A, Snyderman CH, Carrau RL, Gardner P, Mintz A: Endoneurosurgical hemostasis techniques: lessons learned from 400 cases. Neurosurg Focus 2005;19:E7.
26 Shin M, Kurita H, Sasaki T, Tago M, Morita A, Ueki K, Kirino T: Stereotactic radiosurgery for pituitary adenoma invading the cavernous sinus. J Neurosurg 2000;93(suppl 3):2–5.
27 Molitch ME: Medical management of prolactin-secreting pituitary adenomas. Pituitary 2002;5:55–65.
28 Melmed S, Vance ML, Barkan AL, Bengtsson BA, Kleinberg D, Klibanski A, Trainer PJ: Current status and future opportunities for controlling acromegaly. Pituitary 2002;5:185–196.
29 Colao A, Attanasio R, Pivonello R, Cappabianca P, Cavallo LM, Lasio G, Lodrini A, Lombardi G, Cozzi R: Partial surgical removal of growth hormone-secreting pituitary tumors enhances the response to somatostatin analogs in acromegaly. J Clin Endocrinol Metab 2006;91:85–92.
30 Petrossians P, Borges-Martins L, Espinoza C, Daly A, Betea D, Valdes-Socin H, Stevenaert A, Chanson P, Beckers A: Gross total resection or debulking of pituitary adenomas improves hormonal control of acromegaly by somatostatin analogs. Eur J Endocrinol 2005;152:61–66.

Giorgio Frank, MD
Neurosurgical Department
'Bellaria' Hospital
Via Altura 3, IT–40100 Bologna (Italy)
Tel. +39 051 6225 111, E-Mail giorgio.frank@ausl.bo.it

Kassam AB, Gardner PA (eds): Endoscopic Approaches to the Skull Base.
Prog Neurol Surg. Basel, Karger, 2012, vol 26, pp 140–151

Expanded Pure Endoscopic Endonasal Approach for Clival Lesions

Amir R. Dehdashti[a,b] · David A. Omahen[a] · Fred Gentili[a]

[a]Division of Neurosurgery University Health Network, Toronto Western Hospital, University of Toronto, Toronto, Ont., Canada; [b]Department of Neurosurgery, Geisinger Clinic, Danville, Pa., USA

Abstract

Widespread use of the endoscope in transsphenoidal surgery has recently contributed to the extension of approaches beyond the tuberculum sellae for the management of suprasellar, anterior skull base or clival lesions. Based on our experience with the standard purely endoscopic approach to the pituitary fossa, we evolved the use of the expanded pure endoscopic endonasal approach to address clival lesions. Because of their midline location, clival neoplasms are suitable indications for this minimally invasive technique. However, those with significant lateral extension cannot be dealt with by this technique as a sole approach and open transcranial procedures need to be combined with the endoscopic approach. The technique described below incorporates technological advances in endoscopic endonasal surgery, frameless stereotactic guidance and novel skull base reconstruction methods. Our results in terms of tumor removal rate, complications and survival are similar to those reported in previous series. The minimally invasive nature of this approach with comparable results makes the technique very attractive and probably the procedure of choice for selected clival lesions.

Clival lesions are rare tumors that continue to pose significant challenges for skull base surgeons. Their central location and tendency to infiltrate bone makes total removal rarely possible. This is associated with a high incidence of recurrence in some pathologies such as chordoma. Likewise, their proximity to vital neurovascular structures, including cranial nerves and the brainstem, carries significant potential for postoperative morbidity. Despite the difficulty in achieving a surgical cure in the majority of chordomas, radical surgical resection with adjuvant radiotherapy appears to offer the best chance of survival for patients with this tumor [1]. Thus, the optimal operative approach should offer the best chance of radical removal while minimizing the potential for postoperative complications. Benign clival lesions might have a more indolent course and the approach to these lesions should therefore be less aggressive.

The increasing use of the endoscope in transsphenoidal surgery and its application to other lesions of the skull base has opened another chapter in skull base surgery.

The versatility of this minimally invasive technique has widened the boundaries past the pituitary fossa to include regions far beyond the sellar floor. Using the expanded endonasal approach one can readily access, in a minimally invasive way, the entire central skull base from the frontal sinus anteriorly to the clivus and region of the foramen magnum and odontoid process inferiorly. In this chapter, we will present the anatomical and technical nuances of the expanded purely endoscopic endonasal approach for the treatment of clival lesions and report our surgical experience and compare our results to the well established transcranial techniques.

Clivus Anatomy

It is useful to divide the clivus into thirds. The upper third extends from the dorsum sellae and posterior clinoids to the plane of Dorello's canal. The middle third ranges from the petrous apex at Dorello's canal to the pars nervosa of the jugular foramen. The inferior third spans from the pars nervosa to the foramen magnum. The overall distance from the floor of the sella to the inferior extent of the clivus averages 34.5 mm. The whole length is accessible by the expanded endoscopic endonasal approach. The average thickness of the clivus ranges from 9 to 18 mm. The clivus ends an average of 5.8 mm from a line connecting the hypoglossal canals. The upper two thirds of the intracranial portion is adjacent to the pons. The petroclival fissures separate the upper two thirds of the clivus from the petrous temporal bone on either side.

Retroclival Anatomy

Situated between the two layers of dura behind the upper clivus, the basilar venous plexus forms interconnections between the paired cavernous sinuses superiorly, the inferior petrosal sinuses laterally, and the marginal sinus inferiorly. It can span from one third to the entire length of the clivus. Also found laterally between these two layers of dura are the abducent nerves which are found an average of 20 mm apart at their dural emergence. This explains the expected sixth nerve palsy in clival lesions.

Fully opening the dura exposes the vertebrobasilar complex and its branches, the mamillary bodies, the brainstem, the pituitary stalk, the optic apparatus, and cranial nerves III through VI. Aggressive clival lesions (e.g. chordoma and chondrosarcoma) involve the dura in the majority of cases.

Preoperative Evaluation

Preoperative imaging using both CT scan to demonstrate bony anatomy and MRI to provide anatomic relationships of soft tissues is necessary. The position of the optic nerve and carotid arteries must be determined prior to any operative approach. Sphenoid pneumatization and septae should also be evaluated. Noninvasive evaluation of vascular structures using MRA or CT angiography can provide useful information regarding arterial structures.

Surgical Indications

The expanded endoscopic endonasal approach is indicated for centrally located clival lesions. Those with significant lateral extension beyond the cavernous sinus or with posterolateral extension are treated by craniotomy as the only approach or as the first procedure prior to the endoscopic technique. In terms of the evolving use of this approach, an ideal application for the expanded endonasal approach is for the purposes of obtaining a tissue diagnosis. Currently, endoscopic techniques allow biopsy sampling with minimal morbidity and very short hospitalization. Another indication would be for patients undergoing palliative tumor debulking for improvement of quality of life.

Description of the Surgical Approach

Patient Positioning

The procedure takes place with the patient in the supine position with the head fixed in a three-pin Mayfield holder. The head of the bed is elevated 20–30°. The neck is placed in a neutral or slightly flexed position (which improves the view toward the clivus) and is slightly rotated toward the side of the surgeon. Intraoperative image guidance using frameless stereotactic navigation (Stealth, Medtronic®, Jacksonville, Fla., USA) is used routinely and has proven quite reliable. One video monitor is positioned behind the patient's head directly in front of the surgeon's line of vision. A second monitor is placed across from the assistant. The face is prepared and pledgets soaked with epinephrine (diluted 1/1,000) are placed into each nostril while the blood pressure and pulse rate are carefully monitored. Perioperative antibiotics (cefazolin and metronidazole) are used routinely.

Surgical Approach

All patients underwent a pure endoscopic endonasal approach using a 0°, 18-cm-long, 4-mm endoscope throughout the procedure (Karl Storz GmbH & Co., Tuttlingen, Germany). The use of an automatic endoscope irrigating system (ClearVision, Karl Storz) has proven very useful. Two sets of instruments are used.

A standard nasal access set used in endoscopic paranasal sinus surgery is used for the initial and extradural part of the procedure. A second set of low profile instruments and specially designed bipolar forceps are used for the intradural work. It cannot be overemphasized that appropriate instrumentation is essential for this approach. The surgical approach is tailored according to the location and extension of the tumor. A bi-nostril approach is used with the endoscope typically positioned in the right superior nasal cavity by one surgeon who is responsible for maintaining the visual field. This allows a second surgeon to use two hands and an instrument in each nostril for resection of the tumor.

Resection of both middle turbinates is performed. The uncinate processes can be removed bilaterally in selective cases. The posterior half of the nasal septum including the maxillary crest is removed to widely expose the rostrum. After cauterizing both posterior nasal branches of the sphenopalatine arteries, the sphenoid sinus is widely opened and the floor drilled down to the nasopharynx to allow better exposure and bimanual manipulation. By drilling the lateral recess of the sphenoid, the optico-carotid recess and clivo-carotid protuberances are visualized and are important surgical landmarks for the rest of the procedure. At this point, the tumor will often be visible, especially if the clivus is eroded anteriorly. On rare occasions when the lesion is not visible, its location is confirmed by intraoperative navigation, and drilling of the upper clivus can be started. The medial wall of the clival carotids represents the lateral limits of the clival exposure. The floor of the sphenoid is further drilled down to get access to the mid and lower clivus. Inferiorly, the pre-clival fascia is opened with a midline incision and reflected laterally. Resection of the medial pterygoid process can be performed to expose the lateral extension of the lower part of the tumor.

It is not unusual for the tumor to have eroded the dura with intracranial extension. In these cases, the dura is opened in the midline and in a linear fashion to better expose the intradural component of the tumor. This should be done after locating the position of the ICAs on both sides with image guidance and confirming their position with micro Doppler. The tumor is then removed with the same bimanual technique used during microscopic resection, but with a significantly wider field of vision under endoscopic visualization.

In cases of tumor extension to the upper clivus only, the expanded endoscopic endonasal approach consists of exposure of the upper part of the clivus and dorsum sella. A total ethmoidectomy and maxillary antrostomy can also be performed to augment the exposure especially if the tumor presents with more central and inferior extension in the clivus. For tumors extending to the foramen magnum region, the septum is lowered flush with the palate to achieve maximum exposure and bony removal should be extended to the lower part of the clivus.

Reconstruction

Reconstruction represents one of the most challenging steps of the expanded approach. A multilayered reconstruction is favored. A single layer of surgicel or Duragen® is positioned as an inlay to reconstitute the arachnoid barrier. Next, an autogenous fascia lata graft is placed intradurally in an in-lay fashion. A second layer of fascia lata is placed extradurally (out-lay) to cover the dura and bone edges. A thin layer of fibrin glue or Bioglu® is used at the edges and then fat is applied to cover the out-lay fascia. We use a local vascularized nasal septal flap (based on the posterior septal artery) for repair of these defects as described by Hadad et al. [2] and add fascia lata graft over the out-lay. More fibrin glue and Gelfoam are used to cover the whole reconstruction. In an attempt to prevent graft migration and the development of persistent CSF channels, we use a 14-Fr Foley catheter to apply pressure and to hold the repair in place; a modified version of a technique defined by Kassam et al. [3] using a balloon stent. The Foley catheter is left in place for 3–4 days.

Illustrative Cases

Case 1
A 37-year-old man presented with headache. He had a normal neurological examination. Imaging revealed a clival-based lesion with retroclival extension (fig.1a). Gross total resection was obtained using an endoscopic endonasal approach. Figure 1b shows the intraoperative view of the tumor origin in the clivus. The panoramic view of the retroclival structures is shown in figure 1c. Figures 1d–f show the details of closure with the tensor fascia lata on-lay graft, free fat graft, and a Foley catheter balloon to support the closure. Final pathology was that of a chordoma.

Case 2
A 39 year old man presented to his family physician with atypical headaches but no focal neurological deficits. Figures 2a and b show his initial MRI scan which revealed the presence of a large clival chordoma with marked brainstem compression. His CT scan revealed evidence of bony erosion. The patient with treated with a two-stage approach. The first stage was a right-sided far lateral retrosigmoid resection of the exophytic intradural component of the tumor. Figures 2c and d show the residual extradural component. This was subsequently removed using an endoscopic transsphenoidal approach. Figure 2e shows an intraoperative view of the tumor at its origin in the clivus. Figure 2f shows the visualization of the brainstem and retroclival structures possible with this endoscopic approach.

Results of our Experience with the Expanded Endonasal Endoscopic Approach
Prior to 2005, patients with clival lesions were operated using classical skull base approaches (lateral rhinotomy, frontobasal craniotomy, microscopic transsphenoidal, far lateral). Since June 2005, 15 of our patients underwent an expanded purely endoscopic endonasal approach for different clival lesions. All patients underwent radiological assessment of their lesions by computed tomographic scans and magnetic

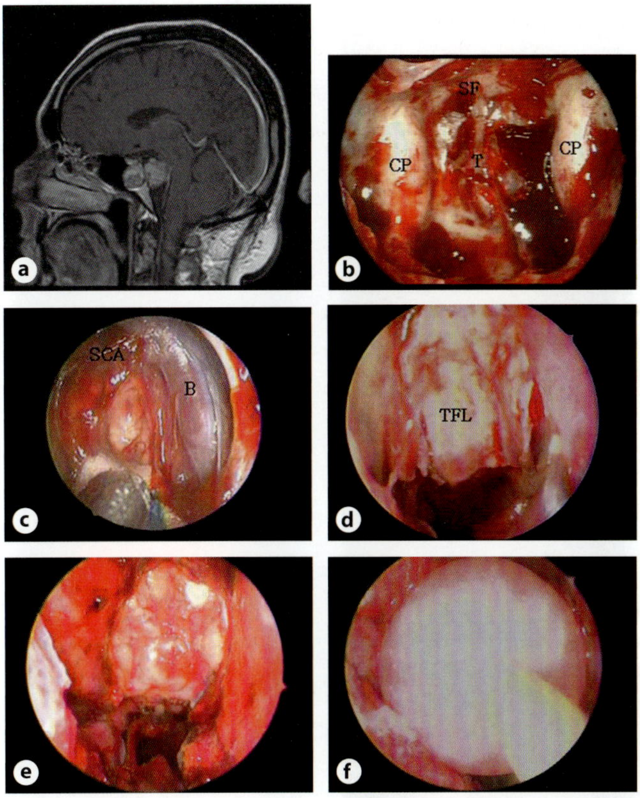

Fig. 1. a. Preoperative T_1-weighted MRI scan with intravenous gadolinium contrast in a 37-year-old with a clival mass. **b** Intraoperative endoscopic view of focal clival chordoma. Tumor is marked with a T. CP = Carotid prominence; SF = sellar floor. **c** Intraoperative view of the retroclival anatomy after tumor resection. The basilar artery is labeled B. SCA signifies the take off of the superior cerebellar artery. **d, e** Final steps of the closure using an autologous tensor fascia lata onlay graft (**d**), followed by a free fat graft (**e**). **f** The balloon of a Foley catheter being used to support the closure from below.

resonance imaging. There were 12 chordomas, 2 ossifying fibromas and one osteogenic sarcoma. Two patients had prior craniotomy for large cranial base chordomas with significant lateral extension. Two patients had a lateral rhinotomy 8 and 10 years before, and one patient had a previous microscopic transsphenoidal surgery 7 years before the current recurrence. All 3 patients with recurrent tumors had radiation after their initial treatment. None of the newly diagnosed patients had radiotherapy prior to surgery.

Radiological Findings. All patients underwent MR imaging and CT scanning prior to surgery. Bony erosions were found on CT scans in all cases. In 9 cases, a centrally located inhomogeneous tumor that was hyperintense on T_2-weighted MR imaging allowed a presumptive diagnosis of chordoma. All cases had moderate-to-significant nonhomogeneous enhancement after contrast injection.

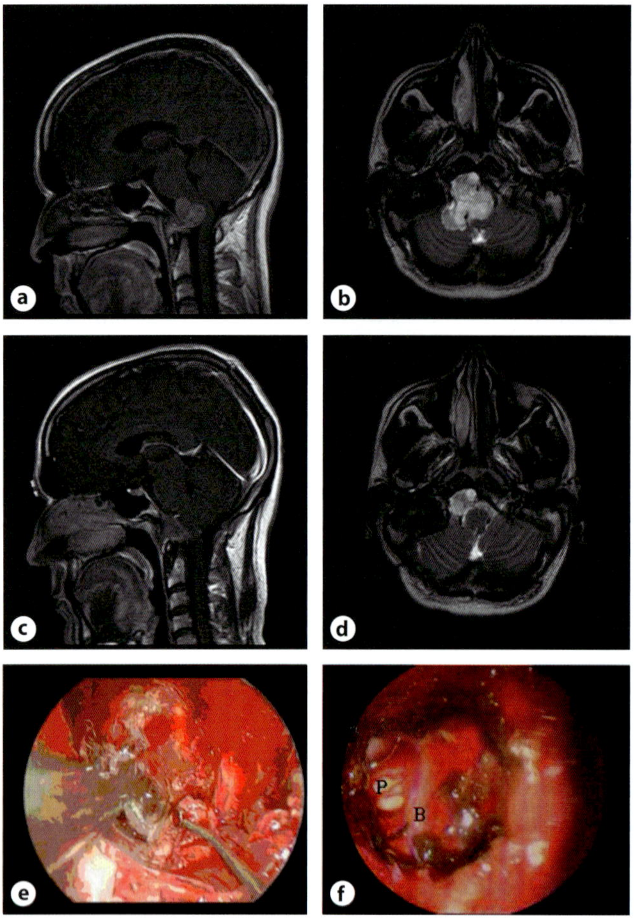

Fig. 2. a, b Preoperative T_1-weighted gadolinium-enhanced MRI scan showing a clival chordoma with a large exophytic intradural extension and marked brainstem compression. The intradural component was initially treated with a retrosigmoid far lateral approach, leaving residual extradural tumour (shown in **c** and **d**). **e** View of the tumor bed at the time of the bimanual binostril endoscopic endonasal approach to the extradural clival portion of the tumor. **f** Endoscopic view of the retroclival structures. The pons is labeled P. B denotes the basilar artery.

Tumor Removal. The extent of tumor removal was evaluated on the basis of surgical findings and postoperative MRIs done immediately and 3 months after the surgery. If during surgery the tumor was removed completely and the immediate MRI did not show any postoperative enhancement, it was classified as a gross total removal. However, we do believe that even in these satisfactory cases, some microscopic cells likely have been left behind in bone, especially in the chordoma cases. Therefore, the gross total removal does not mean cure. We achieved gross total resection in 9 cases (60%, no visible tumor on postoperative MRI) and 6 (40%) had subtotal resection (>80%). The large size and extensive bony involvement, the lateral extension of the lower part of the tumor and the scar tissue in recurrent cases were the main reasons for subtotal resection.

Pre- and Postoperative Clinical Status. Of the 7 patients who presented with preoperative 6th nerve palsy, 4 totally recovered after surgery, 1 showed a partial recovery and 2 remained unchanged. One of these 2 also had chiasm compression and had only partial improvement of vision. The last patient with 6th nerve palsy remained unchanged. Of the 3 patients with lower cranial nerve deficit, two had improvement after the surgery and one showed worsening.

In the patient with brainstem compression and long tract signs, a significant improvement was observed after surgery. One patient with lower cranial nerve deficit and brainstem compression prior to surgery, secondary to extensive recurrent chordoma, developed a postoperative hematoma which necessitated re-exploration and clot removal. This patient presented with new hemiparesis and worsening of her lower cranial nerve deficit and required temporary tracheostomy after surgery.

Complications. There were few complications after surgery. The most serious was one patient with a postoperative hematoma and new neurological deficit. This patient also developed hydrocephalus with the need for temporary external ventricular drainage. Four patients presented with CSF leak, two of which responded well to lumbar drainage. The remaining two underwent successful re-exploration and repeat reconstruction of the skull base with the multilayer closure technique followed by lumbar drainage for 5 days. One patient presented with tension pneumocephalus which required burr hole evacuation.

Discussion

Although complete resection of clival lesions and especially chordomas is desirable, this is often not possible without causing substantial morbidity. In our overall series, only in focal centrally located lesions did we feel we had achieved a total removal. Nonetheless, radical surgical resection with adjuvant radiation therapy is the mainstay of treatment as confirmed by Colli and Al-Mefty in a review of 53 patients with chordomas [1]. Other clival lesions might have a more benign course and the surgical strategy should be modified according to the histopathological features of those lesions. The 5-year survival rates vary between 65 and 79% for chordomas but 10-year survival drops significantly [4, 5]. This emphasizes the importance of minimally invasive techniques for these not curable lesions.

Current State of the Art in Surgical Approaches

With regard to surgical approaches, a variety of craniotomies, standard transsphenoidal and transoral approaches or a combination thereof have been advocated for clival lesions. The choice of the surgical route depends on the location of the tumor, the main extension of the tumor and also the surgical experience and the comfort level of the surgeon. Because clival tumors are, in general, midline tumors that displace the neuraxis dorsally or dorsolaterally, anterior midline approaches, e.g. transbasal, extended frontal [6], transsphenoidal [7], transmaxillary [8], midfacial degloving [9], and transoral [9], are generally preferred. However, lateral extension of clival lesions to the parasellar region, petrous bone and occipital condyle requires a lateral approach to the clivus [10] which may be combined with an anterior approach. Chondrosarcomas, which typically present with more lateral location, are not ideal for the expanded pure endoscopic endonasal technique; we prefer transcranial approaches for the majority of them.

For midline clival lesions, we have come to favor the expanded endoscopic transsphenoidal approach with the aim of decompression of the neuraxis. This minimizes the morbidity associated with more invasive and aggressive approaches and offers better patient comfort.

The use of this approach for clival chordomas and other lesions involving the clivus has evolved over the last couple of decades using microscopic and extended techniques [11–13].

The expanded endoscopic endonasal technique for skull base lesions is a state of the art approach with limited illustration in the current literature. As opposed to the microscopic technique, the endoscope offers a superb panoramic view of the structures and allows excellent visualization of parasellar regions. The avoidance of a nasal speculum with endoscopic technique along with the incorporation of the binostril technique offers a greater amount of flexibility, visibility and maneuverability of the surgical instruments. Moreover, the use of the microvascular ultrasound Doppler probe and computer assisted neuronavigation have significantly improved safety during endonasal endoscopic techniques [14, 15].

Jho [16] reported a series of endoscopic approach to clival lesions in 2001 with good results. Kassam et al. [3], Solares et al. [17] and Cappabianca et al. [18] described the technique and the feasibility in a group of patients with different parasellar and clival pathologies.

Kingdom et al. [19] reported the results of a series of 10 clival lesions approached endoscopically. Pathologic diagnosis was obtained in all cases and included adenocarcinoma, cholesterol granuloma, plasmacytoma, metastases (liposarcoma, renal cell carcinoma), fibrous dysplasia, meningoencephalocele, and teratoma. Frank et al. [20] reported their experience in a series of 11 patients, harboring chordomas (9 cases) and chondrosarcomas (2 cases) of the cranial base. They concluded that this approach is an important adjunct to craniotomy for treatment of such lesions. Recently, our group [21] and Stippler et al. [22] reported experience with pure endoscopic resection of chordomas. The results were considered similar to traditional techniques.

Extent of Resection and Complications

As previously noted, total removal of clival lesions, specifically chordomas, is extremely difficult to achieve and only possible in focal central lesions. In a series of

18 chordomas, operated on with an extended transsphenoidal microscopic approach, a gross total resection was achieved in 12 cases (66%). However, there was an internal carotid injury in 3 of them and new neurological deficit and cranial nerves deficit in 3 other cases [11]. In 1999, Kelley et al. [23] reported a series of 7 cases involving transsphenoidal endoscopic approaches to clival lesions in 7 patients. A definitive diagnosis was obtained in 5. There was one CSF leak and one hemorrhage. In the purely endoscopic series from Frank et al. [20], gross total resection was achieved in 3/9 (33%) of chordoma cases and the major complication was an ICA injury during exposure. Two patients presented with CSF leak and 3 patients in their series died as the tumor recurred at follow-up (range 10–20 months). Stamm et al. [24] published their series of 36 clival region tumors in 2006. As in our series, chordoma was the most common pathology (13/36 lesions). They also treated CSF leaks (6 patients), cholesterol granuloma (6 patients), fungal disease (4 patients), meningoceles (2 patients), mucoceles (2 patients), malignant tumors (3 patients), an angiofibroma, and a teratoma. In order of frequency, their complications included CSF leak, bleeding, orbital hematoma, brain injury, and intrasellar complications.

In our series, gross total resection was achieved in 9 patients (60%) with large but focal lesions and subtotal resection was performed in the 6 other cases (40%). We had 4 patients with postoperative CSF leak, 2 of whom responded well to lumbar drainage and 2 of whom needed re-exploration and repair. We attribute the high rate of CSF leak to the presence of large premesencephalic and prepontine cisterns next to the wide bony opening of the transclival approach.

Feasibility and Safety

Our results are in concordance with previous reports with regards to feasibility, equivalence to other approaches, and the safety of this technique in selective cases of clival lesions [18, 20]. We do not recommend this type of surgery as the only approach for laterally located lesions such as very extensive chordomas or chondrosarcomas. This extension can raise the risk of vascular injury (e.g. carotid tear) without providing safe control of structures in the lateral part of the cavernous sinus. It also might be hazardous for lesions with lateral extension in the lower clival area. Despite being very selective in patient selection for this novel approach, we had a patient with new hemiparesis and aggravation of lower cranial nerve deficit after surgery due to an immediate postoperative hematoma in the prebulbar region in the setting of an extensive recurrent chordoma. The cause of the hematoma could not, however, be related to the type of approach itself.

Limitations of the Expanded Pure Endoscopic Endonasal Approach

The major limitations of this endoscopic approach are significant lateral extension of the tumor, extensive intradural invasion of the tumor, and tumor being primarily centered on the inferior clivus with extension towards the occipital condyle. In these situations, craniotomy offers a better degree of tumor exposure and removal.

Although very large lesions are not a limiting factor in appropriately selected cases, the inability to achieve a gross total removal presents the same problems as it does for any open approach. Dural invasion per se is not a contraindication for endoscopic surgery, but extensive dural involvement poses the same challenges as with craniotomy. In our point of view, brain invasion is considered a contraindication for expanded endoscopic endonasal approach. While this might raise some controversial arguments, we feel that brain invasion is better addressed with transcranial approaches especially when dealing with subpial dissection of the tumor and bleeding. Advances in expanded endonasal approaches might change this policy in the future.

CSF Leak

CSF leak has been a major challenge but the introduction of the nasal septal flap is a promising evolution in the final part of the reconstruction of the clival defect. We did not encounter CSF leakage in more recent cases in our series where this novel technique was used. For recurrent cases, the use of a nasal septal flap is limited, however, because of scar tissue or prior resection of the posterior nasal septum. Fortes et al. [25] advocated the use of a posterior pedicle inferior turbinate flap as an alternative.

Conclusion

The expanded fully endoscopic endonasal approach is a valid alternative to transcranial or transoral operations in the treatment of clival lesions. The main indication is for centrally located neoplasms or as an adjunct to craniotomy for more extensive tumors. Its minimally invasive nature makes it very attractive for selected cases with the potential for minimizing morbidity associated with other extensive approaches and maximizing the patient's comfort. Early results suggest at least equivalency to other techniques, although long term outcomes have yet to be analyzed. This approach should be in the armamentarium of skull bases surgeons and be considered as an important option for the treatment of carefully selected clival tumors.

References

1 Colli B, Al-Mefty O: Chordomas of the craniocervical junction: follow-up review and prognostic factors. J Neurosurg 2001;95:933–943.
2 Hadad G, Bassagasteguy L, Carrau RL, et al: A novel reconstructive technique after endoscopic expanded endonasal approaches: vascular pedicle nasoseptal flap. Laryngoscope 2006;116:1882–1886.
3 Kassam A, Carrau RL, Snyderman CH, Gardner P, Mintz A: Evolution of reconstructive techniques following endoscopic expanded endonasal approaches. Neurosurg Focus 2005;19:E8.
4 Gay E, Sekhar LN, Rubinstein E, et al: Chordomas and chondrosarcomas of the cranial base: results and follow-up of 60 patients. Neurosurgery 1995;36: 887–896, discussion 96–97.
5 Crockard HA, Steel T, Plowman N, et al: A multidisciplinary team approach to skull base chordomas. J Neurosurg 2001;95:175–183.
6 Sekhar LN, Nanda A, Sen CN, Snyderman CN, Janecka IP: The extended frontal approach to tumors of the anterior, middle, and posterior skull base. J Neurosurg 1992;76:198–206.

7 Laws ER Jr: Transsphenoidal surgery for tumors of the clivus. Otolaryngol Head Neck Surg 1984;92: 100–101.
8 James D, Crockard HA: Surgical access to the base of skull and upper cervical spine by extended maxillotomy. Neurosurgery 1991;29:411–416.
9 Crockard HA, Sen CN: The transoral approach for the management of intradural lesions at the craniovertebral junction: review of 7 cases. Neurosurgery 1991;28:88–97, discussion 98.
10 George B, Lot G, Velut S, Gelbert F, Mourier KL: French language Society of Neurosurgery. 44th Annual Congress, Brussels, 1993. Tumors of the foramen magnum. Neurochirurgie 1993;39(suppl 1): 1–89.
11 Couldwell WT, Weiss MH, Rabb C, Liu JK, Apfelbaum RI, Fukushima T: Variations on the standard transsphenoidal approach to the sellar region, with emphasis on the extended approaches and parasellar approaches: surgical experience in 105 cases. Neurosurgery 2004;55:539–547, discussion 47–50.
12 Dusick JR, Esposito F, Kelly DF, et al: The extended direct endonasal transsphenoidal approach for nonadenomatous suprasellar tumors. J Neurosurg 2005; 102:832–841.
13 de Divitiis E, Cappabianca P, Cavallo LM: Endoscopic transsphenoidal approach: adaptability of the procedure to different sellar lesions. Neurosurgery 2002;51:699–705, discussion 707.
14 Di Rocco F, Oi S, Samii A, et al: Neuronavigational endoscopic endonasal sellar and parasellar surgery using a 2-mm-diameter lens rigid-rod endoscope: a cadaver study. Neurosurgery 2007;60(4 suppl 2): 394–400.
15 Gong J, Mohr G, Vezina JL: Endoscopic pituitary surgery with and without image guidance: an experimental comparison. Surg Neurol 2007;67:572–578.
16 Jho HD: Endoscopic transsphenoidal surgery. J Neurooncol 2001;54:187–195.
17 Solares CA, Fakhri S, Batra PS, Lee J, Lanza DC: Transnasal endoscopic resection of lesions of the clivus: a preliminary report. Laryngoscope 2005;115: 1917–1922.
18 Cappabianca P, Frank G, Pasquini E, de Divitiis O, Calbucci F: Extended endoscopic endonasal transsphenoidal approaches to the suprasellar region, planum sphenoidale and clivus; in de Divitiis E, Cappabianca P (eds): Endoscopic Endonasal Transsphenoidal Surgery. Wien, Springer, 2003, pp 176–187.
19 Kingdom TT, Delgaudio JM: Endoscopic approach to lesions of the sphenoid sinus, orbital apex, and clivus. Am J Otolaryngol 2003;24:317–322.
20 Frank G, Sciarretta V, Calbucci F, Farneti G, Mazzatenta D, Pasquini E: The endoscopic transnasal transsphenoidal approach for the treatment of cranial base chordomas and chondrosarcomas. Neurosurgery 2006;59(1 suppl 1):ONS50–57.
21 Dehdashti AR, Karabatsou K, Ganna A, Witterick I, Gentili F: Expanded endoscopic endonasal approach for treatment of clival chordomas: early results in 12 patients. Neurosurgery 2008;63:299–307, discussion 309.
22 Stippler M, Gardner PA, Snyderman CH, Carrau RL, Prevedello DM, Kassam AB: Endoscopic endonasal approach for clival chordomas. Neurosurgery 2009;64:268–277, discussion 277–278.
23 Kelley TF, Stankiewicz JA, Chow JM, Origitano TC: Endoscopic transsphenoidal biopsy of the sphenoid and clival mass. Am J Rhinol 1999;13:17–21.
24 Stamm AC, Pignatari SS, Vellutini E: Transnasal endoscopic surgical approaches to the clivus. Otolaryngol Clin North Am 2006;39:639–656, xi.
25 Fortes FS, Carrau RL, Snyderman CH, et al: The posterior pedicle inferior turbinate flap: a new vascularized flap for skull base reconstruction. Laryngoscope 2007;117:1329–1332.

Amir R. Dehdashti, MD
Department of Neurosurgery
Geisinger Neurosciences Institute
100 North Academy Avenue, Danville, PA 17822 (USA)
Tel. +1 570 214 1722, E-Mail ardehdashti@geisinger.edu

Kassam AB, Gardner PA (eds): Endoscopic Approaches to the Skull Base.
Prog Neurol Surg. Basel, Karger, 2012, vol 26, pp 152–167

Endoscopic Endonasal Approach to the Odontoid and Craniocervical Junction

Paul A. Gardner[a] · Matthew J. Tormenti[a] · Amin B. Kassam[b] · Richard M. Spiro[a] · Daniel M. Prevedello[c] · Ricardo L. Carrau[d] · Carl H. Snyderman[a,e]

[a]Department of Neurological Surgery, University of Pittsburgh, Pittsburgh, Pa., USA; [b]Department of Neurological Surgery, University of Ottawa, Ottawa, Ont., Canada; Departments of [c]Neurological Surgery and [d]Otolaryngology, Ohio State University, Columbus, Ohio, and [e]Department of Otolaryngology, University of Pittsburgh, Pittsburgh, Pa., USA

Abstract

Background: Endoscopic endonasal approaches (EEAs) have been applied for skull base pathologies from the christa galli to the clivus. This approach also provides a natural corridor to the craniocervical junction and odontoid process. **Objectives:** To evaluate the surgical techniques, challenges, advantages and limitations of EEA for craniocervical pathologies. **Methods:** We present the endoscopic endonasal surgical technique for accessing the odontoid process and craniocervical junction. We present the advantages such as avoidance of oral mucosal transgression with its associated increased infection risk and potential swallowing delay and worsening. The caudal limits are discussed as well as methods for predicting them radiographically with the nasopalatal line. Finally, outcomes are presented to further examine the advantages and disadvantages of the transnasal approach. **Conclusions:** The ventral craniocervical junction and odontoid process can be addressed safely and effectively via EEA, without the attendant swallowing issues created by transoral approaches.

Ventral pathology of the craniocervical junction and upper cervical spine is difficult to access due to the surrounding facial structures and skull. The transoral approach has been the standard route employed for such pathology [1–8]. However, there are several potential morbidities with this approach. Transgressing oropharyngeal mucosa introduces oropharyngeal bacteria into the surgical field and often delays initiation of oral intake postoperatively. Rostral pathology, such as odontoid compression associated with basilar invagination, requires a palatal split, whereas a limited jaw opening may require a mandibular split [9], both of which add morbidity and discomfort for the patient. In addition, palatal insufficiency can occur following a transoral-transpalatal approach [10]. In high-risk cases or cases with limited oral access, a tracheostomy may need to be performed in the event of upper airway swelling and obstruction [8, 11]. Finally, surgical tools and retractors may injure the tongue or teeth.

Evolution of Technique

The addition of the endoscope to the trans-sphenoidal approach [12] together with the collaboration between otolaryngologists and neurosurgeons allowed for its expansion to other areas of the skull base [13, 14]. Extension of these approaches caudally to access the odontoid was a natural and relatively simple modification of these techniques [15, 16]. Since the initial report of this approach [16] it has been gaining popularity [17–22].

Advantages and Disadvantages

There are several advantages to approaching the odontoid process through an endonasal route. The confinement of the incision to the nasopharynx spares exposure to the oropharynx and the oropharyngeal flora which are greater in number and virulence than those in the nasopharynx [23]. Patients can resume oral intake immediately after surgery, increasing their comfort without risk of palatal or pharyngeal dehiscence, dysphagia, and nasal regurgitation. In our early series, the only patients who required a tracheostomy were those with pre-existing dysphagia and aspiration [20].

The endoscopic endonasal approach (EEA) also provides natural access to rostral pathology. There is commonly a degree of basilar invagination associated with craniocervical pathology that makes transoral access to the point of maximal compression challenging. The endonasal approach has no such rostral limitation.

Limitations of the EEA to the odontoid include caudal access and the learning curve associated with endoscopic techniques. Pathology extending below the odontoid process, into the body of the axis (C2) can be inaccessible except in the setting of basilar invagination. Thus far, we have not encountered any case of degenerative craniocervical (atlanto-occipital or atlantoaxial) disease that we have not been able to access endonasally. When using an endoscope (2D) instead of a microscope (3D) for visualization, there is a loss of depth perception. This has not proven to be a major obstacle. Initially the EEA may require longer surgical times but this diminishes with experience and is balanced by the previously mentioned advantages.

Indications and Contraindications

The EEA to the odontoid process and craniocervical junction can be applied to a myriad of ventral pathologies. As with any midline approach, it is best for lesions with a midline or paramedian origin that displace neurovascular structures laterally. We have used the approach largely to decompress cervicomedullary stenosis associated with osteo- and rheumatoid arthritis. However, it has also been applied to intradural meningiomas, bony tumors and metastasis at the craniocervical junction.

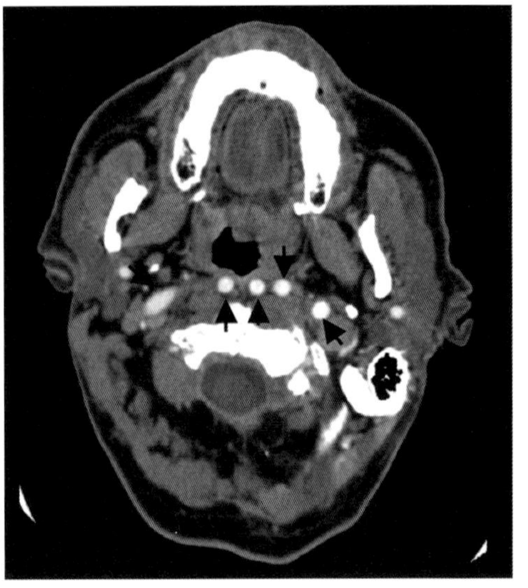

Fig. 1. Axial CT angiogram showing looping, ectatic parapharyngeal internal carotid arteries (ICAs) (arrows) blocking direct access to the odontoid.

It is also a useful approach in pediatric patients. We have used it successfully in the setting of cervicomedullary compression associated with congenital craniocervical abnormalities and basilar invagination. Indeed, given the smaller oral cavities and often limited mouth opening in children the EEA may provide improved visualization and access.

There are few contraindications to an EEA. Active sinus infection, diagnosed by an otolaryngologist, is an absolute contraindication and needs to be fully treated prior to an endonasal surgery where there may be risk of dural compromise. An inadvertent dural breach can lead to severe meningitis in this situation. Treatment of the infection usually delays surgery by only one or two weeks. Pathology with a posterior or posterolateral origin is best treated with a direct posterior approach, especially if a fusion is required. Some patients have very ectatic parapharyngeal internal carotid arteries that can be displaced into the nasopharynx (fig. 1), but as long as this is recognized, it is only a relative contraindication and can be managed by incising the basopharyngeal tissue above the artery and retracting it to access behind it. Other limitations include the hypoglossal nerves posterolaterally and the vertebral arteries and lower cranial nerves intradurally.

We strongly believe that EEAs are best performed by two surgeons, an otolaryngologist and a neurosurgeon, operating together. Most otolaryngologists are very comfortable with sinus endoscopy and can help the neurosurgeon to navigate the anatomy. The EEA to the odontoid is a very deep approach and having an active endoscopist during the entire surgery is important. This helps to maintain visualization, provides the ability to obtain close-up views and assists with the instrumentation. Finally, as with the transoral approach, otolaryngologists are much more experienced and comfortable with the postoperative care and healing of pharyngeal mucosa.

Preoperative Assessment and Evaluation

Physical Examination

Patients with ventral pathology necessitating decompression typically have significant myelopathy. In addition, because of the level of compression, patients usually have some degree of dysphagia, something that should be evaluated preoperatively as it can affect the perioperative course. If there is vocal fold paresis or paralysis, regardless of approach, consideration should be given to a prophylactic tracheostomy. In our experience this condition will only worsen at least transiently with transoral intubation. Again, this is a strong argument for a team approach as the otolaryngologist is more versed in management of the swallowing deficits and the airway. Full neck range of motion should also be assessed preoperatively to determine any restrictions or evidence of instability that may limit surgical positioning.

Radiological Studies

Diseases in and around the odontoid inevitably have bony, neural and vascular associations. Therefore, each condition needs to be evaluated with appropriate imaging. Fine cut CT angiography with sagittal and coronal reconstructions provides bony and vascular imaging while MRI with fine cut T_2 and T_1 postcontrast axial sequences will show neural involvement and degree of pannus formation.

The CT angiogram should be carefully studied to assess the degree of bony involvement, adequacy of surgical access and the course of the ICA (internal carotid artery) in the nasopharynx. In children or patients with congenital anomalies, it is critical to understand the bony anatomy and abnormalities to ensure adequate decompression. In the setting of basilar invagination, the inferior clivus may need to be removed to allow adequate rostral access to the invaginated dens. A midsagittal reconstruction will demonstrate this relationship. It will also allow for a preoperative evaluation of degree of caudal access. The nasopalatine line is a line drawn from the tip of the bony nasal bridge to the posterior hard palate and then extended to the dens and beyond (fig. 2). This gives a simple approximation of the point of maximal caudal access, but does not take into account soft tissue constraints.

If available, intra-operative imaging can be useful to assess the adequacy of decompression and resection. We have an operating suite equipped with a CT scanner, which is ideal for this purpose. Alternatively, intra-operative MRI or AP and lateral upper cervical spine radiographs with instillation of radio-opaque dye into the defect can help to confirm the adequacy decompression.

Patient Education

The patients should be educated perioperatively about the healing process, especially in the setting of dural opening, whether intentional or unintentional. If there are CSF (cerebrospinal fluid) leak concerns, the patient should avoid lifting, bending and straining during the postoperative period. If a vascularized nasal mucosal flap is used

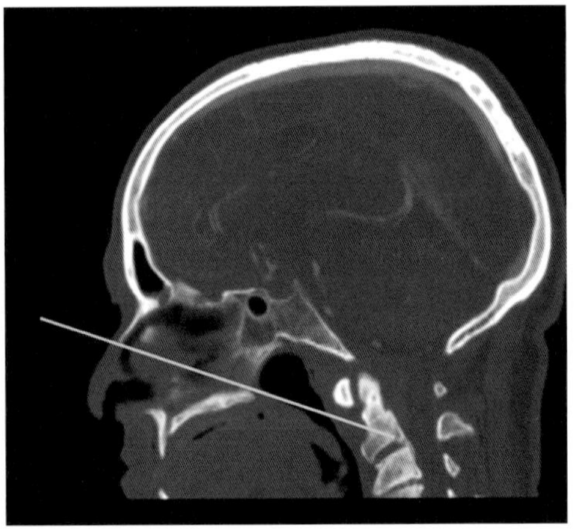

Fig. 2. Midsagittal CT with the nasopalatine line illustrated. This line predicts the caudal extent of endoscopic endonasal access.

for reconstruction, complete healing takes 3–4 weeks. If there is no graft, remucosalization of the defect typically takes 6–8 weeks. Monitoring of the healing and cleaning of the associated crusting can be performed endoscopically in the outpatient setting.

Preoperative Planning

Surgical Approach

When planning an endonasal approach to the odontoid, it is important to ensure that the caudal access will be adequate. As mentioned above, a midsagittal view on a CT that includes the nose and palate can be used to draw the nasopalatine line to the odontoid. This predicts the caudal extent of resection [22]. The actual access typically ends up several millimeters higher than this. Cases in which the nasopalatine line suggests inadequate access should be considered for a transoral, transcervical or posterolateral approach.

Equipment and Instrumention

We perform all endoscopic endonasal cases with intra-operative image guidance. We usually resort to a 'fusion' study where CT angiography and MR imaging are fused by the image guidance system to allow varying levels of bony, soft and neural tissue imaging, the needs for which change throughout the case. Care must be taken to ensure that the patient is in a position during imaging that is similar to that of surgery, as flexion, extension and rotation of the head can all change the accuracy of a cranially registered image guidance system when working in the upper spine.

Rod lens endoscopes (4 mm, Storz Endoscopy, Tuttingen, Germany) are used for all cases. The majority of all endoscopic endonasal cases are performed with a zero-degree endoscope. There are rare situations during an odontoid approach in which an angled endoscope is helpful. Enhanced lateral and perhaps superior and inferior visualization provided by the angled scopes can be helpful to ensure an adequate decompression or to localize critical neurovascular structures.

Traditional sinus instrumentation can be used for much of this approach, including pituitary and ethmoid rongeurs, Cottle periosteal dissectors, suction Bovie electrocautery and through-cutting instruments. However, for the deeper and more delicate dissections, special instrumentation has been developed, including extendable dissectors, fine rongeurs, pistol-grip microscissors and bipolar electrocautery with various blades (Storz Endoscopy, Tuttingen, Germany). Finally, for bony decompression, we use a specially-designed, extended high-speed electric drill with a hybrid, diamond/cutting bit with an extendable tip or a extended, curved tip for improved caudal access (Stryker TPS, Kalamazoo, Michigan) and traditional Kerrison rongeurs.

Hemostatic agents such as morselized gel foam products are delivered via a suction tip with the hole blocked attached to a syringe. Finally, for dural reconstruction or repair, we occasionally use the U-Clip anastomotic device (Medtronic, Inc.). This is a nitinol loop with autocoiling properties, which is triggered upon release from its needle thereby allowing suturing without tying.

Operating Room Set-Up

We perform all cases with both surgeons standing on the patient's right side. The patient is supine with the anesthesia staff and equipment on their left and the scrub nurse standing toward the patient's feet, to the right of the surgeon(s). Either an endoscopic monitor tower or screens on booms from the ceiling are used. Operating rooms with more than one endoscopic monitor screen are preferable, as the screens can be set up at 45–90° angles to one another, one across from each member of the surgical team, to allow a more ergonomic position and allow the surgeon to stand in a neutral, comfortable position. Screens should typically be placed slightly lower than the surgeon's shoulder height as this seems to be the most ergonomic position for long cases, creating less neck and shoulder strain and pain. The image guidance system is set up at the patient's head.

Surgical Technique

Patients are positioned supine on the operating table in a neutral or slightly flexed position. Care should be taken to not overly flex or extend the head of patients who already have neural compression. This can be constantly monitored with somatosensory evoked potentials (SSEPs) during positioning. Slight rotation of the head toward the surgeon improves his or her comfort. Position changes, which may affect the relationship of the head to the cervical spine must be taken into account as they may affect the accuracy of image guidance.

The endoscope is introduced into the right nostril and paranasal sinus structures are identified. The middle and inferior turbinates, choana, nasopharynx and

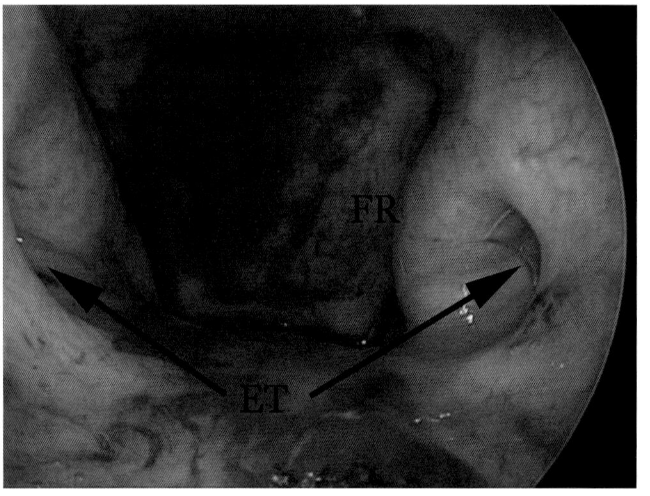

Fig. 3. Initial endoscopic view of the nasopharynx with important landmarks notated. ET = Eustachian tube; FR = fossa of Rosenmuller.

eustachian tubes are all important initial landmarks (fig. 3). The inferior turbinates may be lateralized to allow maximal access. A small portion of the posterior, inferior nasal septum may need to be removed to allow the introduction of instruments from the contralateral nostril without obscuring the endoscopic view when this portion of the septum is displaced over. However, this is often unnecessary and some difficulty with this part should be tolerated as the approach rapidly deepens and this problem becomes insignificant.

The eustachian tubes (ETs) and fossae of Rosenmuller mark the lateral borders of a standard endonasal approach to the odontoid (fig. 3). The ICAs are usually lateral to the ETs and therefore protected if the mucosal work is all done between the ETs. It is important, however, to evaluate the position of the parapharyngeal ICAs preoperatively to avoid inadvertent injury (fig. 1). Image guidance can be used to identify the approximate location of relevant bony structures such as the basion, anterior arch of C1 and body of C2 relative to the superficial pharyngeal structures. Confirmation of caudal access can be assessed at this point. Monopolar electrocautery can be used safely in the midline to remove the nasopharyngeal mucosa and detach the dense basopharyngeal fascia, anterior longitudinal ligament or longus capittis and rectus capittis anterior muscles from the clivus, ring of C1 and body of C2 as necessary. As with any anterior cervical approach, care should be taken laterally to avoid injury to the ICAs. There is no need to create a fascial or mucosal flap. The area will remucosalize on its own within 6–8 weeks.

Once the anterior ring of C1 has been dissected, it can be removed with a high-speed extended drill (fig. 4). As with every endonasal approach, each step of the exposure must be completed to its widest safe extent. Caudal and lateral dissection of mucosa and fascia should be more than anticipated and the same applies to bony resection. The endoscopic magnification combined with the hesitation of inexperience often

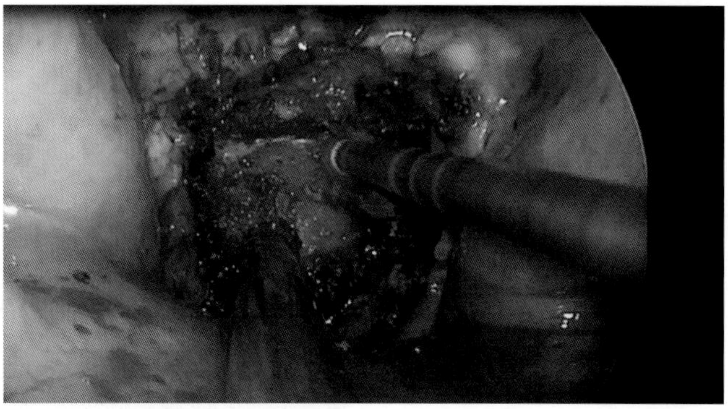

Fig. 4. High speed drill being used to remove the anterior ring of C1 via EEA.

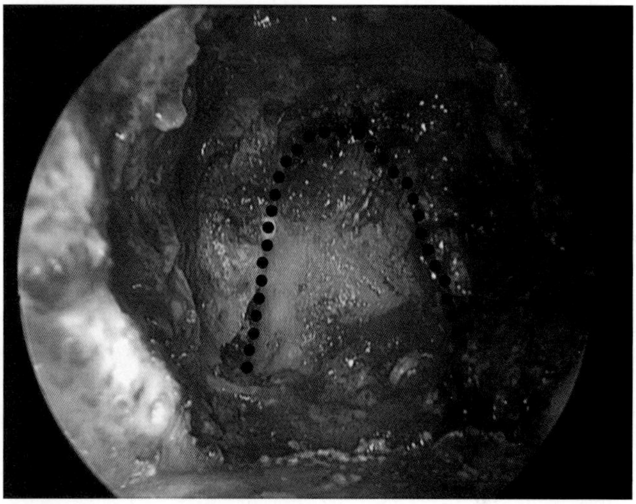

Fig. 5. Endoscopic view following wide removal of the anterior ring of C1. The dens is well visualized prior to removal (dotted line).

leads the surgeon to resect less than is necessary. There is also a natural tendency to 'cone' down with each successive step, leading to a small decompression in the depth. Image guidance is helpful to ensure the adequacy of the initial exposure, the complete exposure of each bony target and its adequate removal. Caudal exposure can be improved by reducing the bony maxillary crest (attachment of the nasal septum) to the level of the hard palate. The anterior ring of C1 should be resected until the curve toward the lateral mass is evident and the entire dens is exposed (fig. 5). Often, in the setting of degenerative disease, there is significant pannus between C1 and the odontoid process. This can be resected with through-cutting sinus instruments, Kerrison rongeurs or even an ultrasonic aspirator.

Once the odontoid process is exposed (fig. 5), it can be carefully removed with a high speed drill. Care should be taken not to remove the 'neck' of the dens, thereby disconnecting the tip of the odontoid from the body of C2. The ligamentous attachments at the apex are very difficult to dissect if the dens is free-floating. The bone can

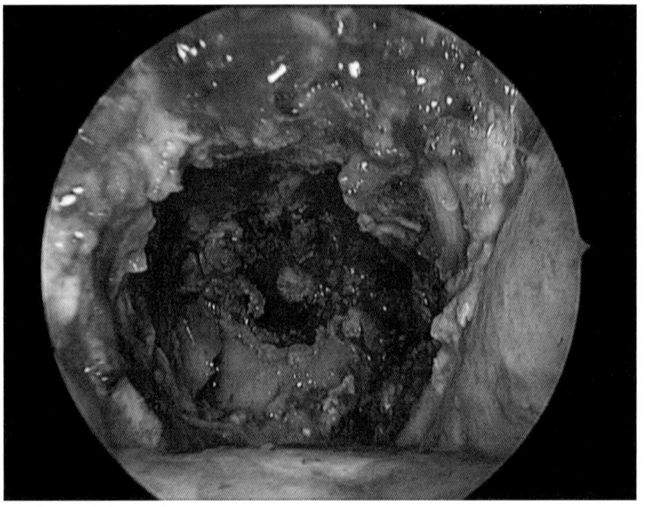

Fig. 6. Endoscopic view following removal of the tip of the odontoid process up to the ligamentous attachments and tectorial membrane.

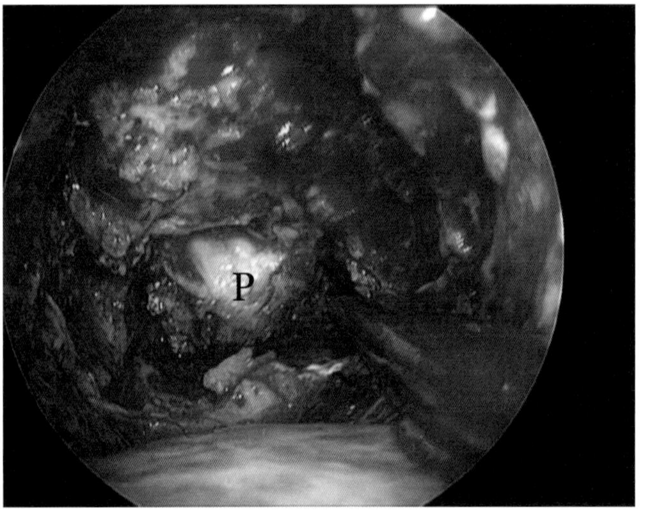

Fig. 7. Endoscopic view showing pannus (P) involving the tectorial membrane.

be drilled down to the ligament, taking care to avoid durotomy (fig. 6). In degenerative cases, there can be significant pannus between the dens and the tectorial membrane, even replacing the membrane in some cases (fig. 7). Again, this can be removed using rongeurs. If there is only bony compression or if there is significant pannus resected and the tectorial membrane is normal or transmits dural pulsations, it is adequate to leave the membrane intact and not risk a durotomy (fig. 8). However, if there is any question, resecting the tectorial membrane to ensure dural decompression is required.

After the intial dissection, odontoid and pannus resection via an EEA is no different than via a transoral approach, it may just require slightly different instruments and entails a different trajectory. A retractor is not used, so resection of the overlying

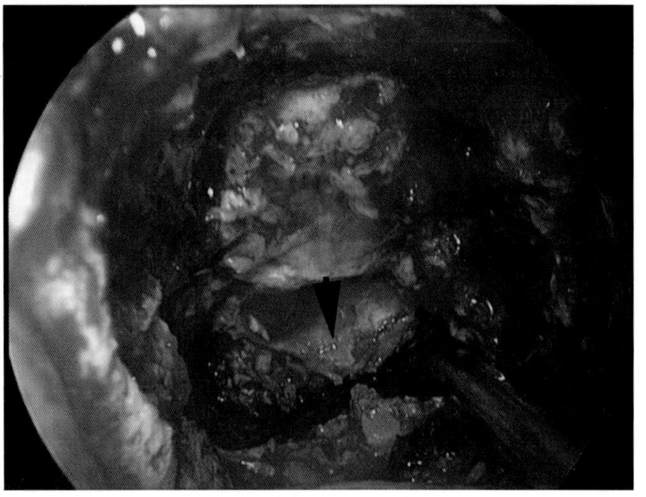

Fig. 8. Endoscopic view of the tectorial membrane (arrowhead) following decompression.

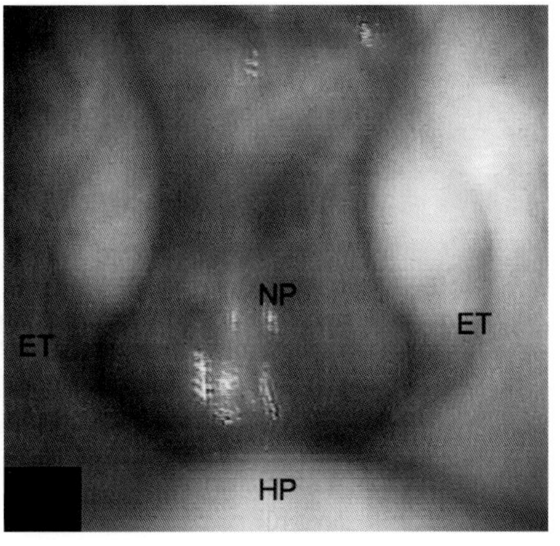

Fig. 9. Endoscopic view of the healed nasopharynx during office postoperative examination. No reconstruction was performed, the healing is a result of normal remucosalization. NP = Nasopharynx; ET = eustacian tube; HP = hard palate.

mucosa and fascia is required. The suction tip can provide some retraction during drilling. Extended suction tips and drills are critical due to the depth of the surgical field.

Reconstruction of the odontoid defect is simple if there is no dural defect. Fibrin glue may help the healing process and remucosalization (fig. 9). Conversely, a dural defect in this area may be difficult to repair. A pedicled septal mucosal flap often does not reach the depth of the defect. An inferior turbinate flap [24] may provide the best vascularized coverage for this area but is difficult to raise. Use of an abdominal fat graft alone or to fill the defect prior to flap placement is a good option given the depth and shape of the defect. The risk of postoperative CSF leak is higher when non-vascularized repair is used (i.e. fat packing alone) [25, 26]. Silastic splints should be sewn to the septum and left in place for 2–3 weeks to prevent synechiae.

Craniocervical Fixation

Most patients with degenerative craniocervical disease are in need of posterior fixation regardless of anterior decompression, as their disease results from instability. Indeed, many patients do not require an anterior decompression, merely a posterior fixation with or without posterior decompression. In those patients who do require anterior decompression (due to irreducible bony compression, severe neural compromise or failed posterior decompression), we typically perform the EEA decompression first. This may add a degree of safety during manipulation or reduction as a part of instrumentation and also may help determine if any additional posterior decompression is needed, or if bony structures can be left in place to aid with fusion. The fixation can be done in the same day if time allows or staged into the following day with the patient placed into a halo in between.

In carefully selected intradural cases, preservation of the atlantoaxial ligamentous complex and occipital condyle joint should allow preservation of stability, something with which we have had success. This should, however, be taken into account when choosing approach, especially for more caudally extending tumors.

Postoperative Care

Postoperative care following an EEA, like the surgery itself, is best done with close collaboration between a neurosurgeon and an otolaryngologist. During the immediate postoperative period, saline nasal sprays keep the mucosa moist during healing. In addition, long-lasting oxymetazoline sprays can be used to relieve nasal congestion during the first week. Nasal instrumentation (nasogastric tubes, etc.) must be avoided unless placed under endoscopic view. If there is a dural breach, positive pressure mask ventilation (CPAP/BiPAP) should be avoided, as this could lead to tension pneumocephalus. Similarly, incentive spirometry, drinking straws and nose-blowing should be avoided.

The silastic nasal septal splints can be removed after 2–3 weeks. Gentle debridement of the surgical site under endoscopic visualization should be performed at 2 weeks and then approximately 6 weeks postoperatively. The surgeon can also inspect for CSF leak and proper healing at this time (fig. 9).

Complications and Outcomes

24 EEAs for disease in and around the odontoid process were performed at our institution between May 2004 and October 2008. The majority of these (19) were for irreducible compression related to degenerative (osteo- or rheumatoid) arthritis. The average

Table 1. Complications and outcomes following EEA for odontoid-related disease

Patient no.	Pathological diagnosis	Gender	Age	Fusion	Complication	Disposition
1	Arthritic pannus	F	73	yes	respiratory failure	SNF
2	Clival meningioma	F	47	no*	none	home
3	Arthritic pannus	M	62	yes	PNA, respiratory failure	home
4	Arthritic pannus	F	77	yes	none	rehab
5	Arthritic pannus	F	74	yes	none	rehab
6	Arthritic pannus	F	96	no	death	death
7	Arthritic pannus	F	74	yes	none	SNF
8	Arthritic pannus	F	69	yes	none	home
9	Chondrosarcoma	F	59	previous	none	home
10	Breast Ca metastasis	F	50	yes	none	rehab
11	Arthritic pannus	M	77	yes	PNA	rehab
12	Arthritic pannus	M	79	yes**	none	rehab
13	Arthritic pannus	M	74	yes**	PNA	rehab
14	Arthritic pannus	M	87	yes	none	rehab
15	Arthritic pannus	F	57	yes	none	rehab
16	Arthritic pannus	M	84	yes	DVT	rehab
17	Arthritic pannus	M	85	yes	none	rehab
18	Arthritic pannus	M	76	yes	durotomy	rehab
19	Arthritic pannus	F	60	yes	none	rehab
20	Arthritic pannus	M	53	yes	none	home
21	Congenital – basilar invagination	M	11	yes	durotomy	rehab
22	Congenital – basilar invagination	F	11	yes	pulmonary edema	home
23	Arthritic pannus	M	75	yes	PNA	home
24	Arthritic pannus	F	71	yes	none	rehab

SNF = Skilled nursing facility. * Limited ligamentous resection – patient symptom-free and stable based on dynamic radiographs. ** Previous fusion redone after EEA.

patient age was 68 (11–96) and there were 13 women and 11 men. Complications and outcomes are listed below (table 1). There were no neurologic complications and no patient worsened with surgery. Two intraoperative durotomies were repaired with fat graft without sequelae. Both were treated with postoperative lumbar drainage.

There was one death. This occurred in a 96-year-old woman who underwent an anterior decompression with planned fusion in the future. She had no intraoperative complication and recovered well. Unfortunately, she died unexpectedly 11 days postoperatively from unknown causes. No patient required tracheostomy for surgery, but 3 required tracheotomy for respiratory failure in the setting of pneumonia. No patient had worsened dysphagia and there was no permanent palatal insufficiency.

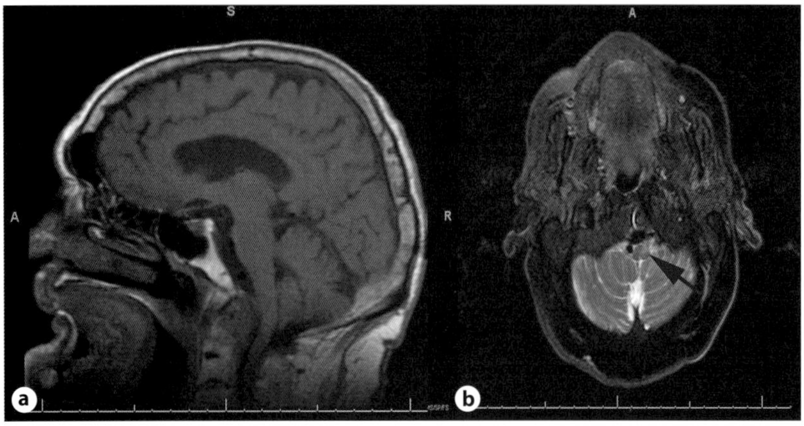

Fig. 10. Preoperative sagittal (**a**) and axial (**b**) MRI showing cervicomedullary compression due to an atlantoaxial synovial cyst. There is T_2 signal change in the left medulla seen on the axial MRI (arrow).

Results – Case Studies

Case 1

A 75-year-old man presents with significant progressive difficulty with gait. He also admits to some difficulties with dysphagia which have worsened to the point that he has limited himself to a pureed diet. Physical examination reveals hyperreflexia, Hoffman's and Babinski's signs and gait instability. He has atrophy of the intrinsic muscles of the hands. His gag is decreased.

The patient was referred to a swallowing expert who performed laryngoscopy which did not show any vocal cord dysfunction. Preoperative MRI shows cervical spondylosis with the greatest compression created by a synovial cyst at the C1–2 joint (fig. 10). He had limited range of motion in his neck. The patient underwent an EEA for odontoid resection followed by posterior cervical decompression and fixation. The patient did well postoperatively but developed a fever and was diagnosed with aspiration pneumonia, successfully treated with antibiotics. His swallowing has subjectively improved at his last postoperative vision and his gait and upper extremity strength have improved (fig. 11).

Case 2

An 11-year-old girl presents with progressive scoliosis. MRI and CT showed syringomyelia associated with platybasia, significant basilar invagination and a Chiari I malformation (fig. 12). Flexion-extension radiographs showed no movement at the craniocervical junction. Attempts at reduction were unsuccessful. The patient underwent an EEA for resection of the lower clivus and dens followed by a posterior suboccipital craniectomy and C1 laminectomy with occipitocervical fusion. She remained

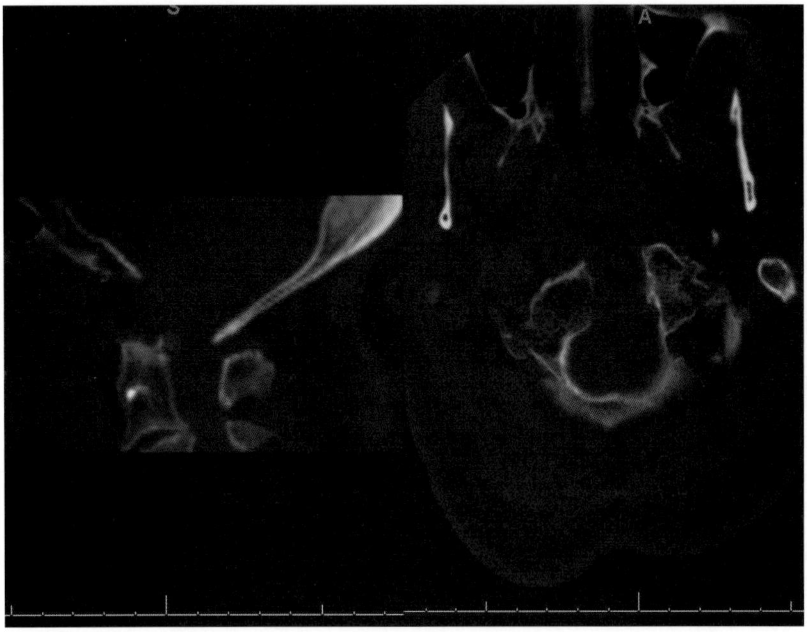

Fig. 11. Postoperative sagittal reconstruction and axial CT showing craniocervical junction decompression.

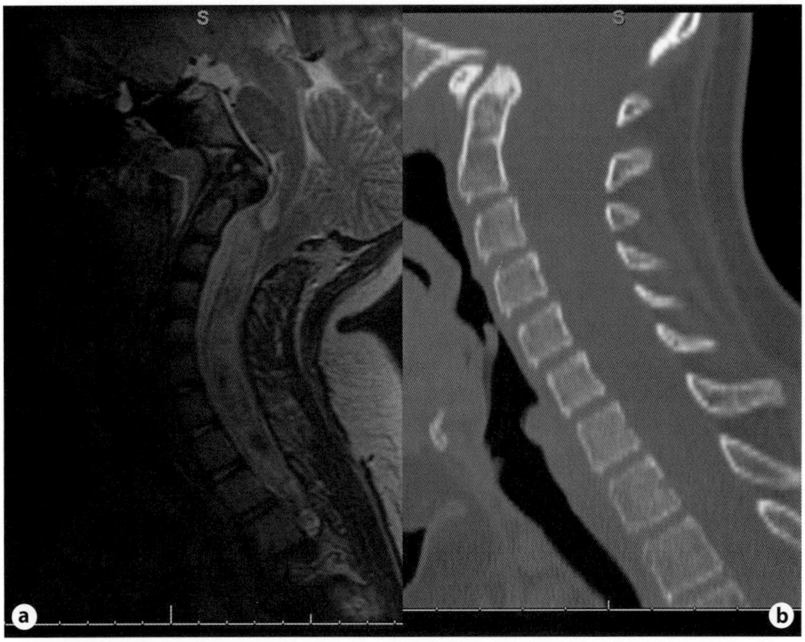

Fig. 12. Preoperative midsagittal T_2-weighted MRI (**a**) and CT reconstruction (**b**) showing severe basilar invagination, platybasia, Chiari malformation and syringomyelia.

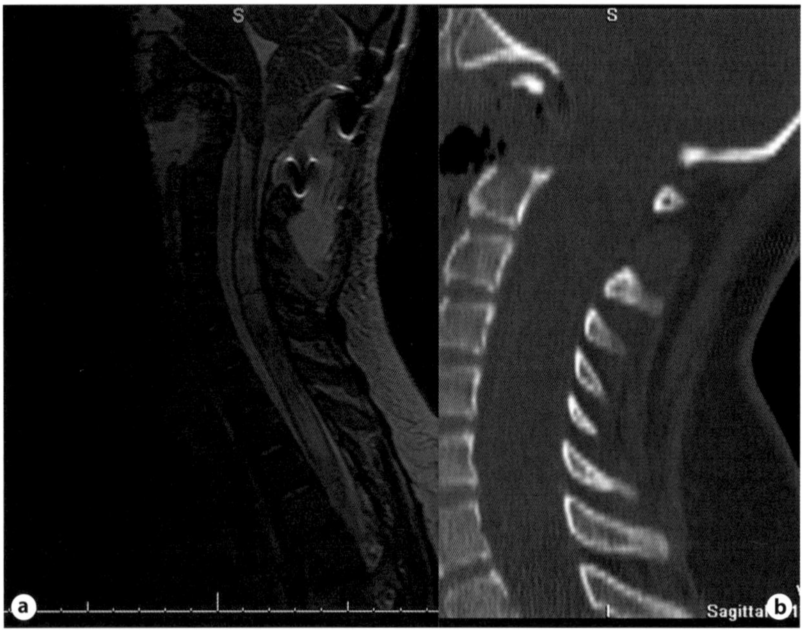

Fig. 13. Postoperative midsagittal T_2-weighted MRI (**a**) and CT reconstruction (**b**) showing good decompression of the craniocervical junction and improvement in syrinx.

intubated for one day due to pulmonary edema but otherwise had an uncomplicated postoperative course. Postoperative imaging reveals a good decompression of the craniocervical junction (fig. 13) and the patient has improved clinically.

Conclusions

The EEA to the odontoid can provide good results with good decompression or resection and low complication rates. It is limited caudally by the fulcrum of the hard palate and the nasal bridge/nostril. It is limited laterally in the soft tissue by the parapharyngeal ICAs, in the bone by the hypoglossal nerves and intradurally by the vertebral arteries and lower cranial nerves. This approach has advantages over the transoral approach in that it avoids an oral mucosal incision and the attendent problems associated with that.

References

1 Crockard HA: The transoral approach to the base of the brain and upper cervical cord. Ann R Coll Surg Engl 1985;67:321–325.
2 Crockard HA, et al: Transoral decompression and posterior fusion for rheumatoid atlanto-axial subluxation. J Bone Joint Surg Br 1986;68:350–356.
3 Greenberg AD, Scoville WB, Davey LM: Transoral decompression of atlanto-axial dislocation due to odontoid hypoplasia: report of two cases. J Neurosurg 1968;28:266–269.
4 Donald PJ, Bernstein L: Transpalatal excision of the odontoid process. Otolaryngology 1978;86:ORL-729–731.
5 Apuzzo ML, Weiss MH, Heiden JS: Transoral exposure of the atlantoaxial region. Neurosurgery 1978;3:201–207.
6 Menezes AH, VanGilder JC: Transoral-transpharyngeal approach to the anterior craniocervical junction: ten-year experience with 72 patients. J Neurosurg 1988;69:895–903.
7 Yang SY, Gao YZ: Clinical results of the transoral operation for lesions of the craniovertebral junction and its abnormalities. Surg Neurol 1999;51:16–20.
8 Menezes AH: Surgical approaches: postoperative care and complications 'transoral-transpalatopharyngeal approach to the craniocervical junction'. Childs Nerv Syst 2008;24:1187–1193.
9 Vishteh AG, et al: Bilateral sagittal split mandibular osteotomies as an adjunct to the transoral approach to the anterior craniovertebral junction (technical note). J Neurosurg 1999;90(2 suppl):267–270.
10 Cantarella G, Mazzola RF, Benincasa A: A possible sequela of transoral approach to the upper cervical spine. velopharyngeal incompetence. J Neurosurg Sci 1998;42:51–55.
11 Landeiro JA, et al: Transoral approach to the craniovertebral junction. Arq Neuropsiquiatr 2007;65:1166–1171.
12 Jho HD, Carrau RL: Endoscopy assisted transsphenoidal surgery for pituitary adenoma (technical note). Acta Neurochir (Wien) 1996;138:1416–1425.
13 Kassam A, et al: Expanded endonasal approach: the rostrocaudal axis. I. Crista galli to the sella turcica. Neurosurg Focus 2005;19:E3.
14 Kassam A, et al: Expanded endonasal approach: the rostrocaudal axis. II. Posterior clinoids to the foramen magnum. Neurosurg Focus 2005;19:E4.
15 Alfieri A, Jho HD, Tschabitscher M: Endoscopic endonasal approach to the ventral cranio-cervical junction: anatomical study. Acta Neurochir (Wien) 2002;144:219–225; discussion 225.
16 Kassam AB, et al: The expanded endonasal approach: a fully endoscopic transnasal approach and resection of the odontoid process: technical case report. Neurosurgery 2005;57(1 suppl):E213.
17 Laufer I, et al: Endonasal endoscopic resection of the odontoid process in a nonachondroplastic dwarf with juvenile rheumatoid arthritis: feasibility of the approach and utility of the intraoperative Iso-C three-dimensional navigation (case report). J Neurosurg Spine 2008;8:376–380.
18 Magrini S, et al: Endoscopic endonasal odontoidectomy in a patient affected by Down syndrome: technical case report. Neurosurgery 2008;63:E373–E374.
19 Messina A, et al: Pure endoscopic endonasal odontoidectomy: anatomical study. Neurosurg Rev 2007;30:189–194.
20 Nayak JV, et al: Experience with the expanded endonasal approach for resection of the odontoid process in rheumatoid disease. Am J Rhinol 2007;21:601–606.
21 Cavallo LM, et al: The extended endoscopic endonasal approach to the clivus and cranio-vertebral junction: anatomical study. Childs Nerv Syst 2007;23:665–671.
22 de Almeida JR, et al: Defining the nasopalatine line: the limit for endonasal surgery of the spine. Laryngoscope 2009;119:239–244.
23 Hull MW, Chow AW: Indigenous microflora and innate immunity of the head and neck. Infect Dis Clin North Am 2007;21:265–282, v.
24 Fortes FS, et al: The posterior pedicle inferior turbinate flap: a new vascularized flap for skull base reconstruction. Laryngoscope 2007;117:1329–1332.
25 Hadad G, et al: A novel reconstructive technique after endoscopic expanded endonasal approaches: vascular pedicle nasoseptal flap. Laryngoscope 2006;116:1882–1886.
26 Kassam AB, et al: Endoscopic reconstruction of the cranial base using a pedicled nasoseptal flap. Neurosurgery 2008;63(1 suppl 1):ONS44–S52, discussion ONS52–53.

Paul A. Gardner, MD
Department of Neurological Surgery, University of Pittsburgh School of Medicine
200 Lothrop Street, PUH, Suite B400
Pittsburgh, PA 15213–2582 (USA)
Tel. +1 412 647 3685, E-Mail gardpa@upmc.edu

Kassam AB, Gardner PA (eds): Endoscopic Approaches to the Skull Base.
Prog Neurol Surg. Basel, Karger, 2012, vol 26, pp 168–181

Endoscopic Reconstruction of Anterior Skull Base Defects

Adam M. Zanation[a] · Ricardo L. Carrau[b] · Carl H. Snyderman[c,d] · Amin B. Kassam[e] · Paul A. Gardner[d] · Daniel M. Prevedello[f] · Arlan H. Mintz[d]

[a]Department of Otolaryngology, Head and Neck Surgery, University of North Carolina, Chapel Hill, N.C., [b]Department of Otolaryngology, Head and Neck Surgery, The Ohio State University Medical Center, Columbus, Ohio, Departments of [c]Otolaryngology, Head and Neck Surgery and [d]Neurological Surgery, University of Pittsburgh Medical Center, Pittsburgh, Pa., [e]Department of Neurological Surgery, University of Ottawa, Ottawa, Ont., Canada; [f]Department of Neurological Surgery, The Ohio State University Medical Center, Columbus, Ohio, USA

Abstract

Over a 10-year interval, major advances in endoscopic technique as well as instrumentation to facilitate the endoscopic endonasal approach (EEA) to the skull base have been reported. The authors describe the evolution of and resulting methods for reconstruction of the skull base following EEA using multilayer, free tissue grafts to the more recent adoption of the vascularized nasoseptal flap. Other options such as the pedicled inferior turbinate flap and temporoparietal fascial flaps are also discussed. Technical aspects of flap harvest and application are discussed as well as risk factors for CSF leak. The high-risk CSF-leak patient is identified, and methods to reduce CSF leak to less than 5% are described.

Over the past 10 years, significant anatomic, technical and instrumentation advances have facilitated the exposure and resection of intradural lesions via a fully endoscopic expanded endonasal approach (EEA). In this report we describe our progressive experience with the reconstruction of the ensuing defects. This chapter describes our sequential learning from our initial free tissue grafting reconstructive techniques advancing to our current vascularized flaps. Outcomes and limitations of the current endoscopic reconstructive techniques are discussed.

The goals of reconstructing defects produced by the EEA are identical to those of reconstructing conventional external approaches, i.e. to completely separate the cranial cavity from the sinonasal tract, eliminate dead space, and preserve neurovascular structures and ocular function [1]. The underlying principle of multilayered reconstruction to re-establish tissue barriers is also the same as traditional open techniques. Using endonasal pedicled vascular flaps and a reconstruction based on the aforementioned principles, we have been able to reduce our postoperative CSF leak rates below 5%, which is comparable with that reported for open cranial base reconstructive techniques.

Endoscopic Reconstruction with Free Tissue Grafts

Prior to the adoption of the nasoseptal flap as our primary reconstructive technique (see below) skull base reconstruction after EEA was limited to the use of free tissue grafts. These techniques were adapted from the experience accumulated with the endoscopic repair of CSF leaks associated with endoscopic sinus surgery and trauma [2] and expanded to repair larger dural defects and defects over high-flow intraoperative CSF leaks. A multilayer approach with complete defect coverage is key to an endoscopic transdural reconstruction.

First, a subdural inlay graft (between the brain and the dura) of collagen matrix (Duragen, Integra Life Sciences) is placed; this helps to obliterate the intradural dead space. Its pliability and texture allows for its safe manipulation around neurovascular structures. This subdural graft should extend beyond the dural margins, ideally by 5–10 mm in all directions. A subsequent inlay graft of acellular dermis (Alloderm) or fascia is placed in the epidural space (between the dura and the skull base). Occasionally, the bony ledges are not adequate to support an inlay graft; therefore, the acellular dermal or fascia graft is placed extra-cranially (at the nasal side of the defect) as an onlay graft. All the edges of the defect should be denuded of mucosa to allow for the revascularization of the graft and to avoid mucocele formation. Alternatively, this graft can be sutured to the dura with nitinol U-clips (Medtronic U-Clips, Memphis, Tenn., USA). Although technically challenging, U-clips provide anchor points to prevent migration of the graft but does not result in a water tight suture line.

While this is an off-label indication for the acellular dermal graft, we found that its handling characteristics, its availability (no need for skin graft harvesting) and ingrowth of the patient's own tissue and rapid epithelialization are advantages that sometimes outweigh its cost. Facial grafts, however, have the advantages of being a homologous graft, being more resistant to infection and may promote faster healing. It is important to use a single graft with dimensions that will extend beyond the defect margins in all direction, and that the graft should be adequately hydrated in normal saline solution prior to its insertion. It is our experience that a thin thickness graft offers the best take although it is somewhat difficult to manipulate endonasally.

Once both grafts are in place, the edges of the Alloderm or fascial graft are bolstered intranasally with oxidized cellulose (absorbable packing), a biological or synthetic glue is sprayed or applied over the edges and absorbable gelatin sponge squares are used to further bolster the reconstruction. These layers of absorbable packing accomplish three goals. First, they fix the grafts in place and protect them from changes in airflow within the nose. Secondly, these layers allow for 'filling' of the concavities and convexities of the skull base to better distribute the pressure of the removable packing. Third, this absorbable packing protects the grafts from movement during removal of the non-absorbable packing 3–5 days postoperatively. We then use the balloon of a 12- Fr Foley catheter or 10-cm expandable sponge packing which will stabilize and bolster the inlay/onlay grafts, further preventing early brain herniation. Placement and inflation of the balloon catheter using 10ml of saline is performed under endoscopic vision. Over inflation may result in compression of intracranial structures. A Foley is avoided if the optic nerves or chiasm are exposed during the dissection as the balloon may exert too much pressure on these structures. Instead, expandable sponge packing is used. Any nasal packing or balloon is removed 3–5 days after the EEA.

For moderate skull base defects, we have also utilized an onlay free mucosal graft harvested from the resected middle turbinate instead of an Alloderm graft. The remainder of reconstructive procedure is as described above. The 'take' of the free mucosal grafts is excellent; however, they are limited by size and the fact that they can only be utilized as onlay grafts. Lastly, abdominal free fat is utilized mainly as a bolster or biologic dressing applied to the multilayered reconstruction. Fat is also utilized to obliterate spaces such as the clival recess or the nasopharyngeal defect after a transnasal approach to the anterior spine. It has the minor added morbidity of an abdominal incision, scar and the potential for infection, hematoma or seroma formation.

Endoscopic reconstruction with multilayered free tissue grafts resulted in postoperative CSF leak rates of 20–30%. All of these leaks were managed with further endoscopic bolstering or revision of the reconstruction and some with the addition of lumbar drainage CSF diversion for 3–5 days (see below for further details). What was clear during the endoscopic revisions was that most of CSF leaks were due to graft migration or CSF fistula formation in the most dependent area of the flap. Most of these leaks were managed with endoscopic revisions and only one of our first 400 EEA patients had to undergo an open reconstruction for a persistent CSF leak. This patient had undergone chemoradiotherapy for a sinonasal malignancy and the remaining blood supply to the nose was inadequate to sustain the take of the grafts. The overall incidence of meningitis in the first 400 EEAs was less than 3%, which is on par with the incidence associated with open skull base techniques. However, a CSF leak rate of 20–30% was too high and vascularized tissue options were sought to reduce this incidence.

Endoscopic Reconstruction with Vascular Pedicled Flaps

Nasoseptal Flap (Hadad-Bassagastegay Flap – HBF)

Over recent years, the use of a vascular pedicle flap has become our preferred skull base reconstruction. The most commonly used technique is a pedicled vascular flap of the nasal septum mucoperiosteum and mucoperichondrium based on the nasoseptal artery, a branch of the posterior septal artery, which is one of the terminal branches of the internal maxillary artery (Hadad-Bassagasteguy flap [HBF]) [3].

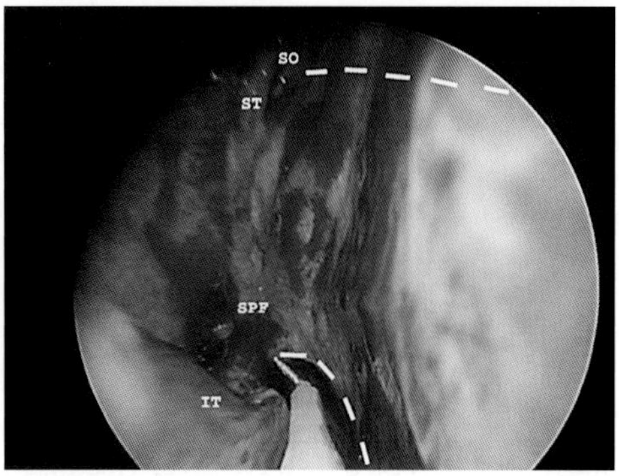

Fig. 1. Planned incisions around the pedicle of the nasoseptal flap. IT = Inferior turbinate; ST = superior turbinate; SO = sphenoid ostium; SPF = mucosa over the sphenopalatine foramen.

The nasal cavity is decongested with oxymetazoline 0.05% on pledgets and the nasal septum is infiltrated with lidocaine 0.5 to 1% with epinephrine 1/100,000 to 1/200,000. The inferior and middle turbinates are outfractured to allow visualization of the entire height of the nasal septum, from the olfactory sulcus to the nasal floor. To facilitate a bimanual technique during the EEA, we usually elect to remove one of the middle turbinates, usually on the right. In addition, resection of the middle turbinate facilitates the visualization of the ipsilateral HBF vascular pedicle and elevation of the flap. The side of the flap (right or left) is determined by several factors. First, if the lesion requires a lateral dissection of the lateral pterygoid recess or the pterygomaxillary fossa then the vascular supply of the flap may be compromised; thus, a flap on the opposite side is utilized. Similarly, lesions that invade the rostrum of the sphenoid or the septal mucoperiosteum will mandate harvesting of the contralateral side. If the lesion is in the midline and no significant lateral dissection is required, then sharp or large septal spurs (creating a risk for perforation of the flap during dissection) may dictate the side of the flap. Lastly, all things being equal, the right side is usually an easier dissection for the right handed surgeon, especially in the setting of removal of the right middle turbinate. The flap is designed according to the size and shape of the anticipated defect, although it is best to overestimate the size and then trim the flap if needed. Two parallel incisions are performed following the sagittal plane of the septum, one over the maxillary crest and the other 1–2 cm below the most superior aspect of the septum (this preserves the olfactory epithelium) (fig. 1, 2a, b) These incisions are joined anteriorly by a vertical incision at a level that is anterior to the anterior head of the inferior turbinate (fig. 2c). These incisions may be modified to account for the specific area of reconstruction or to allow adequate oncologic margins. At the posterior septum, the superior incision is extended laterally and with an inferior slant over the rostrum of the sphenoid sinus crossing it horizontally at the level of the natural ostium (fig. 1). The inferior incision is extended superiorly along the free posterior edge of the nasal septum and then laterally to cross the posterior choana below the floor of the sphenoid sinus. Its elevation starts anterior

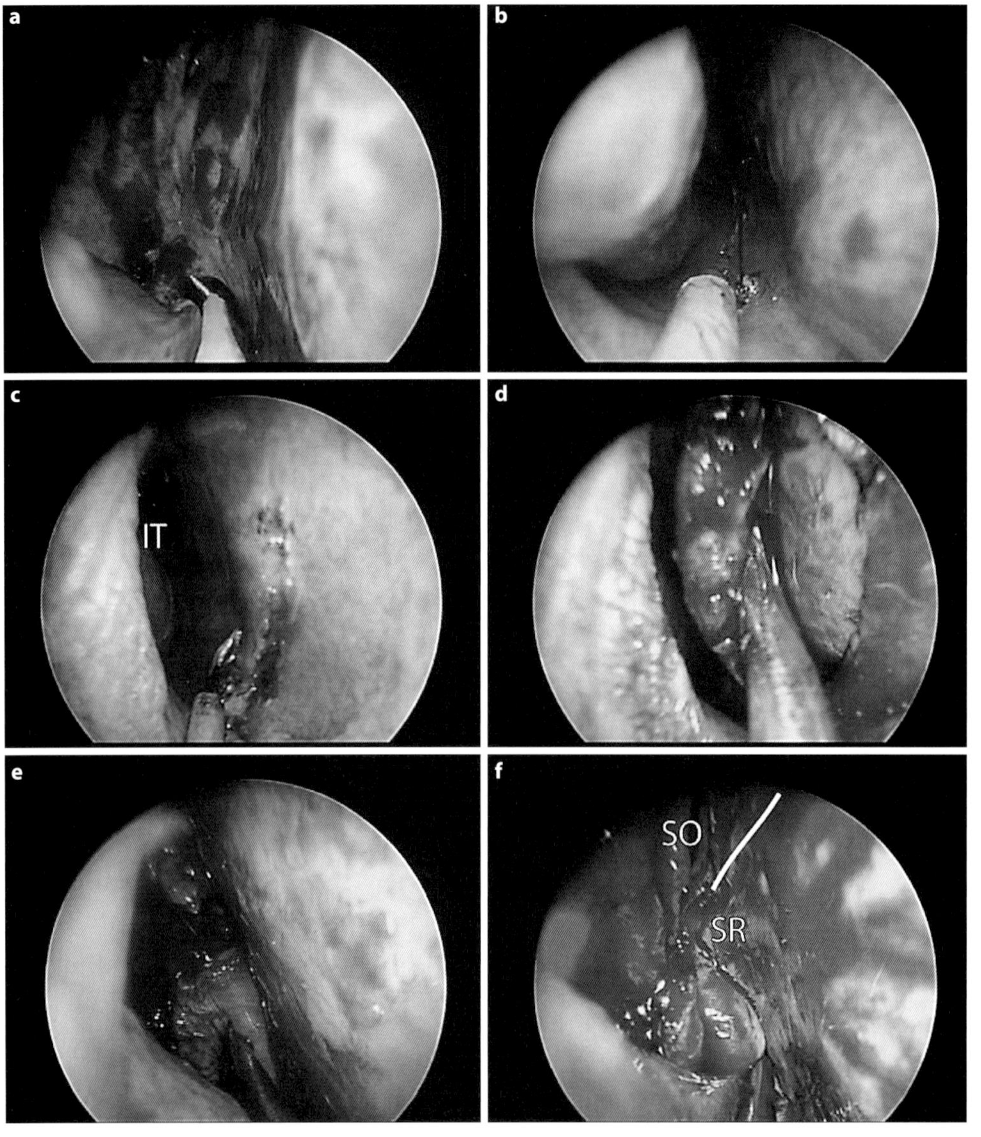

Fig. 2. Intraoperative endoscopic view of dissection of nasoseptal flap (Haddad-Bassagastegay flap). **a** Starting the incision crossing the posterior choana. **b** Continuing the inferior incision along the nasal floor. **c** Connecting the inferior and superior incisions via a vertical incision anterior to the inferior turbinate (IT). **d** Starting to dissect the anterior nasoseptal flap. **e** Continuing to dissect the nasoseptal flap from the underlying septal cartilage. **f** Final posterior dissection of the flap along area of the pedicle over the sphenoid rostrum (SR). The white line represents the area of the superior incision as it continues right below the sphenoid ostium (SO).

with a Cottle dissector or a small suction dissector (fig. 2d, e). It is advantageous to complete all incisions before the elevation of the flap because it becomes difficult to orient the tissue and to maintain it under tension once it has been elevated. Septal incisions may be completed with scissors or other sharp instruments as necessary. Elevation of the flap from the anterior face of the sphenoid sinus is completed with preservation of its posterior septal neurovascular bundle (fig. 2f). The flap is then placed in the nasopharynx or maxillary sinus until it is needed at the end of the procedure for reconstruction. Multiple modifications of the flap regarding length and width are possible. The entire ipsilateral mucoperiosteum and mucoperichondrium may be harvested to cover anterior skull base defects as extensive as those that include the area from the posterior wall of the frontal sinus to the sella turcica and from orbit to orbit. A wide flap may be harvested extending the incision to include the mucoperiosteum of the floor of the nose. A radioanatomic study of the HB flap compared the relative size of the anterior skull base to the size of the potential nasoseptal flaps; results showed that most anterior skull base defects should be able to be completely covered with the HB flap (fig. 4) [4]. Bilateral flaps are conceptually possible; however, they are rarely utilized and could compromise the septal cartilage. During surgery, it is important to be careful with bone removal lateral to the pterygoid canal so that the vascular pedicle is not injured.

Once the extirpative portion of the procedure is complete (fig. 3a), a multilayer cranial base repair is performed (fig. 3). An inlay collagen matrix (Duragen, Integra Life Sciences) is placed as described above (fig. 3b). The HB flap is then placed as an onlay, over the bone edges of the cranial base defect (fig. 3c). All mucosa is removed around the defect before the flap is placed to prevent nonhealing or mucocele formation. After the collagen graft and flap are in place, the edges of the flap are bolstered intranasally with oxidized cellulose absorbable packing (fig. 3d); Duraseal (Confluent Surgical Inc., Waltham, Mass., USA) is then placed (fig. 3e). It is critical to separate the grafts from the packing using some type of nonadherent material such as absorbable gelatin sponge or absorbable gelatin film as this will prevent traction on the grafts when the packing is removed (fig. 3f). In addition, shifting of the underlying inlay/onlay grafts may occur during the placement of the packing; thus, the surgeon must be vigilant and the packing should be placed under direct visualization with the endoscope. Packing is either a Foley balloon or expandable packing sponges as described above. Sealants are never used between the grafts or under the flap as this prevents direct tissue contact and healing. Packing is kept in place for 3–5 days.

After adopting the nasoseptal flap for the reconstruction of EEA defects, our postoperative CSF leak rates dropped considerably [3] to less than 5%, a rate that compares with the those of traditional open techniques. Advantages of the HB flap as a reconstructive option include that a second approach or incision is not necessary and the flap can be harvested endoscopically. A major drawback of the HBF is that its need must be anticipated prior to embarking on the resection, as the vascular pedicle of this flap is frequently compromised during the sphenoidotomy and posterior

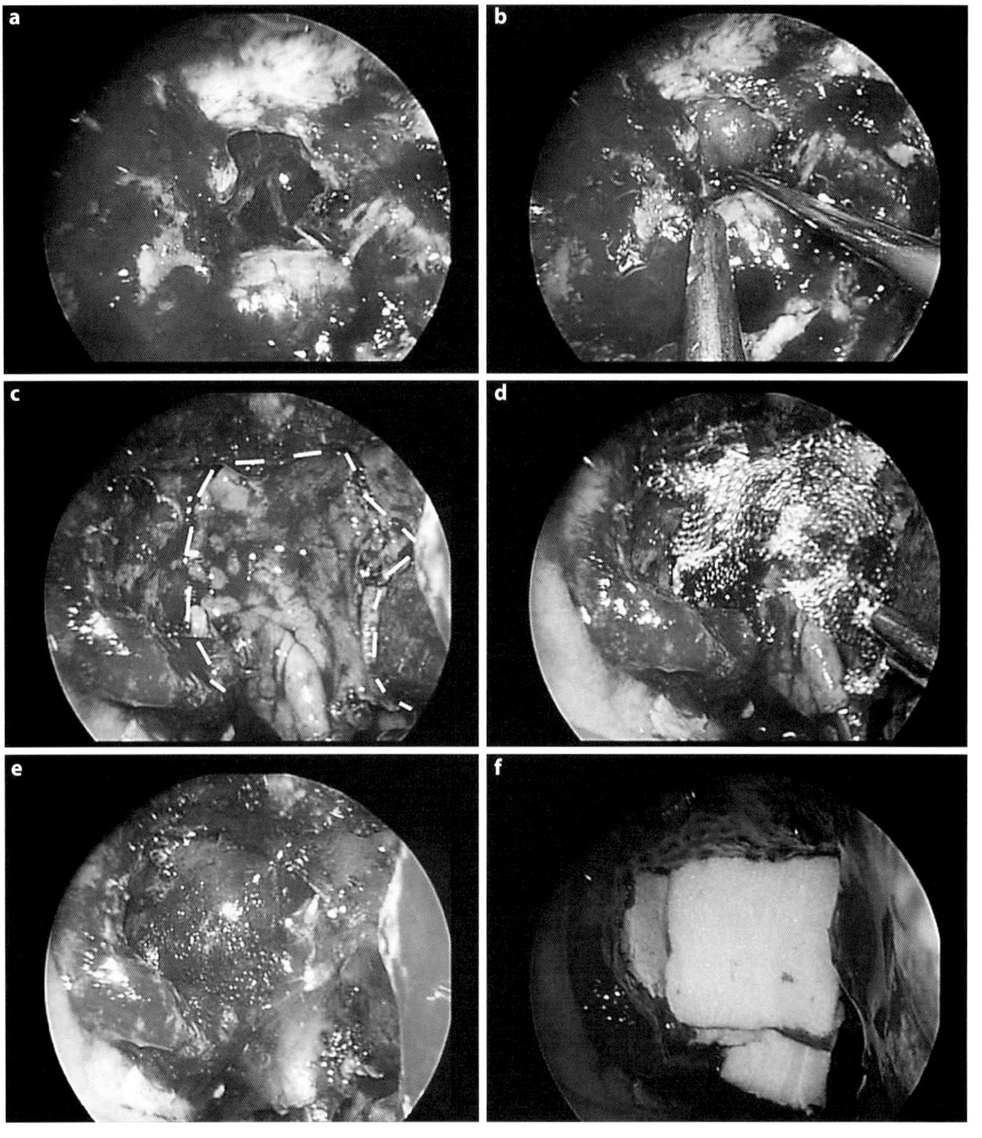

Fig. 3. Intraoperative endoscopic view of placement of a nasoseptal flap (Hadad-Bassagastegay flap). **a** A transsellar and transplanum skull base defect over the area of the suprasellar cistern. **b** A collagen matrix inlay graft. **c** Placement of the nasoseptal flap over the entire defect and over the denuded surrounding bone. **d** The edges of the flap are bolstered intranasally with oxidized cellulose absorbable packing. **e** Duraseal placement. **f** Absorbable gelatin sponge placed. This will prevent traction on the repair when the nonabsorbable packing is removed.

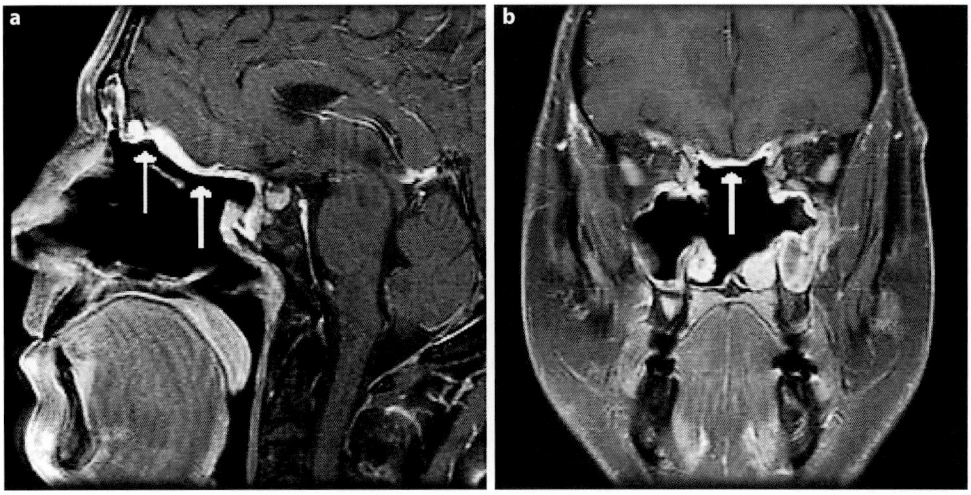

Fig. 4. Postoperative sagittal (**a**) and coronal (**b**) T_1 with contrast MRI an anterior transcribiform skull base resection with excellent enhancing HB flap reconstruction (arrows).

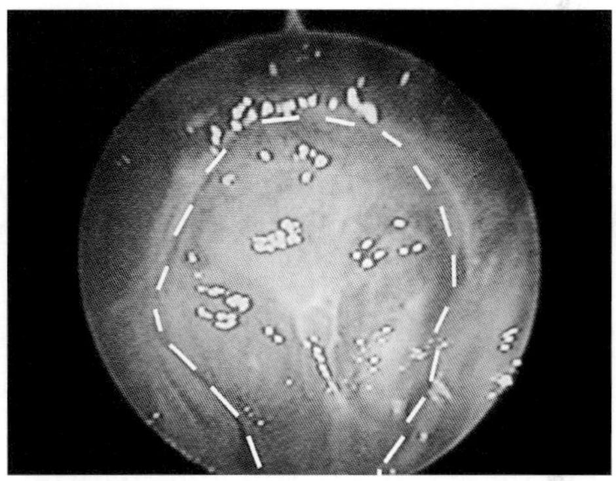

Fig. 5. Endoscopic view of a healed nasoseptal flap over a transsellar and transclival defect.

septectomy. In addition, if a revision procedure is necessary, the flap may have been used previously or the pedicle previously damaged; therefore, two other pedicled flap options have been described and are reviewed below. In revision cases, the HB flap can be dissected from the defect and reused. Healing of the intranasal dissection and nasoseptal flap reconstruction is usually completely healed in 6–12 weeks (fig. 4, 5).

Posterior Pedicle Inferior Turbinate Flap

In patients with prior septectomy or prior wide sphenoidotomies, the HBF blood supply may have been interrupted and this option cannot be used. Other options such as free grafting, or other local or regional vascular pedicle flaps have to be considered. The posterior pedicle inferior turbinate flap (PPITF) is based on the inferior turbinate artery, a terminal branch of the posterior lateral nasal artery (PLNA), which arises from the sphenopalatine artery (SPA) [5]. For the design and harvesting of the PPITF, the anatomic course of the PLNA has to be understood (reviewed in 5) The PNLA runs in a descending vertical or anteroinferior course over the perpendicular plate of the ascending process of the palatine bone, giving a branch medially to supply the middle turbinate. As the artery courses inferiorly, it enters the inferior turbinate on the superior aspect of its lateral attachment, 1.0–1.5 cm from its posterior tip [6]. Some have found that the artery may lie within the bone (50%), within the soft tissue (14%), or following a mixed pattern (36%) [7]. The artery runs for some distance (mean of 1.2 cm) before piercing the bone and soft tissue and splitting off into two to six branches [7].

The nasal cavity is decongested and the lateral nasal wall, just anterior to the inferior turbinate, is injected with a solution of lidocaine 1% with epinephrine 1/100,000. We harvest the PPITF (after completion of the EEA) ipsilateral to the defect whenever possible to minimize the distance of the pedicle to the defect. Initially, the inferior turbinate is gently medialized to better expose the entire medial surface of the inferior turbinate. Given that this flap is substantially smaller than the HB flap, it is best to harvest the entire turbinate to assure adequate coverage (fig. 6a) A wider flap may be harvested by extending the lower incision to include the lateral mucoperiosteum of the turbinate and even the middle meatus. It is best to first identify the SPA as it exits the sphenopalatine foramen and follow it distally to identify the PLNA. The flap will be based solely on this vascular pedicle. Two parallel incisions are performed endoscopically following the sagittal plane of the inferior turbinate, the superior one just above the inferior turbinate and the inferior one following the caudal margin of the turbinate (fig. 6a). A vertical incision, placed over the anterior head of the inferior turbinate, connects the two previous incisions (fig. 6b). Next, the mucoperiosteum is elevated starting at the anterior aspect of the inferior turbinate. A variable amount of bone may be elevated also, depending on the ease of dissecting the mucoperiosteum from the underlying bone. Care must be taken to avoid injuring the vascular pedicle as it enters at the superior aspect of its lateral attachment, approximately 1.0 and 1.5 cm from its posterior tip. In addition, it is important to preserve the LNA as it descends vertically over the ascending process of the palatine bone. It may course anteriorly to the posterior wall of the maxillary sinus; therefore, this should be considered when extending the maxillary antrostomy posteriorly. Once harvested, the flap is gently unrolled and mobilized to cover the skull base defect (fig. 6c). The PPITF can be applied directly to dura or denuded bone or may be used over a fat graft. It is critical, however, that the vascularized flap be in direct contact with the margins of the defect and to remove any nonvascularized tissue between the margins of the defect and the flap. A biological glue is applied over the flap, absorbable gelatin sponges are placed and sponge nasal packing or the balloon of a 12-Fr Foley catheter is inserted to hold the PPITF against the defect. Silicone nasal splints are used to protect the denuded lateral wall and are left in place for 10–21 days. According to an anatomical analysis of the anteriorly based inferior turbinate flap, the mucosal surface area of this flap is

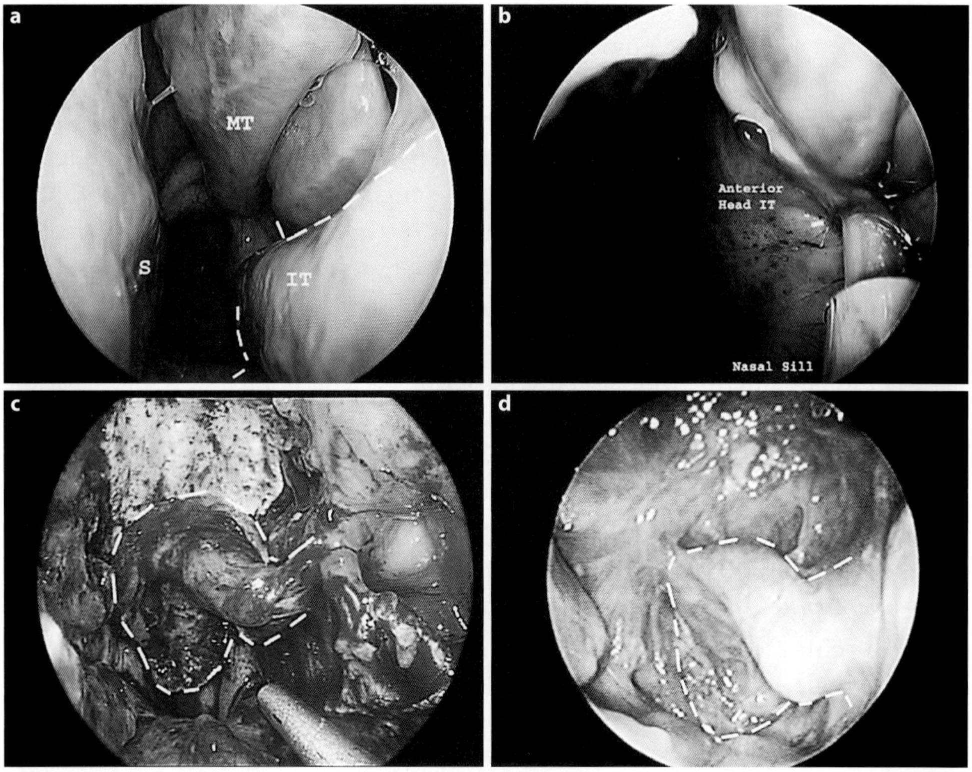

Fig. 6. Intraoperative endoscopic view of a posterior pedicle inferior turbinate flap. **a** Two parallel incisions are performed endoscopically following the sagittal plane of the inferior turbinate, the superior one just above the inferior turbinate and the inferior one following the caudal margin of the turbinate. IT = Inferior turbinate; MT = middle turbinate; S = septum. **b** A vertical incision, placed over the anterior head of the inferior turbinate, connects the two previous incisions. **c** Posterior pedicle inferior turbinate flap placed over a clival defect. **d** Healed posterior pedicle inferior turbinate flap.

approximately 4.97 cm^2 (2.8 cm length with 1.7 cm width) [8]. Bilateral flaps can be harvested to cover larger defects.

The limitations of this flap are a shorter length and the arc of rotation, as compared to the HB flap. It is best suited for posterior defects of the sella or parasellar and mid-clival areas. The flap size limits its use for distant anterior skull base reconstruction. Another disadvantage of using the PPITF is the formation of crusting over the inferior turbinate bone in the postoperative period. Mucosalization of the donor site was observed after a period of 3–4 weeks [5] (fig. 6d).

Temporoparietal Fascial Flap

The temporoparietal fascia flap (TPFF) has been used extensively in various head and neck reconstructive procedures and its anatomy is well described. This section will describe the use of the TPFF in endoscopic skull base reconstruction [9]. This flap is utilized when no viable endonasal options are available for reconstruction.

The temporoparietal fascia (TPF) is a strong fascial layer that is connected to the overlying fibrous septae of the subcutaneous tissue above. The blood supply for the TPF comes from the superficial temporal artery (STA), which is one of the terminal branches of the external carotid artery. It courses through the retromandibular parotid gland, crosses the posterior root of the zygomatic process, and becomes incorporated into the temporal fascia at the level of the zygomatic arch. The average diameter of the vessel is 2.73 mm over the zygomatic arch, and the mean distance between the STA and the tragus is 16.68 mm [10]. In most patients, the STA divides into an anterior frontal and a posterior parietal branch at the level of the zygomatic arch (61–88%); however, the bifurcation point can be superior to the arch (4–26%) or inferior to the arch (7–12%) [10, 11]. One or two veins accompany the STA, which lies just deep to them [10]. The frontal branch of the facial nerve courses just under the TPF after it crosses the superficial surface of the zygomatic arch [12]. The TPF is 2–3 mm in thickness over the parietal region and extends in a fan-like manner from the preauricular region, comprising a surface area as large as 17 × 14 cm [13].

Harvesting and transposition of the TPFF into the nasal cavity is performed after the EEA dissection is complete so the defect size is known. It may be harvested from either side of the scalp, but we most commonly utilize the side ipsilateral to the defect. Previous incisions over the area of the flap may alter the laterality of the harvesting.

If not performed previously as a part of the EEA, an anterior and posterior ethmoidectomy and a large maxillary antrostomy are performed. Then, the SPA and posterior nasal artery are clipped at the level of the sphenopalatine foramen. A retrograde dissection of the SPA serves to remove the posterior wall of the maxillary sinus thus exposing the pterygopalatine fossa (PPF). Part of the lateral wall of the maxillary sinus is removed also to open a wide communication with the infratemporal fossa (ITF). The descending palatine artery is identified in its inferior vertical trajectory from the internal maxillary artery (IMA) and is dissected from its canal. This allows the inferior and lateral displacement of the contents of the upper PPF, therefore exposing the pterygoid plates. The pterygopalatine ganglion may be preserved, but the vidian nerve has to be divided to allow the displacement of the ganglion. Then, the anterior aspect of the pterygoid plates is reduced with a high-speed drill to enlarge the space for the transposition of the TPFF. Now we have full access into the ITF and the IMA should be completely mobile at the pterygomaxillary fissure.

A TPFF is harvested from the ipsilateral side using a conventional technique. A hemicoronal incision is carried down to the level of the hair follicles. Care must be taken to avoid injuring the pedicle during the hemicoronal incision as the STA lies directly under the skin within the subcutaneous tissue. Dissection of the TPF from the subcutaneous tissue effectively elevates the flap. Once enough surface area is exposed, the fascia is incised at its lateral margins and is elevated from the cranium and deep temporal fascia down to its pedicle. The superficial layer of the deep temporal fascia is incised vertically, and the fascia is separated from the muscle following this plane of dissection inferiorly to elevate the periosteum from the surface of the zygomatic arch. This creates a wide tunnel beneath the superficial layer of the deep temporalis fascia that will accept the passage of the pedicle without compression. To help the transposition of the TPFF, a lateral canthotomy incision is used to expose and separate the temporalis muscle from the lateral orbital wall and from the pterygomaxillary fissure. This creates a tunnel that communicates the temporal, the infratemporal fossa, and the endoscopic transpterygoid approach. This soft tissue tunnel is sequentially dilated by passing a guide wire into the nose under endonasal endoscopic visualization and then advancing percutaneous tracheotomy dilators over the wire. After an adequate tunnel is created, the dilators are removed, and the flap is tied to the external end of the guide wire. As the nasal end of the guide wire is pulled out through the nostril, it pulls the flap through the tunnel into the nasal cavity. The mobilization of the flap through the tunnel is assisted with external manipulation. It is important to avoid a rotation of the flap because this may compromise its blood supply. The external incisions are closed with a running nylon stitch after insertion of a suction drain. The reconstruction of the skull base begins with the placement of an inlay graft of a collagen matrix. The edges of the defect are refreshed, and the TPFF is placed over the defect. A sealant may be used after the flap is in position. The flap is then covered with absorbable gelatin sponges, and a sponge packing is placed to stabilize the flap. We remove the packing 3–5 days later.

Advantages of the TPFF include a large tissue area, vascularized tissue from a non-radiated field in the setting of sinonasal or skull base radiotherapy, and a pliable flap with sufficient thickness for ample reconstruction. Disadvantages of this technique include the need for an external approach and a surgical scar, risk of alopecia, risk to the frontal branch of the facial nerve, and the need for associated EEA access to the to the infratemporal fossa.

High CSF Leak Risk Patient Factors

1 Body habitus of the patient: high body mass index is associated with higher intracranial pressure.
2 Pathology being treated, especially craniopharyngiomas and lesions involving the arachnoid cisterns.
3 Entry in arachnoid cisterns or ventricles.
4 Site and size of the defect. Defects in the anterior cranial base are much more likely to leak than clival defects.
5 Cushing's patients with extrasellar ACTH-secreting tumors, likely due to the poor state of tissue healing in these patients.

6 Patients with no vascularized tissue reconstructive options due to prior surgery or chemoradiation therapy.

Lumbar CSF Drainage

Lumbar spinal drains are not routinely utilized in the postoperative period. If a patient has a postoperative leak, they are taken directly back to the operating room for endoscopic re-exploration and repair of the leak. If at this time, the patient is noted to have a high flow leak, a spinal lumbar drain is considered. CSF diversion is usually continued for 3–5 days, averaging up to 10 ml/h. This is preferable to leaving the lumbar drain open to gravity, since excessive CSF drainage may occur with changes in patient position. Rarely, patients have CSF leaks that persist even after endoscopic re-exploration and repair and spinal lumbar drain. In these situations, the CSF pressure is measured and if high-pressure hydrocephalus is noted permanent CSF shunting is considered.

Conclusions

Advances in endoscopic skull base reconstruction must match the ever-increasing size and complexity of lesions that are approached and resected endoscopically. The principles of multilayer reconstructions and the routine use of vascularized flaps in expanded endonasal surgery have reduced postoperative CSF leak rates to less than 5%. Future advances will help us to understand and manage patients with high risk for a postoperative CSF leak, especially those patients who have been previously irradiated and patients that require revision surgery.

References

1 Neligan PC, Mulholland S, Irish J, Gullane PJ, et al: Flap selection in cranial base reconstruction. Plast Reconstr Surg 1996;98:1159–1166.

2 Hegazy HM, Carrau RL, Snyderman CH, et al: Transnasal endoscopic repair of cerebrospinal fluid rhinorrhea: a meta-analysis. Laryngoscope 2000; 110:1166–1172.

3 Hadad G, Bassagasteguy L, Carrau RL, Mataza J, Kassam A, Snyderman CH, Mintz A: A novel reconstructive technique after endoscopic expanded endonasal approaches: vascular pedicle nasoseptal flap. Laryngoscope 2006;116:1882–1886.

4 Pinheiro-Neto CD, Prevedello DM, Carrau RL, Snyderman CH, Mintz A, Gardner P, Kassam A: Improving the design of the pedicled nasoseptal flap for skull base reconstruction: a radioanatomic study. Laryngoscope 2007;117:1560–1569.

5 Fortes FS, Carrau RL, Snyderman CH, Prevedello D, Vescan A, Mintz A, Gardner P, Kassam A: The posterior pedicle inferior turbinate flap: a new vascularized flap for skull base reconstruction. Laryngoscope 2007;117:1329–1332.

6 Padgham N, Vaughan-Jones R: Cadaver studies of the anatomy of arterial supply to the inferior turbinate. J Royal Soc Med 1991;84:728–730.

7 Hadar T, Ophir D, Yaniv E, Berger G: Inferior turbinate arterial bloody supply: histologic analysis and clinical implications. J Otolaryngol 2005;34:46–50.
8 Murakami CS, Kriet D, Ierokomos A: Nasal reconstruction using the inferior turbinate mucosal flap. Arch Facial Plast Surg 1999;1:97–100.
9 Fortes FS, Carrau RL, Snyderman CH, Kassam A, Prevedello D, Vescan A, Mintz A, Gardner P: Transpterygoid transposition of a temporoparietal fascia flap: a new method for skull base reconstruction after endoscopic expanded endonasal approaches. Laryngoscope 2007;117:970–976.
10 Moore KL, Dalley AF: Clinically ORIENTED ANATOMY, ed 5. Baltimore, Lippincott Williams & Wilkins, 2006, pp 788–798.
11 Pinar YA, Govsa F: Anatomy of the superficial temporal artery and its branches: its importance for surgery. Surg Radiol Anat 2006;28:248–253.
12 Casoli V, Dauphin N, Taki C, et al: Anatomy and blood supply of the subgaleal flap. Clin Anat 2004;17:392–399.
13 David SK, Cheney SL: An anatomic study of the temporoparietal fascial flap. Arch Otolaryngol Head Neck Surg 1995;121:1153–1156.

Ricardo L. Carrau, MD, FACS
Department of Otolaryngology, Head & Neck Surgery
Director of the Comprehensive Skull Base Surgery Program
The Ohio State University Medical Center
456 West 10th Avenue, Cramblett Hall, Suite 4A
Columbus, OH 43210-1282 (USA)
Tel. +1 614 293 8074, Fax +1 614 293 3193, E-Mail Ricardo.Carrau@osumc.edu

Kassam AB, Gardner PA (eds): Endoscopic Approaches to the Skull Base.
Prog Neurol Surg. Basel, Karger, 2012, vol 26, pp 182–190

Management of Complications of Endonasal Cranial Base Surgery

Carl H. Snyderman[a,b] · Harshita Pant[c] · Paul A. Gardner[b] · Ricardo L. Carrau[d] · Daniel M. Prevedello[e] · Amin B. Kassam[f]

Departments of [a]Otolaryngology and [b]Neurological Surgery, University of Pittsburgh, Pittsburgh, Pa., USA; [c]Department of Medicine, University of Adelaide, Adelaide, S.A., Australia; Departments of [d]Otolaryngology and [e]Neurological Surgery, Ohio State University, Columbus, Ohio, USA; [f]Division of Neurosurgery, University of Ottawa, Ottawa, Ont., Canada

Abstract

Endoscopic endonasal surgery of the cranial base is maximally invasive surgery and poses many of the same risks as traditional skull base approaches. Preliminary data demonstrates that serious complications can be avoided through a strong foundation in endoscopic skull base anatomy, adherence to principles of surgical dissection, and a dedicated surgical team with proper training and experience. Surgical complications may be categorized by severity, location, organ system or tissue type, and time period. Advances in reconstruction have decreased the incidence of CSF leaks to less than 5%. Major complications such as vascular injury are rare and can be managed using endoscopic techniques. Nasal morbidity is acceptable.

You cannot prevent the birds of sorrow from flying over your head,
but you can prevent them from building nests in your hair.
(Chinese proverb)

The prevention and management of complications is an integral part of surgical practice. Even with the greatest vigilance, complications are inevitable in any surgical endeavor. Although endonasal skull base surgery is often considered less invasive than traditional open approaches, it shares many of the same risks and has the potential for catastrophic complications. Without proper training, the risk of neurological or vascular injury may actually be increased.

Paradigm shifts in surgery progress through different stages. In the first stage, the feasibility of the surgery is assessed and new techniques are introduced and refined. Once feasibility has been demonstrated, the safety of the surgery is critically examined. When a new surgical technique or technology is introduced, there is often a rise in complication rates as the new procedure is adopted. With increased experience, complication rates drop to baseline. A direct comparison of complication rates may not be possible since the types of complications seen with different surgical approaches or techniques may be qualitatively different. If complication rates are acceptable, the final phase of development is the assessment of outcomes (recurrence, survival, quality of life, etc).

The feasibility of endonasal skull base surgery has been amply demonstrated with the description of surgical modules that provide access to the entire ventral skull base for the removal of extracranial and intracranial pathology [1–12].

Our own experience with over 1,300 completely endoscopic endonasal skull base procedures has shown that complex surgeries can be performed with minimal morbidity and few serious complications. In some cases, the evolution of techniques has resulted in a dramatic decline in postoperative complications (CSF; cerebrospinal fluid leaks) [13].

Classification of Complications

A uniform classification scheme for perioperative complications does not exist for skull base surgery. Surgical complications may be categorized by severity (major and minor), location (intracranial [neurosurgical] and extracranial [otolaryngological]), organ system or tissue type (systemic, vascular, neurological, infectious, etc.), and time period (intra- and postoperative). In this chapter, we will use a variety of classifications for the discussion of complications and their management.

From the otolaryngologist's perspective, potential complications of the endonasal approach predominantly include loss of sinonasal airway (synechiae) or function (chronic rhinitis, sinusitis, mucocoele, septal perforation, etc.), cranial nerve injury (trigeminal hypesthesia/anesthesia, anosmia, etc.), and epistaxis (external carotid artery branches). Although many of these complications may seem minor, they can have a significant impact on quality of life. Neurosurgical complications are generally more serious and include infection (meningitis, brain abscess), CSF leak, cranial nerve injury (sensory and motor cranial nerves, visual loss), loss of pituitary function, brain injury and vascular injury (stroke, hemorrhage). Systemic complications may also occur and they range from a simple superficial phlebitis to major complications, such as pulmonary embolism, myocardial infarction and death.

Prevention of Complications

The prevention of complications starts with a strong foundation in endonasal skull base anatomy. The skull base is a 'black box' filled with critical neural and vascular structures. The sphenoid sinus is at the epicenter and is the starting point for most endonasal procedures due to its important anatomical relationships and familiarity.

The most important anatomical relationships concern the internal carotid artery (ICA). For the endonasal skull base surgeon, the ICA can be divided into anatomical segments: parapharyngeal (extracranial), petrous (horizontal), paraclival (vertical), parasellar (cavernous), and supraclinoid. Anatomical landmarks exist for each segment (table). Surgeons should be familiar with anatomical variations and the risks they pose, especially in the sphenoid sinus (conchal pneumatization, multiple lateral septations, Onodi cell).

The other cornerstone of prevention is proper training. We have proposed a training program for endonasal skull base surgeons that is both incremental and modular [see chapter by Snyderman and Mintz, this vol.]. It has five levels of training that are predicated on multiple factors including the familiarity of the anatomy, technical difficulty, potential risk of neural and vascular injury, extent of intradural dissection, and type of pathology. Mastery of each level is recommended before proceeding to the next level. The levels are designed to apply to all endonasal surgeons, irrespective of their specialty.

Perioperative antibiotic prophylaxis with a 3rd or 4th generation cephalosporin is started immediately preoperatively and continued postoperatively as long as nasal packing is in place. Antiseptic preparation of the nasal cavity is not performed due to potential toxicity. Untreated sinusitis is an absolute contraindication to endonasal skull base surgery due to the high risk of meningitis with a dural opening. Intraoperatively, neurophysiological monitoring of cortical and brainstem function is performed when there is potential for brain or vascular injury. Electromyographic monitoring of cranial nerves is also performed when there is dissection in proximity to the cranial nerves (cavernous sinus, middle fossa, jugular foramen, occipital condyle). Image guidance is used to identify anatomical landmarks and assess the extent of resection (tumor margins). An intraoperative computed tomography (CT) scanner provides updated information for image guidance and can detect complications such as intracranial hemorrhage in a timely manner.

Intraoperative Complications

The greatest advance in cranial base surgery has been the concept of team surgery. Team surgery is instrumental in the prevention and the management of intraoperative complications. Endoscopic skull base surgery is true team surgery in that multiple disciplines are working simultaneously and neither specialty can accomplish the goals of surgery independently. The benefits of a co-surgeon include improved visualization (especially during a crisis), increased efficiency, shared problem solving ('co-pilot'), and modulation of individual enthusiasm.

Proper surgical technique is essential to avoid disastrous complications such as vascular injury. Bimanual dissection allows the surgeon to use standard microsurgical techniques. Tumors are not pulled out; rather, the central portion of the tumor is debulked to collapse the tumor and careful extracapsular dissection is then performed with visualization of neighboring vascular and neural structures. Bleeding during surgery can be minimized with a combination of strategies: ligation of feeding vessels (ethmoidal arteries), bipolar electrocautery, removal of bone with a diamond drill bit, direct application of hemostatic materials, and frequent hot water irrigation.

Endoscopic reconstruction of large dural defects has been one of the greatest challenges of endonasal skull base surgery [see chapter by Zanation et al., this vol.]. The introduction of the septal mucosal flap has dramatically decreased the incidence of postoperative CSF leaks and provides vascularized coverage of large defects (craniofacial resection). When a septal mucosal flap is not available due to prior surgery or tumor involvement, a pericranial scalp flap or temporoparietal fascia flap can be employed. Reasons for failure of reconstruction are myriad and include high CSF flow defects (dissection in arachnoid cisterns or 3rd ventricle), increased CSF pressure (hydrocephalus), inadequate reconstructive material, inadequate placement of flap, inadequate recipient bed, and disruption of repair. A good repair is the most important aspect of preventing CSF leaks and consequently intracranial infection and systemic complication.

The most dreaded intraoperative complication is a vascular injury. Venous bleeding from the cavernous sinus is expected and can be effectively controlled with the application of hemostatic materials and other techniques described above. Venous bleeding from the basilar plexus can be very brisk and may require staging of a transclival surgery. In the first stage, the overlying bone is removed and the dura fully exposed. The surface of the dura is cauterized with bipolar electrocautery or the plexus packed with hemostatic agent to effect thrombosis of the basilar plexus. If blood loss or surgical time becomes prohibitive, surgery can be staged. At the second stage of surgery (1–2 days later), the dura can be opened with minimal bleeding. Arterial bleeding can be divided into small and large vessel hemorrhage. Small perforating vessels (1 mm diameter) may be important contributions to the brainstem and optic chiasm. If a vessel is injured, packing of the wound or extensive electrocautery is to be avoided. Special bipolar tips allow selective cauterization of the vessel. If this is not possible, warm water irrigation (40°C) for several minutes is often effective. If this doesn't work, gentle application of a hemostatic material with a cottonoid is performed. Multiple exchanges of the cottonoid may be necessary to achieve hemostasis.

With pituitary surgery, the ICA is most susceptible to injury at the medial optic-carotid junction where the parasellar ICA courses medially. Other risk factors for ICA injury include prior surgery or radiation therapy, anatomical variations, and tumor encasement or displacement of the ICA. If there is an injury to the ICA, the goals of treatment are to maintain cerebral perfusion, obtain focal control of the hemorrhage, and transport the patient to angiography for definitive management of the injury. Contrary to common practice, the blood pressure should not be lowered to decrease bleeding since this may result in cerebral hypoperfusion. Neurophysiological monitoring is invaluable in this situation to reflect cerebral perfusion and establish thresholds for blood pressure. Immediate treatment options include bipolar electrocauterization, compressive packing, direct suture repair, clip reconstruction, and ligation of the vessel. If there is a very small laceration or avulsion of an arteriole from the wall of the ICA, this can be sealed with careful use of bipolar electrocautery. If the injury is substantial, the hemorrhage is directed up the suction to maintain visualization while focal packing (cottonoid) at the site of the vascular injury provides temporary control. If this is effective and neurophysiologic monitoring stable, additional packing can be placed while the patient is transferred to angiography for definitive management. If packing does not control the bleeding, it is best to get further control prior to transfer. While the vessel is compressed with focal packing, additional bone can be removed to better expose the vessel proximal and distal to the site of injury. Although direct suture repair is possible, it is technically difficult and may not be a realistic option. With adequate exposure vessel preservation can be attempted through aneurysm clip reconstruction (e.g. Sundt-Keys clips). Otherwise, the vessel can be occluded with additional packing or placement of aneurysm clips. If packing is used, it needs to be focal so that bleeding is controlled and blood is prevented from tracking through a craniotomy defect intracranially. The patient is then transported to radiology for angiographic assessment and treatment. Preservation of blood flow with a covered stent is technically difficult in the region of the cavernous sinus and currently not FDA approved; therefore, permanent occlusion with coils is often the preferred option. Assessment of collateral blood flow is then performed to assess the risk of ischemic stroke and the potential need for revascularization (bypass).

Postoperative Complications

Immediate postoperative complications such as intracerebral hemorrhage, hematoma, or pneumocephalus are screened for with a postoperative CT scan of the head obtained within hours of surgery. If the extent of residual tumor is the primary concern, MRI is obtained. With the availability of an operating room with a built-in CT scanner, we have begun assessing patients before they leave the operating room. In some cases, this allows us to resect additional tumor with an updated image guidance scan. We have detected two unforeseen complications: subdural hematoma in an elderly female presumably due to rapid shift caused by the loss of CSF and an epidural hematoma from head pin placement in a pediatric patient. In both cases, early identification allowed surgical treatment while the patient was still in the operating room with subsequent good outcomes.

Most postoperative complications are relatively minor and are a direct consequence of the transnasal route: chronic rhinitis with crusting, minor epistaxis, transient anosmia, and sinusitis. Within 3–4 months, healing is usually complete and nasal symptoms return to baseline. A transpterygoid approach implies the sacrifice of the vidian nerve, which results in a loss of emotional tearing on the ipsilateral side. Although most patients don't complain of a dry eye, this is a concern in elderly patients and those with loss of ophthalmic trigeminal branch (V1) function. Injury to the descending palatine nerve results in palatal hypesthesia.

Infectious complications are surprisingly rare despite the absence of a 'sterile' operative field. Even though the nasal passages and sinuses are considered 'clean-contaminated', the bacterial load is not nearly as great as with transoral approaches. Other factors that may contribute to the low rate of infection include frequent intraoperative irrigation with saline, reconstruction with vascularized tissues, and prompt treatment of postoperative CSF leaks. A CSF leak may not become apparent until nasal packing is removed 5–7 days following surgery. If clear watery rhinorrhea is noted in the postoperative period, this is confirmed with nasal endoscopy and testing of the fluid for beta-2-transferrin. In most cases, the patient is returned promptly to the operating room where the leak is repaired. An additional fascial or fat graft or repositioning of the septal flap is usually sufficient and nasal packing is replaced. A lumbar spinal drain may be used for 3–5 days.

Any significant postoperative epistaxis warrants close examination. Endoscopic examination of the nasal cavity may reveal the bleeding source. Bleeding from a branch of the sphenopalatine artery (on the side opposite the septal flap pedicle) can be quite significant and is best dealt with surgically with electrocauterization or endoscopic ligation of the sphenopalatine artery. If there is concern that the hemorrhage could be a sentinel bleed form the ICA due to surgery or radiation necrosis, angiography should be performed. Follow-up angiography is essential anytime there is an intraoperative vascular injury due to the risk of a delayed pseudoaneurysm and rupture. A pseudoaneurysm can present weeks to years following a vascular injury.

Incidence of Complications

We have reviewed our experience with our first 800 completely endoscopic endonasal procedures performed from July 1998 to June 2007 at the University of Pittsburgh Medical Center with regards to major complications. There were 399 men (49.9%) and 401 women (50.1%), with a mean age of 49 years of age (range 3 to 96 years). The two most common tumor types were pituitary adenomas (39.1%) and meningiomas (11.8%).

Intraoperative complications such as vascular or neural injuries were rare. We encountered seven major vascular complications (0.9%). One patient suffered an avulsion of a P1 perforator during the resection of a craniopharyngioma. Two patients suffered an internal carotid artery (ICA) injury and one suffered avulsion of the ophthalmic artery. All three injuries were controlled intraoperatively before transferring the patients to the endovascular suite for additional control or sacrifice of the vessel. None of these 4 patients suffered a new permanent deficit, though the patient with the PCA branch injury suffered a stroke with a severe aphasia which took almost a year to recover.

The other 3 patients suffered permanent neurological deficits as a result of a vascular complication (0.4%). One of these 3 patients suffered an avulsion of a frontopolar artery (A2) during the resection of an olfactory groove meningioma, which was controlled intraoperatively. Later, the patient suffered a frontal lobe hemorrhage from a pseudoaneurysm which was controlled sacrificing A2 and the recurrent artery of Huebner leading to a permanent right hemiparesis and cognitive deficit. Another patient suffered a delayed postoperative pontine hemorrhage after an episode of hypertension following the resection of a clival chordoma with brainstem involvement. This led to permanent quadriplegia. The third patient suffered an injury of the internal maxillary artery during the dissection of an infratemporal fossa encephalocele resulting in an acute subdural hematoma that required multiple craniotomies. This patient has a permanent mild weakness (4/5) of the left upper limb.

Fourteen patients (1.8%) suffered neurological injury intraoperatively, with 4 (0.5%) permanent and 6 (0.8%) transient cranial neuropathies, and 4 cases of transient hemiparesis (0.5%).

Fifteen patients developed delayed postoperative neural complications (1.9%), 6 of which were permanent (0.6%). All of these patients were examined after surgery and did not have the deficit that was later encountered. Four patients developed partial new visual loss on a severe preoperative visual loss. Three of them had the deficit interpreted as perioperative optic nerve hypoperfusion. Seven additional patients suffered delayed visual deterioration that recovered once the causative agent was addressed. One patient developed an anterior fossa encephalocele (secondary to progressive hydrocephalus) and the vision improved after ventriculoperitoneal shunt. Four patients developed a postoperative intrasellar hematoma without permanent sequelae. These patients had undergone surgery for recurrent large pituitary tumors and developed apoplexy within residual tumor. They were re-operated and the clot evacuated resulting in recovery of their vision. Two additional patients developed visual deterioration as a result of the compressive effect of the nasal balloon packing which improved upon removal of the balloon packing. One child developed proptosis due to a retrobulbar hematoma after the resection of a juvenile nasopharyngeal angiofibroma requiring orbital decompression without any permanent sequelae. Five patients suffered postoperative seizures (0.6%).

The most common complication overall was postoperative cerebrospinal fluid (CSF) leak, occurring in 15.9% of the patients. Only 1 patient required a transcranial repair, all of the rest were managed via repeat endonasal repair. Our incidence of postoperative CSF leaks decreased significantly with the adoption of vascularized tissue reconstruction of the skull base (<6%). Fifteen patients suffered intracranial infections with confirmed bacterial growth in cultures (1.9%). Thirteen of these 15 patients were successfully treated, and suffered no sequelae. One patient died of meningitis and secondary status epilepticus. Another patient developed a suprasellar abscess following the resection of an epidermoid tumor and currently remains severely incapacitated.

Finally, 23 patients (2.9%) suffered major postoperative systemic complications. Seventeen patients were successfully treated leaving no sequelae, while 6 died as a result of the complications (0.7%). Overall, 7 patients died during the 30-day perioperative period, 6 due to systemic illness and one due to infection (overall mortality 0.9%).

These 800 cases represent a wide variety of pathological diagnoses and endonasal surgical approaches. Interestingly, major complications, such as vascular injuries, were not relegated to our early experience. We attribute this to a cautious start and a gradual increase in case complexity as we gained experience working as a team and mastered hemostatic and reconstructive techniques.

Conclusions

Any new surgical technique has the potential for significant increases in rates of complication. This can be offset by proper vigilance of outcomes and careful attention to the learning curve. This is especially true of complex surgery such as endoscopic endonasal skull base surgery. The complications associated with this surgery are the same as with traditional approaches for some tumors with respect to intricately associated neurovascular structures. However, other potential complications are much different. Scalp, facial, skull and wound complications are traded for sinus and nasal problems. The sixth cranial nerve, with its medial to lateral course, may be at greater risk with an anterior and medial approach (endonasal) compared with the seventh nerve, which, with its intricate lateral course, which may be at higher risk with lateral/petrous approaches.

Careful and honest appraisal of complications of endoscopic endonasal surgery has led to the use of some of the most critical techniques (such as the use of the nasal septal mucosal flap) and development of critical instrumentation (such as pistol-grip microinstruments and aneurysm clip appliers). Continuation of such critical review will surely be the key to understanding the final place of these approaches in the management of skull base disease.

References

1 Alfieri A, Jho HD, Tschabitscher M: Endoscopic endonasal approach to the ventral cranio-cervical junction: anatomical study. Acta Neurochir (Wien) 2002;144:219–225.

2 Cook SW, Smith Z, Kelly DF: Endonasal transsphenoidal removal of tuberculum sellae meningiomas: technical note. Neurosurgery 2004;55:239–246.

3 Carrau R, Kassam A, Snyderman C, Duvvuri U, Mintz A, Gardner P: Endoscopic transnasal anterior skull base resection for the management of sinonasal malignancies. Operative Tech Otolaryngol 2006;17:102–110.
4 Frank G, Sciarretta V, Calbucci F, Farneti G, Mazzatenta D, Pasquini E: The endoscopic transnasal transsphenoidal approach for the treatment of cranial base chordomas and chondrosarcomas. Neurosurgery 2006;59:ONS50–57.
5 Kassam A, Snyderman C, Carrau R, Gardner P, Hirsch B, Mintz A: Endoscopic, expanded endonasal approach to the jugular foramen. Operative Tech Neurosurg 2005;8:35–41.
6 Kassam A, Snyderman CH, Carrau RL, Gardner P, Mintz A: Endoneurosurgical hemostasis techniques: lessons learned from 400 cases. Neurosurg Focus 2005;19:E7.
7 Kassam A, Snyderman CH, Mintz A, Gardner P, Carrau RL: Expanded endonasal approach: the rostrocaudal axis. I. Crista galli to the sella turcica. Neurosurg Focus 2005;19:E3.
8 Kassam A, Snyderman CH, Mintz A, Gardner P, Carrau RL: Expanded endonasal approach: the rostrocaudal axis. II. Posterior clinoids to the foramen magnum. Neurosurg Focus 2005;19:E4.
9 Kassam AB, Gardner P, Snyderman C, Mintz A, Carrau R: Expanded endonasal approach: fully endoscopic, completely transnasal approach to the middle third of the clivus, petrous bone, middle cranial fossa, and infratemporal fossa. Neurosurg Focus 2005;19:E6.
10 Kassam AB, Mintz AH, Gardner PA, Horowitz MB, Carrau RL, Snyderman CH: The expanded endonasal approach for an endoscopic transnasal clipping and aneurysmorrhaphy of a large vertebral artery aneurysm: technical case report. Neurosurgery 2006;59:ONSE162–165.
11 Kassam AB, Prevedello DM, Thomas A, et al: Endoscopic, endonasal pituitary transposition for transdorsum sellae approach to the interpeduncular cistern. Neurosurgery 2008;62(suppl 1):57–72.
12 Kassam AB, Snyderman C, Gardner P, Carrau R, Spiro R: The expanded endonasal approach: a fully endoscopic transnasal approach and resection of the odontoid process: technical case report. Neurosurgery 2005;57:E213.
13 Kassam AB, Prevedello DM, Thomas A, Gardner P, Mintz A, Snyderman C, Carrau R: Endoscopic endonasal pituitary transposition for a transdorsum sellae approach to the interpeduncular cistern. Neurosurgery 2008;62(3 suppl 1):57–72.
14 Kassam AB, Thomas A, Carrau RL, Snyderman CH, Vescan A, Prevedello D, Mintz A, Gardner P: Endoscopic reconstruction of the cranial base using a pedicled nasoseptal flap. Neurosurgery 2008; 63(suppl 1):ONS44–52.

Carl H. Snyderman, MD, MBA
Department of Otolaryngology
UPMC
200 Lothrop Street, EEI 500, Pittsburgh, PA 15213 (USA)
Tel. +1 412 647 8186, E-Mail snydermanch@upmc.edu

Kassam AB, Gardner PA (eds): Endoscopic Approaches to the Skull Base.
Prog Neurol Surg. Basel, Karger, 2012, vol 26, pp 191–203

Endoscopic Approaches to the Cerebellopontine Angle

Daniel R. Pieper[a] · Dennis Bojrab[b]

[a]Michigan Head and Spine Institute, [b]Michigan Ear Institute, Novi, Mich., USA

Abstract

With the introduction of modern endoscopic procedures, the application of the endoscope now includes skull base surgery. However, the utilization of skull base endoscopy has been limited to those procedures accessible through the endonasal approach. In cerebellopontine angle (CPA) surgery the endoscope has historically been limited as an adjunct to the microscope rather than the primary source of visualization. These limitations are attributable directly to the inability to stabilize the endoscope to allow bimanual surgery, overheating from the light source and lack of instrumentation. We describe our experience utilizing the endoscope as the sole source of visualization. We have overcome many of the aforementioned obstacles, and introduce our operative set-up and equipment recommendations. We describe our indications and contraindications for the procedure's use. We present the results of our first 37 patients and describe the nuances of the procedure for a spectrum of CPA pathology including microvascular decompression, neurectomy and neoplasm resection. Despite a steep learning curve, our experience suggests endoscopy for CPA surgery provides improved surgical visualization which enhances neurovascular preservation at the time of surgery. The clinical outcomes in our patient population have resulted in decreased postoperative deficits, decreased operative time and decreased length of stay.

Max Nitze is credited for designing the first surgical endoscope in 1879. His crude invention of multiple lenses illuminated by a light at the tip was sustained by the ongoing passion of improved visualization and magnification in surgery [1]. The use of endoscopy in the cerebellopontine angle (CPA) was first described by Doyen in 1917 for a trigeminal neurectomy [2]. However, the technology of the lenses and light source significantly limited the endoscope's utility. With the introduction of the operating microscope in the 1960s, there was little interest in pursuing this crude endoscopic technology as the microscope provided superior lighting and magnification as compared to the endoscopes of the day. The microscope provided superior

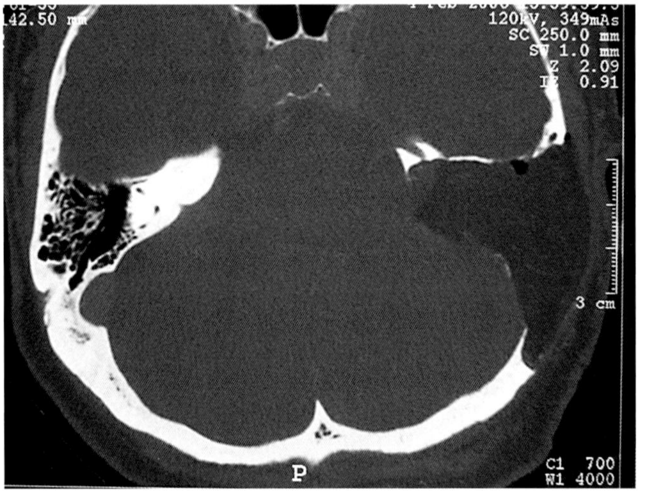

Fig. 1. Postoperative axial CT following a left translabyrinth approach.

illumination and magnification especially to the deep, dark recesses of the skull base.

Advancements in the field of microsurgical techniques have allowed the surgeon to compensate for the microscope's inability to see around corners by creating linear corridors of site. Mobilizing the cerebellum and creating larger cranial openings allowed these corridors for the light source to illuminate the field in a linear fashion from a light source located outside the surgical field to the final target (fig. 1).

Despite the technical advancements of illumination and image resolution, endoscopy was limited to intraventricular and endonasal procedures. It was not until the 1990s that the endoscope was introduced as an adjunct to enhance visualization of the CPA. Since then, a limited but growing number of authors have reported their results using the endoscope as an adjunct to the microscope for CPA pathology [3–11]. The microscope's ability to hold a constant position without the aid of an assistant, thus allowing the surgeon bimanual dexterity, has limited the utilization of the endoscope in microsurgery to date. Shahanian and coworkers [12, 13] were the first to describe a fully endoscopic approach to the CPA for microvascular decompressions (MVD) in trigeminal neuralgia and hemifacial spasm. Since 2005, we have expanded the use of the endoscope in the CPA not only for MVDs but for neurectomies, fenestration of cysts and resection of extra-axial neoplasms without the aid of an operating microscope.

The benefit of performing CPA surgery completely endoscopically is decreased tissue manipulation/retraction while enhancing the visualization of the CPA structures (fig. 2). Endoscopic dissection obviates the need for the use of a retractor, thereby limiting the need to sacrifice venous structures when retracting the cerebellar hemisphere (fig. 3). The wider field of view provided by the endoscope allows essentially unrestrained visualization of the CPA from cranial nerve (CN) IV at the level of the

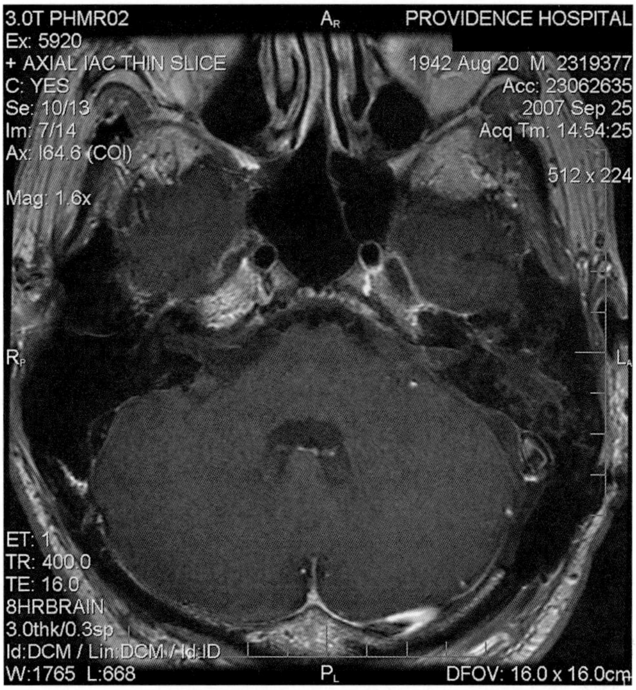

Fig. 2. Postoperative MRI T_1 sequence with gadolinium 24 h following endoscopic resection of a left side vestibular schwannoma. Note the absence of any postoperative changes to the cerebellum or CPA.

incisura to the superior aspect of the cervical cord using the same 14-mm access (fig. 4). This provides the patient with decreased operative time, decreased pain, decreased cerebellar symptoms, decreased cranial neuropathies, and decreased hospital days and recovery time.

Indications

We have utilized CPA endoscopic techniques for MVDs of CN V, VII, and VIII; however, there is no contraindication for its use in MVDs or cranial neurectomies of any cranial nerve in the CPA. The technique has been utilized for the resection of extra-axial lesions of the CPA including petrous meningiomas, epidermoid tumors, and cranial nerve neoplasms. Due to the absence of retraction and the enhanced image quality and illumination, the risk of postoperative cranial neuropathies, especially hearing loss, has been substantially reduced, especially in vestibular neuroma resection.

Despite its inherent advantages, we limit the use of CPA endoscopy based on the preoperative radiographic anatomy. Absence of the interpeduncular and/or prepontine cisterns due to mass effect or elevated intracranial pressure is considered a contraindication to endoscopic CPA surgery (fig. 5). In cases where accessing the cisterna magna is necessary to create a relaxed environment, it is our recommendation that an

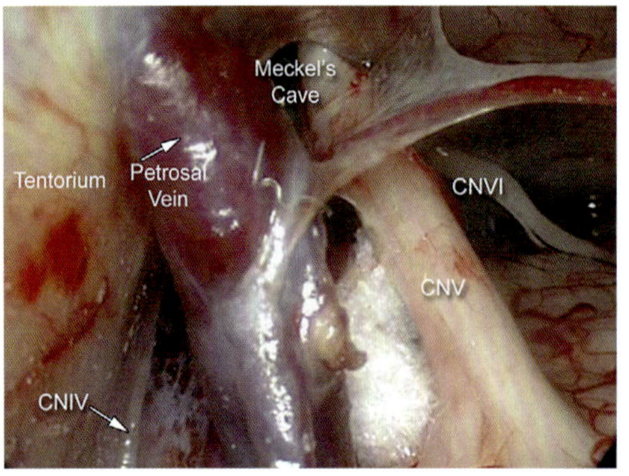

3

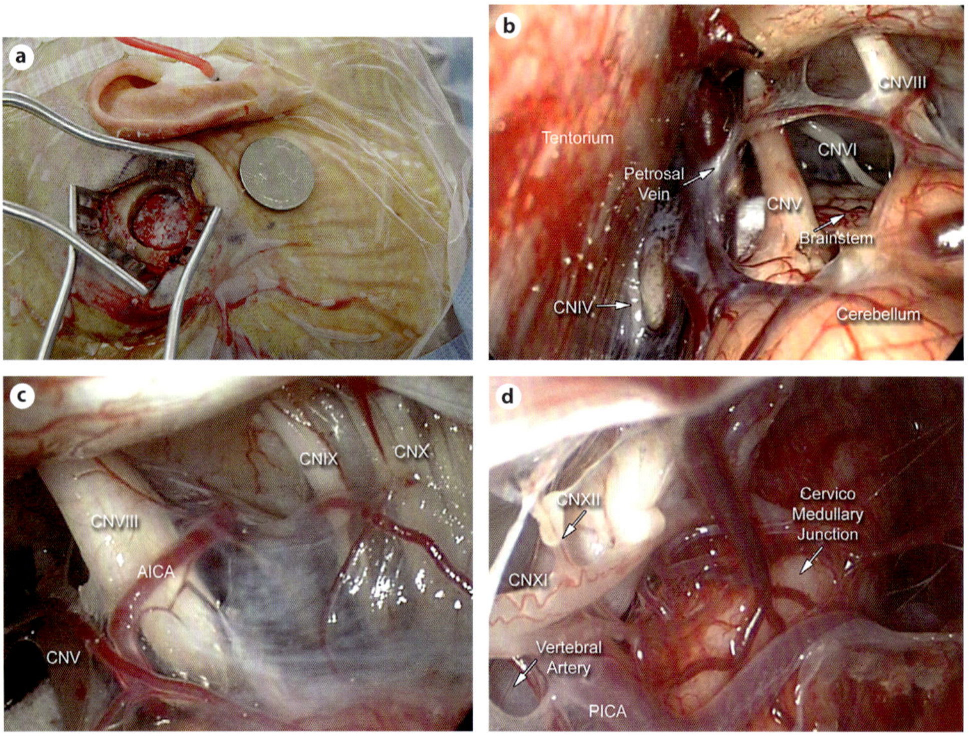

4

Fig. 3. Preservation of the petrosal vein following an endoscopic right CN V MVD.

Fig. 4. a Postauricular incision and 14-mm craniectomy for the endoscopic left CPA approach. **b** Endoscopic visualization of the CPA identifying the CN IV just below the incisura obscured by arachnoid, petrosal vein, CN V, CN VI and the CN VII/VIII complex at the brainstem. **c** Endoscopic visualization of the CPA identifying the CN VII/VIII complex and CN IX/X rootlets at the jugular foramen. **d** Endoscopic visualization of the CPA through the foramen magnum identifying CN XII, the origin of CN XI, cervical rootlets, vertebral artery with the origin of PICA and the cervicomedullary junction.

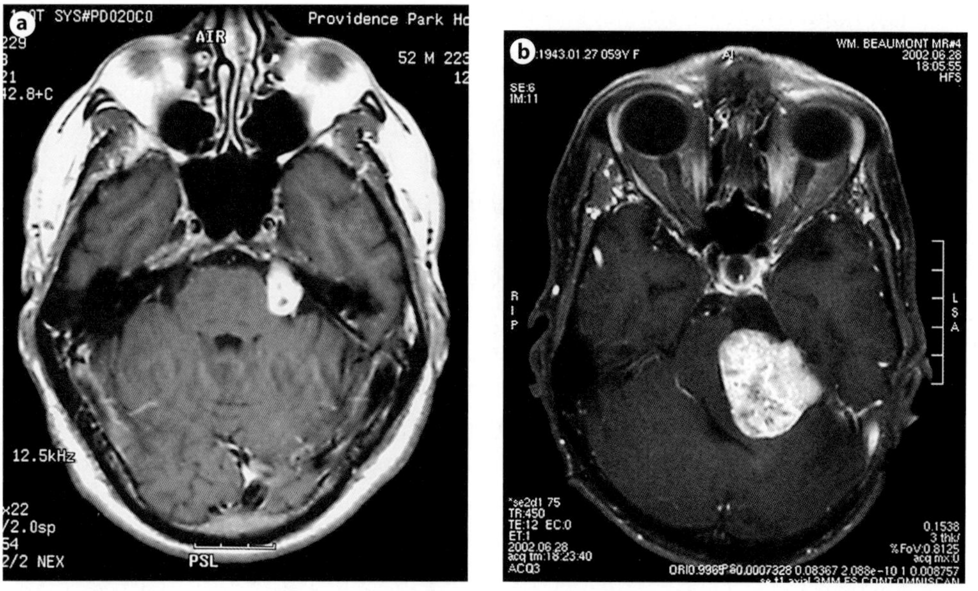

Fig. 5. a Preoperative MRI axial T_1 with gadolinium identifying a CN V neoplasm in the left CPA. The prepontine cistern is patent with minimal mass effect noted. This patient underwent endoscopic resection of this tumor. **b** Preoperative MRI axial T_1 with gadolinium identifying a vestibular schwannoma in the left CPA. There is significant mass effect of the brainstem and fourth ventricle. This neoplasm was resected by an open procedure and was not a candidate for an endoscopic CPA approach due the significant increased posterior fossa pressure. This would preclude a safe cannulation of the CPA endoscopically.

open procedure should be considered, as cannulating the cisterna magna blindly is unnecessarily risky with the consequences of an unintended potentially devastating and possibly fatal event.

Another dilemma facing endoscopy of the CPA is the loss of depth perception when visualizing the procedure on a 2-D monitor. This factor is especially enhanced in the CPA as compared to other skull base sites as every instrument introduced or removed free-handed can potentially come into contact with a major neurologic structure including the cerebellum, brainstem, veins and arteries of the posterior circulation and cranial nerves.

Equipment

Unlike endonasal endoscopy where the surgical field can accommodate two surgeons and four hands working in coordination on either side of the patient's head, the limited space afforded to the lateral suboccipital region precludes this luxury. Additionally, the precision of the CPA requires the surgeon to utilize both hands simultaneously which precludes the surgeon from holding the endoscope during the dissection.

This last point is one of the major reasons to date that the endoscope has been relegated to visual adjunct during CPA surgery. That being said, the majority of endoscope holders are clumsy, multi-jointed apparatus that are not easily adjusted. These holders are adequate for most of the endonasal and intraventricular approaches as the depth of field is usually stable once the surgical site is reached. This, however, is not the case in CPA surgery where the surgical field and field depth are ever-changing and require the surgeon to constantly change trajectory, especially during tumor resections. We have overcome this hurdle with the use of a multi-jointed pneumatic arm which, like most operating microscopes, can be unlocked and fully mobile throughout all planes of motion and then relocked into a stable configuration with the depression and release of a single button. This allows the surgeon to position and reposition the entire apparatus with one hand (fig. 6).

Light source heat injury is another concern related to endoscopy. The introduction of a xenon light source has substantially improved illumination especially in areas like the CPA. Unfortunately, this enhanced illumination is at the cost of increased heat generation, especially relevant given the proximity of the endoscope to neural structures of the CPA. This nuance is diminished in microsurgery because of the distance of the microscope form these structures. We have overcome this obstacle by incorporating a thin sleeve over the endoscope which allows for intermittent irrigation of the system, thereby cooling the tip and minimizing heat transfer.

Unlike microsurgery where the surgical instruments work in series along the optical trajectory of the microscope lens, the surgeon must now learn to work in parallel with the endoscope. Unfortunately, this precludes the use of bayoneted instruments. Additionally, unlike the intraventricular and endonasal endoscopic procedures which allow the surgeon some degree of rotational movement about the point of entry, the point of entry and the trajectory of the instrument is limited in the CPA by the cerebellum, petrous bone and incisura. These limitations necessitated the introduction of an entirely different microsurgical instrument set based on the principle of rotational pistol-grip instruments (fig. 7), as well as straight-shafted dissectors which in some cases incorporate real time neurophysiologic monitoring capabilities (fig. 8).

Procedure

Set-Up

The monitor for the endoscope must be placed in a direct line of site for the surgeon (fig. 6a). The scrub nurse is typically located to the surgeon's dominant side. The electrical devices are typically placed at the patient's feet and the neurophysiologic monitors placed oppositely in order to better shield them from electrical noise signals. The pneumatic arm is secured to the bedframe directly opposite the surgeon and positioned to provide ease of access from both an inferior and superior trajectory. The patient's head is immobilized to avoid any movement of the patient during

6
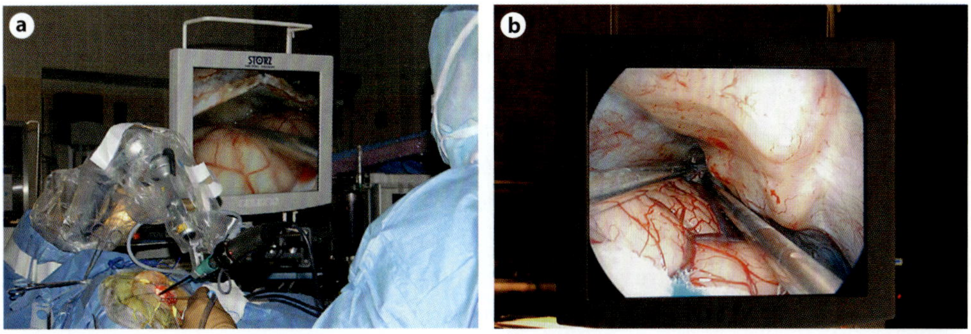

7
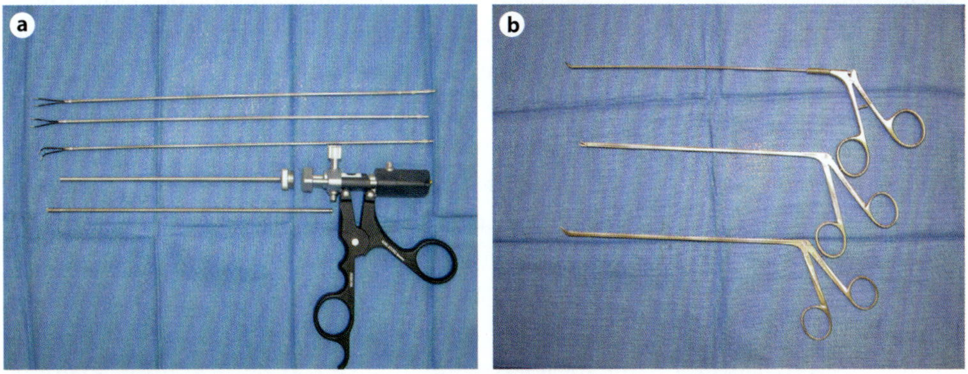

8
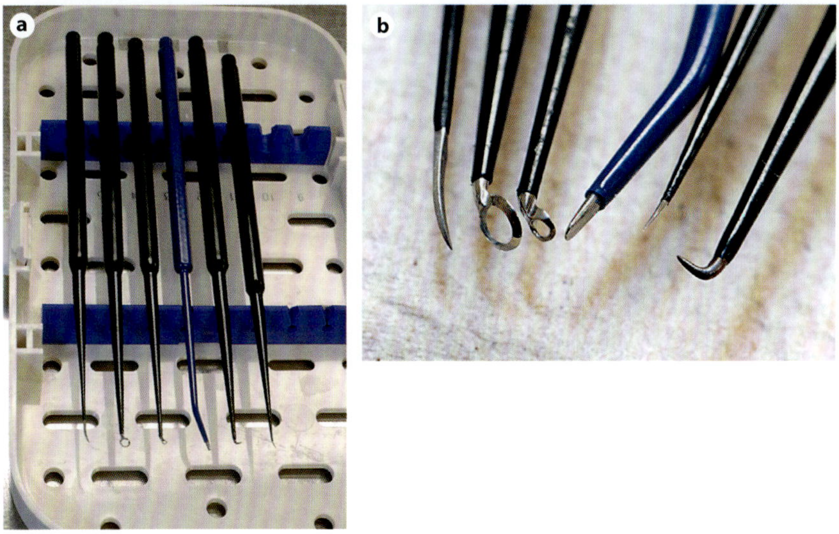

Fig. 6. **a** Operative field set-up of the endoscopic CPA approach. The endoscope is held in position by the pneumatic arm. **b** Bimanual microsurgical technique is illustrated which is made possible by the rigid fixation of the pneumatic arm.

Fig. 7. **a** Rotational pistol grip bipolar system and attachments used for the endoscopic CPA approach. **b** Endoscopic pistol-grip scissor set including straight, angled and rotational scissors.

Fig. 8. **a** Monitored straight-shaft dissectors used for endoscopic CPA surgery. **b** Close-up of the tips of the monitored dissector set.

the procedure. This point is emphasized because we do not typically use paralytics to allow intraoperative facial nerve monitoring. The endoscope, once cannulated into the posterior fossa, is poised in close proximity to the brainstem and any inadvertent head movement could cause the endoscope to impale the brainstem. The head is typically elevated to 30° above the horizontal. The patient is administered 1–2 g/kg of mannitol followed by 20 mg of furosemide at the initiation of the anesthetic, unless contraindicated, and the $PaCO_2$ reduced to 28 mm Hg.

Monitoring electrodes are placed depending on the planned neural elements to be monitored. We typically use facial nerve and brainstem auditory evoked response (BAER) monitoring. In some instances, we may also utilize endotracheal tube monitoring electrodes, SSEP, CN XI and XII electrodes as well. Prior to incision, the presumed locale of the transverse-sigmoid sinus (TS) junction is identified. The superior nuchal line, which localizes the transverse sinus, is a line drawn between the root of the zygoma and the external occipital protuberance. The sigmoid sinus lies parallel and just lateral to the posterior mastoid groove. The intersection of the superior nuchal line and posterior mastoid groove delineates the approximate location of the TS junction.

Approach

The approach remains the same for approaching the CPA regardless if the anatomic site of interest or pathology (MVD verses neoplasm). A 2.5–3.0 cm oblique incision is then made at the locale of the TS junction. A 14-mm craniectomy is performed identifying the edge of the TS junction (fig. 9). A curvilinear dural incision is made paralleling the TS junction. A 4-mm, 0°, rigid endoscope is cannulated along the cerebellum either along the tentorium (if accessing the interpeduncular cistern) or along the ventral aspect of the cerebellum (if accessing the prepontine cistern). The petrosal veins are identified and either mobilized or cauterized/transected to access the CSF cisterns. The CN VII/VIII complex will be encountered prior to the prepontine cistern arachnoid. Once CSF is released, the cerebellum will adequately relax to allow visualization of the ventrolateral brainstem and associated CN root entry zones. The 0° endoscope is primarily used during active dissection within the CPA in order to minimize inadvertent injury to neurovascular structures. The 30° endoscope is utilized for ventral inspections of the CN root entry zones and internal auditory canal (IAC).

Microvascular Decompressions (Fig. 10)

A thorough 360° inspection of the root entry zone should be performed prior to the formal MVD in order to account for all potential vascular entities. Prior to the MVD, the offending vessels should be dissected from the surrounding arachnoid bands to allow adequate mobility during the MVD. Adequate mobilization prior to placement of the pledget will minimize inadvertent vascular injury. Should bleeding be encountered during mobilization of the vessel, the endoscope should not be withdrawn as this will preclude visualization and make recannulation of the CPA more difficult. Copious irrigation, identification of the source and control with either bipolar cautery or gentle pressure must occur prior to the continuation of the procedure. In the case of CN VII MVD, a pre- and poststimulation threshold is recommended in order to evaluate the integrity of the nerve prior to closure. An electrical recording of CN VII at a direct stimulation threshold of 0.05 mA is generally consistent with a favorable facial nerve response.

Vestibular Neurectomy (Fig. 11)
The image quality achieved with modern endoscopes when partnered with high-definition monitors and HD capable cameras surpasses the detail visualized by the operating microscope. As such, the delineation of the nerve allows identification of the vestibular and cochlear portions of the CN. CN VII and nervus intermedius should be identified prior to the neurectomy to avoid injury. During the neurectomy, continuous BAER monitoring is performed to assess the cochlear nerve.

Tumor Resection (Fig. 12)
The minimal size of the endoscope coupled with greater maneuverability allows the surgeon access to the entire CPA from the incisura through the foramen magnum. The endoscope allows enhanced visualization of the neural structures splayed along the tumor capsule. This allows for early identification of the cochlear nerve in hearing preservation cases. The ability to visualize structures ventral to the tumor prior to removal allows identification of CN VII earlier, minimizing risk to the facial nerve. Finally, the use of a 30° endoscope enhances visualization out along the IAC which minimizes the amount of bone removal at the porous acousticus when compared to a typical retrosigmoid microsurgical approach. As there is no need for retractors in endoscopic CPA surgery, tension applied to the neural structures, especially the CNs, is minimized as well.

The disadvantages of the procedure remain mostly in the limited instrumentation. Tumor removal instruments (i.e. CUSA) are limited due to the presence of the endoscope as they are not intended as parallel instruments. The same difficulty is encountered with many of the drill systems. However, as the field of endoscopy expands, there is little doubt that these challenges will be addressed.

Results

Having performed both endonasal and CPA endoscopic cases at essentially the same time in my career, the learning curve for CPA endoscopy is considerably greater. Additionally, obtaining a level of comfort with the endoscope is paramount prior to cannulating the CPA. Our initial experience was confined to MVDs. This self-imposed limitation was essential for multiple reasons:

9

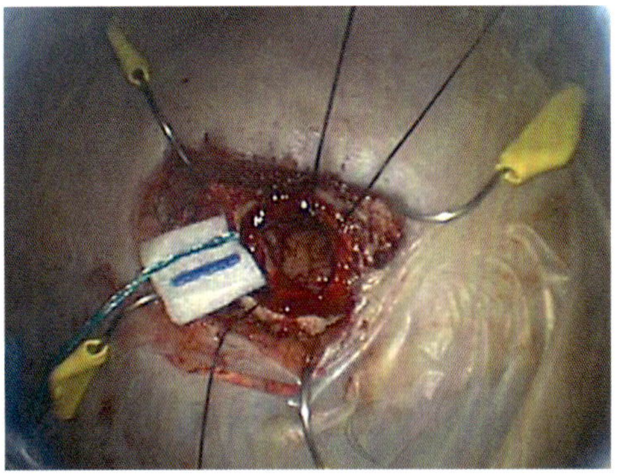

10

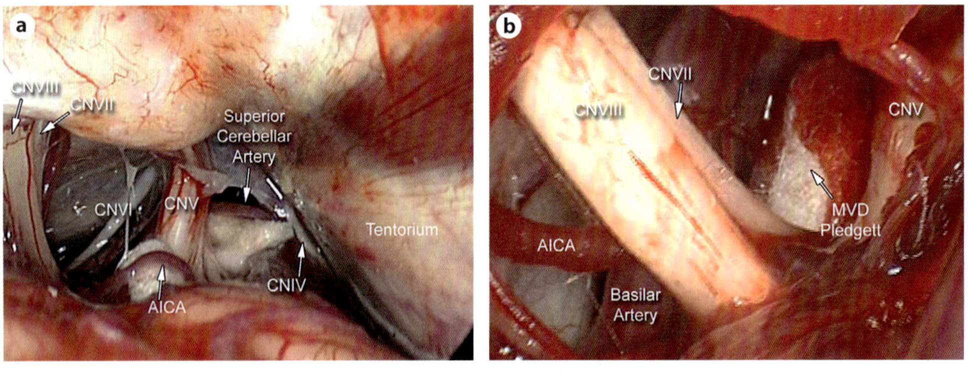

11

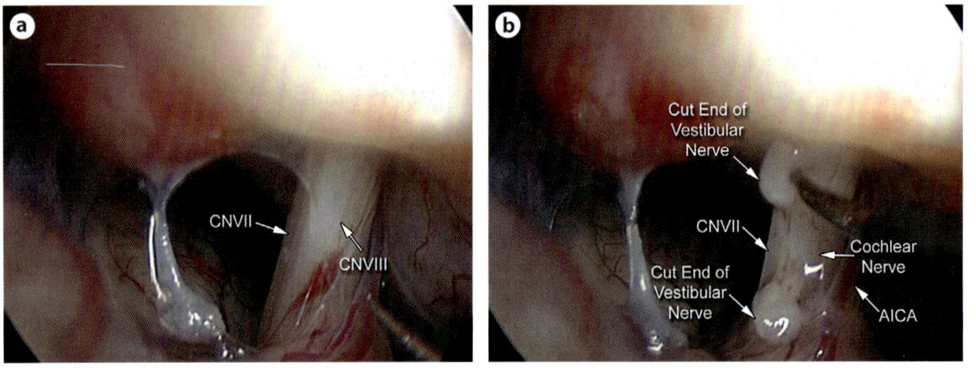

Fig. 9. Dural opening used for the endoscopic CPA approach. A 13-mm cotton patty is placed for reference.

Fig. 10. **a** Endoscopic view of the left CPA following MVD of CN V. CN VII/VII complex is identified to the left, CN VI in the background entering Dorello's canal and 2 pledgets placed at the CN V root entry zone decompressing vessels from the superior cerebellar artery ventrally and AICA dorsally. **b** Endoscopic view of the CN VII/VIII complex following MVD for hemifacial spasm. CN VII is identified ventral to the CN VII complex with the Teflon pledget in place.

Fig. 11. **a** Endoscopic view of the right CN VII/VIII complex. CN VII is identified ventrally. The vestibular nerve is differentiated from the cochlear nerve prior to sectioning. **b** The vestibular nerve has been sectioned while preserving the cochlear nerve to the right and the facial nerve ventrally.

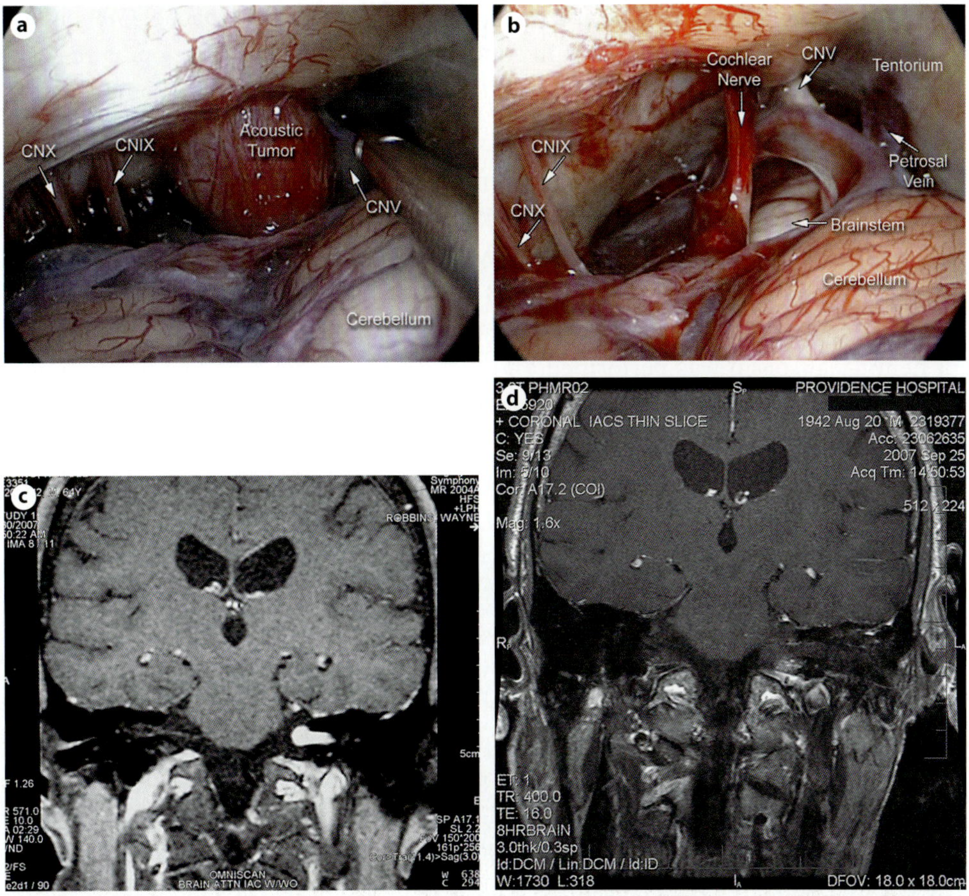

Fig. 12. **a** Endoscopic view of a left sided vestibular schwannoma. CN IX/X are to the left. CN VII is identified along the superior pole of the tumor. **b** Endoscopic view following resection. **c** Preoperative MRI axial T_1 gadolinium enhanced image of this patient showing extension of the tumor throughout the length of the IAC. **d** Postoperative MRI axial T_1 gadolinium enhanced image of the patient showing complete resection of the tumor.

1 Familiarity with accessing the CPA endoscopically: Initially, we used a retractor system. The retractor was used from a historical perspective and from a presumed safety standpoint to avoid contact with the cerebellum during the introduction and withdrawal of instruments to the operative field. We subsequently realized that the retractor severely limited our movements and compromised an already small field. Once all external retractors were removed, dissection of the CPA and associated basilar cisterns was significantly improved.

2 Lack of instrumentation: Complete conversion from a bayoneted instrument system to a rotational pistol grip system was difficult. The lack of readily available instruments and the lack of interest by instrument companies required a complete revision of the surgical instrument tray.

3 Lack of adequate cautery was, and remains, the most difficult aspect of CPA endoscopy. With the increased interest in endoscopy, the interest in developing the necessary instrumentation is growing, but the technology is lagging in comparison to the endoscopic imaging capability.

Over the first 2 years since the inception of endoscopy into our skull base surgical practice, we have performed 37 cases of CPA endoscopy. During the same period of time we performed 223 open cases for CPA pathology. MVD for trigeminal neuralgia was performed on 20 patients of which 18 obtained complete relief without medication and 2 had a good outcome, but still required a smaller dose of medication. MVD for hemifacial spasm was performed on 6 patients of whom 5 had complete remission. Vestibular neurectomy or decompression was performed on 3 patients, all of whom had resolution of their preoperative vertigo. We have performed 8 tumor resections during this period of time; however, as discussed, tumor resections were not attempted until later in the series. Tumors encountered have included meningiomas (3), epidermoid (2), acoustic (3), and trigeminal schwannomas (1). Hearing was preserved in all but 1 of the 37 patients (97%). One patient had substantially diminished hearing without an identifiable BAER at the time of surgery and no discernable plane of dissection could be appreciated during surgery between the tumor and the cochlear nerve. One patient had a slight, transient high-frequency sensorineural hearing loss after a CN VII MVD which improved 6 months postoperatively.

Both operative time (OT) and length of stay (LOS) were considerably decreased overall. Initially, the OT was increased due to the steep learning curve and lack of instrumentation. Currently, the OT for MVDs and neurectomies is around 70 min. The OT for cranial nerve neoplasms is typically 90–110 min. The LOS was decreased to 1–2 days for pathology not involving the CN VII/VIII complex, and 2–3 days for pathology involving the CN VII/VIII complex. This discrepancy was attributed to presence or absence of vertigo postoperatively. Complications were minimal. There was one superficial wound infection and one CSF leak which did not require surgery.

Conclusion

Recent advancements made in the field of endoscopy have increased its utility in the realm of skull base surgery. Improved image quality, enhanced illumination and the introduction of new instrumentation have allowed its use in CPA surgery. Although the steep learning curve may discourage its widespread application, the advantages of the procedure, in our opinion, outweigh this concern. Based on personal experience of over 1,500 cases of open CPA surgery, I have found that, despite my initial reluctance and lack of familiarity with endoscopy prior to 2005, the improvement of surgical exposure and clinical outcomes from neural preservation to LOS supports its utilization in my practice.

References

1 Mouton, WG, Bessell JR, Maddern, GJ: Looking back to the advent of modern endoscopy: 150th birthday of Maximilian Nitze. World J Surg 1998;22: 1256–1258.

2 Doyen E: Surgical Therapeutics and Operative Techniques. London, Balliere, Tindall & Cox, 1917, vol I, pp 599–602.

3 Goksu N, Bayaz L, Kemalog Y: Endoscopy of the posterior fossa and dissection of acoustic neuroma. J Neurosurg 1999;91:776–780.

4 Jarrahy R, Berci G, Shahinian HK: Endoscopic-assisted microvascular decompression of the trigeminal nerve. Otolaryngol Head Neck Surg 2000;123:218–223.

5 King WA, Wackym PA, Sen C, Meyer GA, Shiau J, Deutsch H: Adjunctive use of endoscopy during posterior fossa surgery to treat cranial neuropathies. Neurosurgery 2001;49:108–116.

6 Magnan J, Chays A, Lepetre C, Pencroffi E, Locatelli P: Surgical perspectives of endoscopy of the cerebellopontine angle. Am J Otol 1994;15:366–370.

7 Miyazaki H, Deveze A, Magnan J: Neuro-otologic surgery through minimally invasive retrosigmoid approach: endoscope assisted microvascular decompression, vestibular neurotomy, and tumor removal. Laryngoscope 2005;115:1612–1617.

8 Rak R, Sekhar L, Stimac D, Hechl P: Endoscope-assisted microsurgery for microvascular compression syndromes. Neurosurgery 2004;54:876–883.

9 Teo C, Nakaji P, Mobbs RJ: Endoscope-assisted microvascular decompression for trigeminal neuralgia: technical case report. Neurosurgery 2006;59(suppl 2):ONSE489–490.

10 Wackym PA, King WA, Barker FG, Poe DS: Endoscope-assisted vestibular neurectomy. Laryngoscope 1998;108:1787–1793.

11 Wackym PA, King WA, Poe DS, Meyer GA, Ojemann RG, Barker FG, Walsh PR, Staecker H: Adjunctive use of endoscopy during acoustic neuroma surgery. Laryngoscope 1999;109:1193–1201.

12 Eby JB, Cha ST, Shahinian HK: Fully endoscopic vascular decompression of the facial nerve for hemifacial spasm. Skull Base 2001;11:189–197.

13 Jarrahy R, Eby JB, Cha ST, Shahinian HK: Fully endoscopic vascular decompression of the trigeminal nerve. Minim Invas Neurosurg 2002;45:32–35.

Daniel Pieper, MD
Associate Professor Neurosurgery
Oakland University William Beaumont School of Medicine
Keystone Medical Center, Suite 100
46325 12 Mile Rd.
Novi, MI 48377 (USA)
Tel. +1 248 440 2162, E-Mail pieperd@usa.net

Kassam AB, Gardner PA (eds): Endoscopic Approaches to the Skull Base.
Prog Neurol Surg. Basel, Karger, 2012, vol 26, pp 204–221

Endoscope-Assisted Skull Base Surgery

Manoel A. de Paiva Neto[a,c] · Joshua R. Dusick[b] ·
Nasrin Fatemi[a] · Daniel F. Kelly[a]

[a]Brain Tumor Center, John Wayne Cancer Institute at Saint John's Health Center, Santa Monica, Calif., and [b]Division of Neurosurgery, University of California at Los Angeles David Geffen School of Medicine and UCLA Department of Neurosurgery, Los Angeles, Calif., USA; [c]Disciplina de Neurocirurgia, Universidade Federal de Sao Paulo, SP, Brazil

Abstract

The direct endonasal transsphenoidal approach to the sella with the operating microscope was first described over 20 years ago. Over the last decade, this minimally invasive technique has evolved into an effective skull base approach for pituitary adenomas and many other parasellar tumors. This expansion of the endonasal technique has resulted largely from development of refined instrumentation and greater use of endoscopy. By taking advantage of the expanded panoramic vision provided by the endoscope, one can visualize areas of the skull base not possible with the operating microscope. Our use of endoscopy has increased over time, particularly for extended endonasal transsphenoidal cases. In a total of 900 endonasal microscopic approaches performed since 1998, endoscopic assistance was utilized in 20% of all cases and in 66% of the last 100 cases. In 129 extended endonasal procedures for parasellar pathology, endoscopy was used in 63% of cases overall and in 84% of the last 25 cases. In 109 extended procedures for tumor removal in 97 patients (including 22 pituitary adenomas, 18 meningiomas, 17 craniopharyngiomas, 14 clival chordomas, and 26 other lesions), endoscopic assistance was used in 64% of these procedures. Total or near-total (>90%) tumor removal was achieved in 70% of patients operated with endoscopic assistance compared to only 41% of those operated without endoscopic assistance ($p = 0.003$); other factors including prior surgery, prior radiotherapy and cavernous sinus invasion were also strongly associated with subtotal tumor removal ($p < 0.01$). From our experience and that of others, it is becoming increasingly clear that endoscopy is essential for achieving maximal and safe endonasal removal of parasellar tumors that extend beyond the confines of the sella. Herein we describe the technique of endoscopic-assisted endonasal skull base surgery, its advantages, clinical applications and potential pitfalls.

Transsphenoidal surgery was initially described a century ago by Schloffer, Cushing and Hirsch [1]. The procedure emerged in the microsurgical era in the early 1970s with the advent of the operating microscope and the technique of selective adenectomy as described by Hardy [2]. Additional experience by many in the 1970s and 1980s further improved the safety and efficacy of transsphenoidal surgery [3–6]. Subsequent modifications were developed to minimize patient discomfort associated with the sublabial approach [7, 8], most notable of which was the direct endonasal approach described by Griffith and Veerapan [9] in 1987 and later by Cooke and Jones [10] in 1994. The evolution of the endonasal approach into a versatile skull base approach for parasellar pathology has resulted largely from better instrumentation, surgical navigation and, most importantly, endoscopy [11–17]. The expanded visualization provided by the endoscope facilitates parasellar tumor removal not possible with the tunnel vision of the operating microscope [18]. We began using endoscopic assistance 10 years ago and have increasingly found it useful for removal of many pituitary adenomas as well as other parasellar tumors such as Rathke's cleft cysts, meningiomas, craniopharyngiomas, chordomas, sphenoid sinus carcinomas, and epidermoid tumors [17, 19–22]. Herein, we describe the technique of endoscope-assisted endonasal skull base surgery, discuss complication avoidance and include a summary of patient outcomes and pathologies treated.

Surgical Technique

Patient Preparation

Endonasal transsphenoidal surgery for parasellar tumors is performed as originally described by Griffith and Veerapen [9] with additional modifications as described below and in our recent publications [17, 19, 20, 22]. Preoperative antibiotics (typically cefazolin) are given and continued for 24 h. In patients with normal preoperative adrenal function, no peri-operative glucocorticoids are administered. Those with adrenal insufficiency or borderline adrenal function are given 100 mg of intravenous hydrocortisone.

Patient Positioning and Room Set-Up

After induction of anesthesia, the endotracheal tube emerges from the left corner of the mouth and anesthesia equipment is positioned to the left of the patient. An arterial line and Foley catheter are placed. The patient is placed supine with the head resting freely in the horseshoe head-holder and angled approximately 30° towards the left shoulder as originally described by Laws [23], which allows the surgeon to stand comfortably on the patient's right side. The head is typically inclined in a neutral plane (0°) relative to the floor for most sellar lesions. For patients with tumors exhibiting marked suprasellar extension, 10–15° of neck extension is used and for clival or infrasellar lesions, 10–15° of neck flexion is used. The nostrils and perinasal area are prepped with betadine. Topical or injected mucosal decongestants are not used. The right lower abdominal area is prepped for an abdominal fat graft if needed.

Surgical Navigation
Surgical navigation for trajectory guidance is recommended for all extended endonasal surgeries. Although C-arm fluoroscopy is simple and effective for giving reliable trajectory guidance in the sagittal plane, frameless stereotactic surgical navigation based on either a preoperative MRI or CT provides more useful information. It is particularly recommended in patients undergoing extended approaches to the planum, cavernous sinus or clival regions and for patients undergoing re-operations who often have markedly distorted anatomical landmarks.

Endoscopic Equipment and Set-Up
The endoscope video monitor and tower are placed above the patient's head on the patient's left side to allow for comfortable viewing by the surgeon and his/her assistant who will be standing on the patient's right side. Rigid 4-mm endoscopes (18 cm in length) with 0, 30 and 45° angled lenses should be available. An endoscope holder can also be used and can be positioned with the insertion device fixed to the left-most cephalad aspect of the operating table.

Surgical Instrumentation
Given the narrow endonasal working space, all instruments should be as low-profile as possible with angled or bayoneted handles to minimize visual obstruction and maximize instrument maneuverability. Cottle dissectors, microdissectors, ring curettes and microblades are on bayoneted handles, while microscissors and tumor forceps are single-shaft, pistol-grip constructions to minimize visual obstruction. High-speed drills and ultrasonic aspirators should also be of the lowest possible diameter with angled hand-pieces. A micro-Doppler probe is recommended for all cases to help localize the cavernous carotid arteries prior to dural opening [24]. As emphasized in figure 1, the endonasal speculums used during the skull base exposure and tumor removal portion of the procedure should be short, ideally 60 mm, with a trapezoidal-up or trapezoidal-down construct (Mizuho America, Inc.) to maximize suprasellar or infrasellar exposure, respectively, and to allow effective use of the endoscope [25].

Initial Approach and Sphenoidotomy
As previously described, the initial approach is performed with the operating microscope and a hand-held speculum [17, 19, 22]. Although in some instances of skull base tumors a binarial approach is needed, the initial primary nostril of approach should be based upon tumor location as defined by the patient's preoperative MRI. For tumors projecting more to one side of the sella, the contralateral nostril provides the best exposure across the midline to the contralateral parasellar region. This rule applies even in the great majority of patients with septal deviation. In patients with relatively midline tumors, the right nostril is used given that the surgeon stands on the patient's right side and this affords a more comfortable operating position. A relaxing alar incision, although used occasionally early in our experience to accommodate

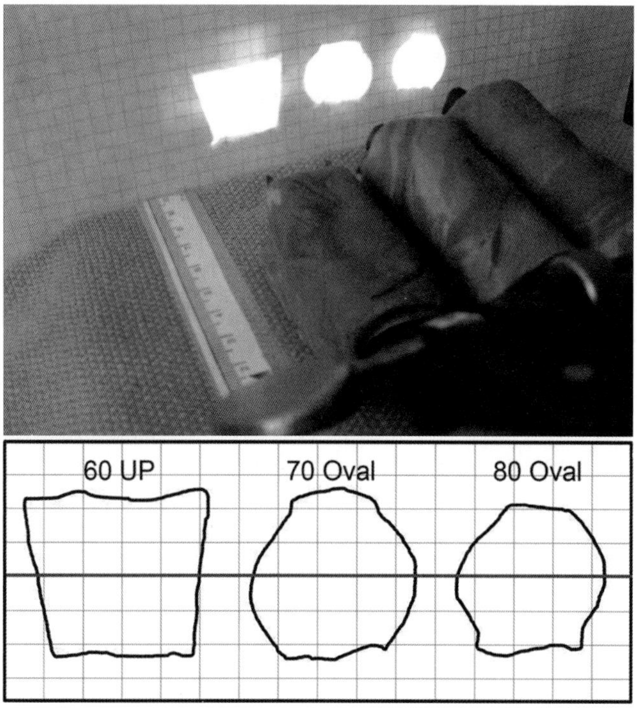

Fig. 1. **a** The clay model used to simulate the endonasal approach to the parasellar area. The 3 speculums (60-mm up-angled trapezoidal, 70-mm oval and 80-mm oval) were positioned with the proximal end of each speculum 100 mm from the target surface and a distal end internal diameter opening of 16 mm. A penlight was placed at the entry of each speculum and the light illumination area at the target was hand-traced. **b** With the 60-mm up-angled trapezoidal speculum (60 UP), the overall area of illumination increased by 31 and 76% compared with the 70 oval and 80 oval mm speculums, and the superior half of the illuminated field increased by 41 and 81%, respectively. Reproduced with permission from Fatemi et al. [25].

the endonasal speculum, has not been used in over 550 cases given the availability of smaller and thinner speculums.

The hand-held speculum is passed into the nostril along the trajectory of the middle turbinate. Care should be taken to minimize trauma to the anterior and mid-nasal septum as well as the turbinates. The speculum blades gently displace the middle turbinate laterally and pass further into the nasal cavity to expose the junction of the keel of the sphenoid and the posterior nasal septum. The posterior septal mucosa is then cauterized with a bipolar in a vertical swath and a vertical mucosal incision is made extending for approximately 2 cm with a Cottle elevator. The mucosa is elevated and reflected laterally to expose the midline sphenoid keel and ipsilateral sphenoid ostium, which is typically superior-lateral to the equator of the keel at the '10 o'clock' or '2 o'clock' position. The posterior septum is then displaced off the midline by the tips of the speculum to allow exposure of the contralateral side of the keel and sphenoid ostium. Once the sphenoid keel and ostia are exposed, the hand-held speculum is replaced by the self-retaining endonasal speculum. The distal speculum blades should straddle the keel and the nasal end of the speculum should be flush with the nostril. To gain full advantage of the short speculum, 1–2 cm of posterior nasal septum is removed as well as any excessive bone and soft tissue along the lateral aspect of the exposure.

A wide and tall sphenoidotomy is next performed with pituitary and Kerrison rongeurs or a high-speed drill. The extent of bony removal is in part dependent upon tumor location as described further below; however, in general, sphenoid bone and mucosal removal should extend beyond the lateral edges of the ostia bilaterally and should allow visualization of the tuberculum sellae and sellar floor. To maximize instrument maneuverability during the endoscopic phase of the procedure, as described below, bone should be removed up close to the ethmoid roof and down to a level flush with the sphenoid sinus floor. Given that the sphenopalatine arteries run in the posterior inferior nasal mucosa at a position of approximately 8 and 4 o'clock, it is best to displace this mucosa laterally with the speculum or to cauterize it prior to removing it to avoid injuring the artery with a Kerrison or pituitary rongeur.

Parasellar Exposure for Planum, Suprasellar, Cavernous Sinus and Clival Lesions

The optimal degree and direction of the sphenoidotomy and the extent of sellar and parasellar bone removal is highly dependent upon the lesion being addressed and the goals of the surgery. As previously described, several important modifications are employed for reaching suprasellar, infrasellar and cavernous sinus lesions [19–22]. In all cases, after the sphenoidotomy, the sella turcica and intrasphenoidal bony septations should be identified and their locations correlated with those seen on the patient's preoperative MRI. Particular note should be made on the coronal images of where these septations reach the posterior wall of the sphenoid sinus relative to the carotid arteries, pituitary gland and tumor, and on sagittal views where such septations reach the planum or sella. Septations ending on the sellar face are removed with a rongeur down to the sella; those that end over a carotid artery should be removed with care and excessive torquing of bone fragments should be avoided. The bony sellar face is then removed from cavernous sinus to cavernous sinus and from the sellar floor inferiorly to the tuberculum sella superiorly with a Kerrison rongeur or in some instances a high-speed diamond bit drill.

Carotid Localization

Prior to dural opening, the cavernous carotid arteries should be definitively localized. Their course can often be visualized directly but further confirmation is recommended with surgical navigation and/or a micro-Doppler probe (10-MHz ES-100X MiniDop® with NRP-10H bayonet probe, Koven, St. Louis, Mo., USA or 20-MHz Surgical Doppler, Mizuho America, Beverly, Mass., USA). The probe is placed initially at the edge of the bony opening perpendicular to the dura [24]. Typically, as the probe

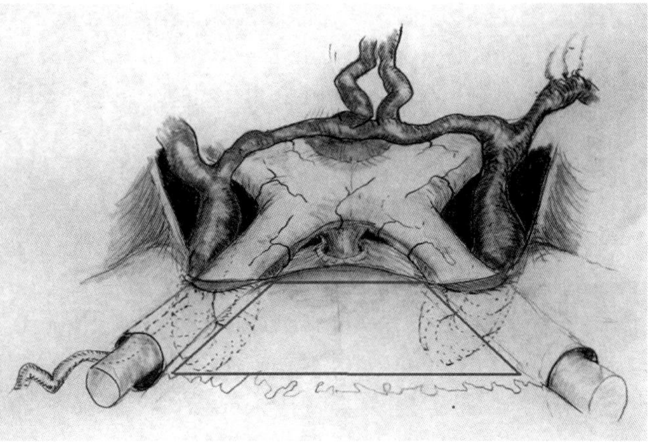

Fig. 2. View from superior and anterior showing the close anatomical relationship of the optic canals and cavernous carotid arteries at the level of the tuberculum sellae and posterior planum sphenoidale.

is angled more laterally, aiming under the bone edge, the carotid flow will become louder. The probe is then moved superiorly and inferiorly to further determine the course of the carotid which typically courses more medially in the superior parasellar area. The carotids typically have their most medial course superiorly near the tuberculum sella just before they pass into the subarachnoid space. If no Doppler flow is evident, then additional bone can be removed laterally to maximize sellar exposure. If audible flow is still not evident, consideration should be given to whether there is a technical problem with the probe, which can occur on occasion.

Suprasellar and Planum Lesions

In cases such as tuberculum sellae meningiomas, craniopharyngiomas, and supraglandular Rathke's cleft cysts, the tuberculum sellae and a portion of the posterior planum is removed. In particular, tuberculum sella meningiomas under 30–35 mm in maximal diameter and without far lateral extension and craniopharyngiomas extending into the retrochiasmal space are ideal for an endonasal removal. A 60-mm up-angled endonasal trapezoidal speculum is used as the working channel to maximize suprasellar exposure (fig. 1). A low-profile high-speed drill (Micromax; Anspach, Palm Beach Gardens, Fla., USA) with a 2- or 3-mm diamond bit is used to remove the tuberculum sella and posterior planum. Care should be taken not to extend the bony opening too far lateral at the level of the optic canals which are the width limiting structures at this level, typically being only 14–18 mm apart at this level (fig. 2). Immediately inferior to the optic canals, the width-limiting structures are the cavernous carotid arteries and their initial intracranial portions, which on average are 14–17 mm apart [26, 27]. Depending on the nature and exact location of the tumor, the initial dural opening is either made in the sellar dura or then extended above and through the diaphragma sellae or only above the diaphragma sellae. The initial dural opening is made with a straight micro-blade and then extended as needed with the use of a right angle micro-hook blade or curved micro scissors which allow the cutting force of the blade to be directed away from the sellar and cavernous sinus structures [24]. When the dural opening extends across the diaphragma sellae, bleeding from the superior circular sinus (also known as the anterior intercavernous sinus) is controlled with Surgifoam (Ethicon Inc., Johnson & Johnson Co., Piscataway, N.J., USA) or Gelfoam and bipolar cautery. After the initial opening, angled micro-dissectors are used to separate the dura from the underlying tumor and pituitary gland (fig. 3). The dural opening is then enlarged superiorly, inferiorly and laterally as needed with the use of a right angle microhook blade or curved microscissors. Laterally, the opening should generally extend to within 1–2 mm of the medial wall of the cavernous sinus. Low pressure cavernous sinus venous bleeding is generally easily controlled using Surgifoam or Gelfoam (Pfizer Inc., New York, N.Y., USA), as needed.

As shown in figure 3, since most of these suprasellar lesions are rather fibrous, rubbery or partially calcified, they require sharp dissection with curved and straight micro-scissors along arachnoid planes. In patients with intact pituitary hormonal function, such as those with supra-glandular Rathke's cleft cysts and tuberculum sellae meningiomas, preservation of hormonal function is typically possible. However, preserving function is more difficult in patients with craniopharyngiomas, particularly those that engulf the pituitary stalk. After tumor debulking, the tumor capsule is dissected away from arachnoid attachments using sharp dissection and gentle traction. Tumor remnants densely adherent to the infundibulum, optic apparatus or perforating vessels should be left behind to avoid new neurological or pituitary hormonal deficits.

Clival Lesions

Given that most clival chordomas have their epicenter medial to the cavernous carotid arteries, they can typically be effectively removed or debulked through an endonasal approach. As we recently described, to remove such chordomas in the infrasellar and cavernous sinus regions, a wide sphenoidotomy is carried to the floor of the sphenoid sinus [22]. This bony removal is performed with rongeurs or a high-speed drill. A 60 mm down-angled endonasal trapezoidal speculum is used as the working channel. Given the tendency of clival chordomas to distort the course of the petrous, vertical and cavernous portions of the carotid arteries, the micro-Doppler probe and surgical navigation are used to help localize these vessels before and during tumor removal. Given the invasive nature of such chordomas, complete tumor removal is rarely possible but effective tumor debulking is typically possible in the sellar, infrasellar and medial cavernous sinus regions. In cases of intradural chordoma extension, the dura is opened further to maximize tumor removal under both microscopic and endoscopic visualization [22].

Cavernous Sinus Lesions

For removal of tumors with extensive cavernous sinus invasion, such as clival chordomas or invasive adenomas, one can approach these lesions from the contralateral nostril or from the ipsilateral nostril after resecting the ipsilateral middle turbinate. By removing the middle turbinate, the lateral speculum blade can expand more widely, allowing greater removal of the sphenoid keel and providing exposure lateral to the ipsilateral cavernous carotid artery. For tumors with extensive bilateral involvement, a binarial approach can be used.

For tumors with obvious or possible cavernous sinus invasion, one should attempt to visualize the medial cavernous sinus wall. A microscopic view of the cavernous sinus contralateral to the nostril of approach can often be achieved provided enough lateral sellar bone has been removed and a short endonasal speculum is in position. Under direct visualization, in some instances, what appeared to be cavernous sinus invasion on MRI may only be tumor compression of the medial cavernous sinus wall [28]. However, in many cases, after the sellar tumor has been removed, a defect in the medial cavernous sinus wall is seen. Tumor in the medial cavernous sinus can often be removed or at least effectively debulked using gentle suction and angled ring curettes which have smooth outer edges. Given the potential for injury to the cavernous carotid and the abducens nerve lateral to the carotid, aggressive curetting or grasping of tumor tissue along or lateral to the carotid artery should be avoided.

Endoscopic Assistance to Maximize Tumor Removal

Once tumor removal is as complete as possible with the microscope, the 0, 30 and 45° angled endoscopes are utilized to further assess for residual tumor and the location of key neurovascular structures not seen with the restricted vision of the microscope. In the majority of such cases, the endoscope will reveal additional tumor. Removal of such tumor remnants can often be performed directly under endoscopic visualization using angled suctions, tumor grasping forceps or ring curettes, or with microscopic visualization and angled ring curettes. Endoscopic visualization is best done with a 3-hand technique in which the assistant holds and drives the endoscope and the surgeon holds the suction and a ring curette or tumor grasping forceps. Alternatively, one can use the endoscope holder as the third hand but this provides less maneuverability and flexibility compared with a surgical assistant. To further maximize maneuverability of the endoscope and minimize instrument congestion within the nasal cavity, the speculum is removed which then allows a binarial approach with the endoscope placed in one nostril and the other instruments placed in the contralateral nostril [11–14].

Skull Base Reconstruction and CSF Leak Repair

As recently described [29], skull base reconstruction and CSF leak repair is tailored to the size of the CSF leak and bony and dural defect. As shown in figure 4, in most patients undergoing a transplanum removal of a suprasellar craniopharyngioma or a tuberculum sellae meningioma, a large grade 3 defect is usually created. This multi-layered repair includes a suprasellar and intrasellar abdominal fat graft, a layer of collagen sponge followed by a buttress of titanium mesh or a Medpor plate placed in the intrasellar extradural space with extension of the buttress to the anterior edge of

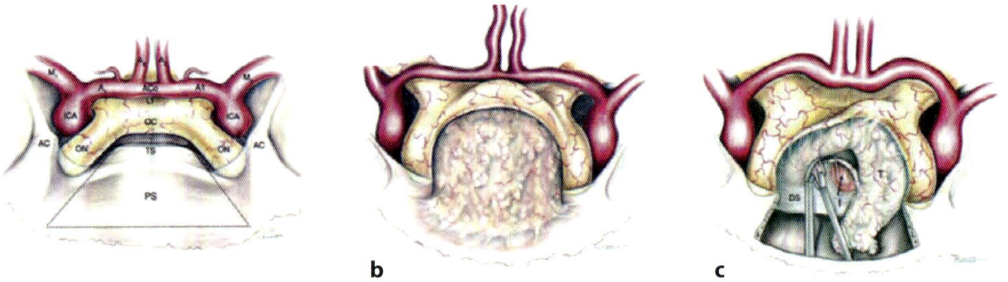

3 a **b** **c**

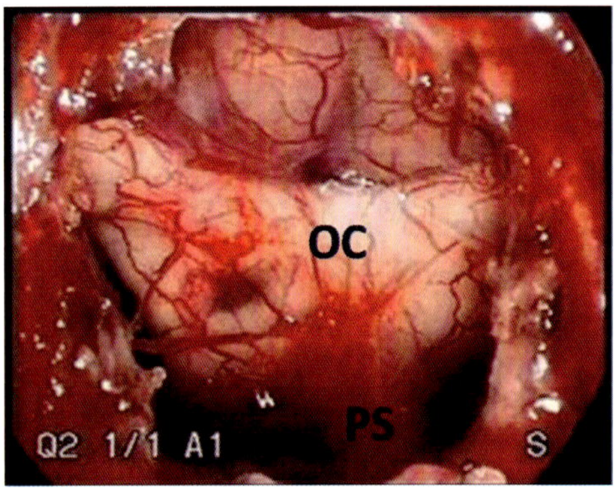

4

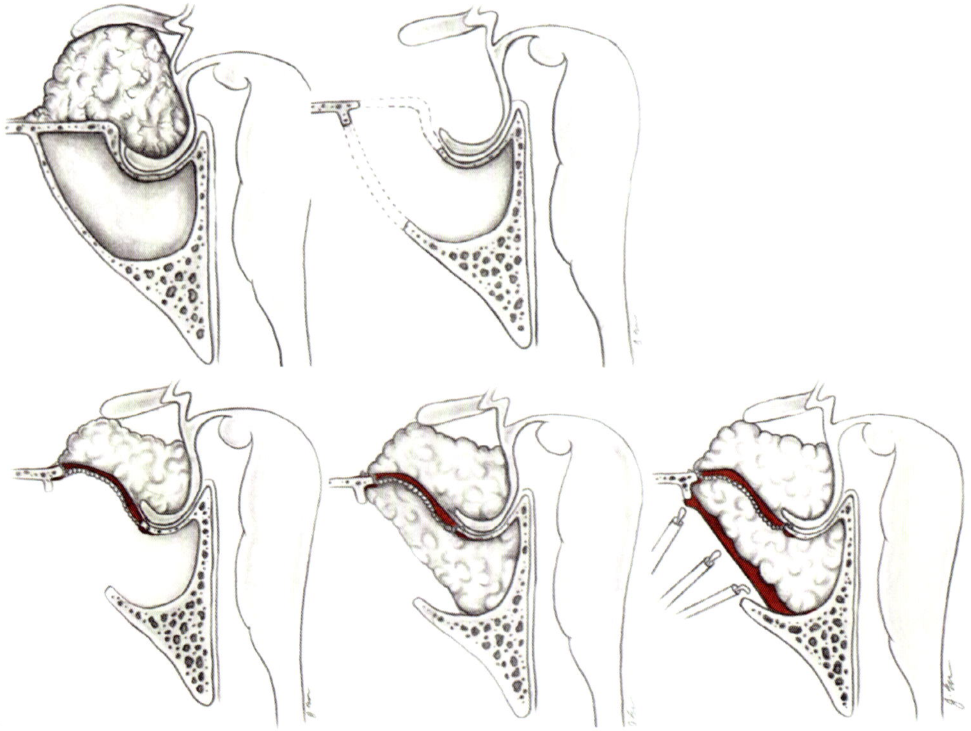

5

the defect in the posterior planum. Additional fat is placed over the planum and sellar defect followed by another layer of collagen; the construct is held in position with BioGlue (fig. 5). A similar multilayered repair is performed for grade 3 clival defects. It is important to note that use of BioGlue in this repair paradigm is not for stopping egress of CSF per se but more to prevent migration of the construct materials (fat and collagen) away from the sella [30]. To further assess the adequacy of the repair, prior to placing BioGlue, the anesthesiologist is asked to perform a Valsalva maneuver to raise the patient's intracranial pressure; should there be CSF streaming around the repair or movement of the buttress, the repair should be revised. For these grade 3 defects, typically seen with extended suprasellar or transclival approaches, a lumbar drain is typically placed for CSF diversion (8–10 ml/h) for 48 h.

Closure

Once sellar reconstruction is complete, the endonasal speculum is removed and the hand-held speculum is used to explore both nasal cavities with the microscope. Mild venous oozing from along the nasal septum, inferior turbinate or middle turbinate is controlled with Surgifoam or the bipolar. Effective nasal hemostasis will minimize the amount of blood the patient will swallow during the first few hours after surgery and will help minimize nausea and vomiting. The middle turbinate on the side of the approach, which is out-fractured by the speculum at the start of the procedure, is medialized toward the nasal septum to reduce the risk of a maxillary sinus mucocele. Finally, the nasal septum is returned to the midline. Nasal packing is not placed. To minimize chances of a postoperative CSF leak, nasal epistaxis or intrasellar bleeding, excessive coughing on the endotracheal tube should be avoided during extubation and blood pressure should be carefully monitored and controlled in the early postoperative period.

Fig. 3. Illustrations of the extended approach from the vantage point of the frontal fossa demonstrating the extent of bony and dural removal along the posterior planum sphenoidale and the tuberculum sellae for the extended approach (**a**), a typical tuberculum sellae meningioma extending out along the proximal planum sphenoidale and causing chiasmal elevation (**b**), and transsphenoidal resection of a meningioma showing the need for sharp dissection and grasping forceps to help define arachnoid planes between the tumor and optic apparatus (**c**). Note the optic canals are the width-limiting structure for the bony and dural opening. A_1 = 1st segment of anterior cerebral artery; A_2 = 2nd segment of anterior cerebral artery; AC = anterior clinoid process; DS = diaphragma sellae; I = infundibulum; ICA = internal carotid artery; LT = lamina terminalis; M_1 = 1st segment of middle cerebral artery; OC = optic chiasm; ON = optic nerve; PS = planum sphenoidale; T = tumor; TS = tuberculum sellae; dotted lines = area of bony resection for extended approach. Reproduced with permission from Dusick et al. [19].

Fig. 4. Intraoperative 45° endoscopic view after complete resection of a small tuberculum sellae meningioma showing the dural defect, optic chiasm (OC) and pituitary stalk (PS).

Fig. 5. Grade 3 repair: Illustration of: tuberculum sellae meningioma (**a**), after tumor removal and before repair (**b**), intrasellar and suprasellar fat placed followed by a layer of collagen sponge (red) placed over fat (**c**), placement of titanium mesh buttress in intrasellar extradural space, wedged inferiorly in bony lip of sella and wedged superiorly in bony defect of posterior planum sphenoidale (**d**), and additional fat placed over mesh in sphenoid sinus followed by another layer of collagen sponge then tissue glue (**e**). Reproduced with permission from Esposito et al. [29].

Postoperative Care

Patients undergoing removal of craniopharyngiomas, meningiomas or any others with a grade 3 intraoperative CSF leak and lumbar drain placement are admitted to the ICU. In patients with grade 3 leaks, prior to opening the lumbar drain and before going to the ICU, a postoperative head CT or MRI is obtained to assess the degree of immediate postoperative pneumocephalus, the status of the skull base repair and for residual tumor. For the first postoperative night, patients are given a humidified face tent and decongestants are available upon request. Saline nasal spray is provided for a week after surgery and used based on patient preference. The Foley catheter is typically removed on the morning of postoperative day one and patients are encouraged to ambulate. All patients with pituitary-related lesions are followed in-hospital by an endocrinologist. Patients are monitored for diabetes insipidus based on urine output and urine specific gravity. Adrenal function is monitored by measuring AM serum cortisol and ACTH levels on postoperative days 1 and 2 unless they are already on glucocorticoids.

As previously described, all endonasal surgery patients undergo a 'tilt test' to assess for occult CSF rhinorrhea either on postoperative day 2 or on the day their lumbar drain is discontinued which is typically the morning of postoperative day three [29]. Most patients without a lumbar drain can be discharged home on postoperative day 2 while those with a lumbar drain are discharged home on postoperative day 4.

All patients have a serum sodium level checked on postoperative days 4 or 5 to assess for delayed hyponatremia. The first postoperative visit is within 2–3 weeks of surgery and a follow-up visit occurs 3 months after surgery, including in most patients, a complete pituitary hormonal evaluation. The first follow-up MRI is usually performed at 3 months after surgery.

Personal Experience

Endoscopic-Assisted Endonasal Surgery

Patient Population

Since July 1998, a total of 829 patients have undergone a total of 900 operations for tumor removal or primary CSF leak repair by the senior author (D.F.K.). Of these, 16% had prior surgery, either transcranial or transsphenoidal, at an outside institution. Pathology included 75% pituitary adenomas, 7% Rathke's cleft cysts, 3% craniopharyngiomas, 3% parasellar meningiomas, 2% clival chordomas, and 10% other neoplasms or primary CSF leaks. The endoscope was first used in 1998 and overall has been employed in 182 cases, including 63% of extended cases and 13% of non-extended cases ($p < 0.001$). Use of endoscopy has increased over time being used in 66% of the last 100 cases in the series overall and 21 (84%) of the last 25 extended endonasal cases.

Table 1. Extended endonasal series for tumor removal

Pathology (n = 97)	
Pituitary adenoma	22
Meningioma	18
Craniopharyngioma	17
Chordoma	14
Rathke's cleft cyst	7
Epidermoid	5
Sphenoid sinus carcinoma	4
Schwannoma	4
Lymphoma	2
Encephalocele	2
Metastatic breast cancer	1
Solitary fibrous tumor	1

Extended Approach Cases and Endoscopy

Over an 8-year period, we have performed 129 extended endonasal procedures for tumor resection (n = 109), tumor biopsy (n = 12), cyst decompression (n = 5), and CSF leak repair (n = 3). Of the 109 extended procedures for tumor removal in 97 patients (including 12 re-operations for residual or recurrent tumor), pathology included 22 pituitary adenomas, 18 meningiomas, 17 craniopharyngiomas, 14 clival chordomas, 7 suprasellar Rathke's cleft cysts, and 19 other various pathologies (table 1). In 70 (64%) of these 109 procedures for tumor removal, endoscopic assistance was used. Total or near-total (>90%) tumor removal was achieved in 70% of patients operated with endoscopic assistance compared to only 41% of those operated without endoscopic assistance ($p = 0.003$) (table 2). Other significant factors associated with achieving only a subtotal resection were prior surgery, cavernous sinus invasion and preoperative radiotherapy ($p < 0.01$ for each comparison).

Complications in Extended Approach Cases

Surgical complications for the overall series of 129 extended endonasal procedures are shown in table 3. The one mortality in this series occurred in a 57-year-old man with a spontaneous CSF leak arising from an encephalocele of the left middle fossa extending into the far lateral sphenoid sinus. The patient had pre-existing cardiopulmonary disease and a history of methamphetamine abuse. His CSF leak was repaired uneventfully with endoscopic assistance. However, he developed respiratory distress and died of a likely pulmonary embolus nine days after surgery.

There were two carotid artery injuries, both in patients with cavernous sinus lesions. In one (previously described) with a cavernous sinus schwannoma, a small puncture wound was likely created in the cavernous carotid artery; the bleeding was

Table 2. Total/near total tumor (>90%) removal by pathology in relation to use of endoscopy in 107 procedures

Pathology	n*	Endoscopic-assisted	Microscopic only	p value†
Adenoma	25	13/19 (68%)	0/6 (0%)	0.005
Craniopharyngioma	20	11/17 (65%)	2/3 (66%)	1
Chordoma	20	5/6 (83%)	10/14 (71%)	1
Meningioma	18	10/13 (77%)	0/5 (0%)	0.006
Others	26	10/15 (67%)	4/11 (36%)	0.23
Total	109	49/70 (70%)	16/39 (41%)	0.003

* Per procedure.
† Fisher's exact test, Pearson's χ^2 test.

Table 3. Surgical complications in 129 extended endonasal procedures

Complication	n (%)
Mortality	1 (0.8)
Carotid artery injury	2 (1.6)
New permanent neurological deficit	2 (1.6)
Postoperative hematoma	1 (0.8)
Postoperative CSF leak	7 (5.4)
Bacterial meningitis	2 (1.6)
Re-operation for excessively large fat graft	2 (1.6)
Delayed epistaxis needing embolization	2 (1.6)

stopped uneventfully and her subsequent cerebral angiogram was normal [24]. In the other patient with a sphenoid sinus carcinoma, the right petrous carotid was injured during tumor removal and bleeding was controlled with a muslin gauze, a fat graft and gentle pressure. His immediate postoperative angiogram showed a carotid occlusion but with good collateral circulation; the patient had no new neurological deficits. In this particular case, in retrospect, the Doppler probe was clearly malfunctioning as the area of the carotid injury was explored with the Doppler immediately prior to the carotid injury and no arterial pulse was audible.

The two permanent neurological deficits included delayed monocular blindness eight days after endonasal tumor debulking in a 66-year-old man with a sphenocavernous meningioma who had undergone prior transcranial surgery and radiotherapy and had pre-existing ophthalmoplegia in the affected eye. The other neurological deficit was mild visual hemi-field worsening in a 72-year-old woman after complete removal of a tuberculum sellae meningioma who had presented with bitemporal hemianopsia.

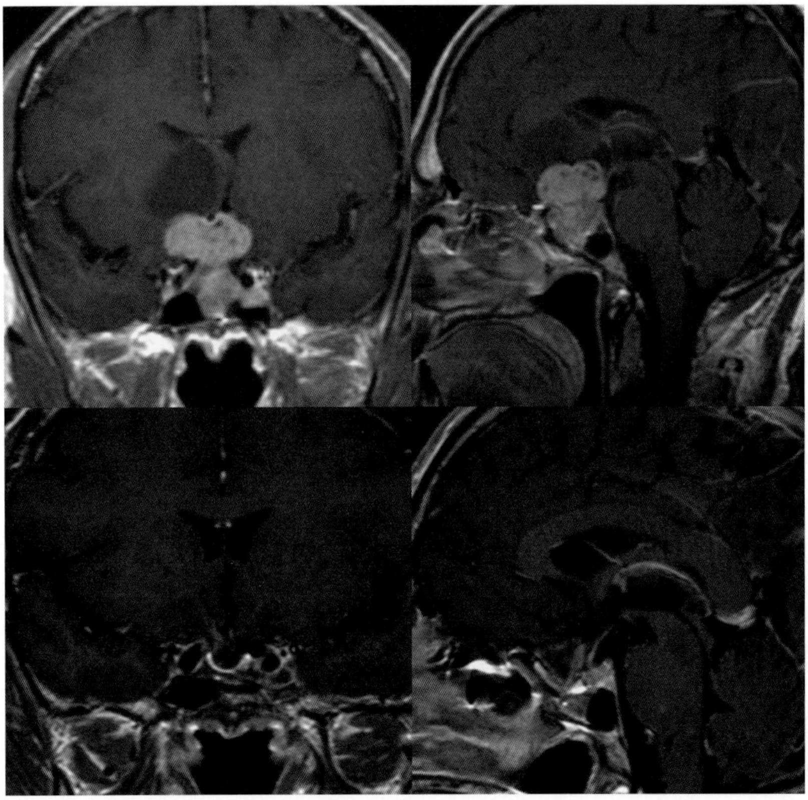

Fig. 6. Preoperative (upper row) and 24-month postoperative (lower row) T_1 post-gadolinium MRI after endonasal removal of a giant solid and cystic macroadenoma.

There were 7 (5.4%) postoperative CSF leaks. Of the 5 major pathologies treated, the postoperative CSF leak rate was highest in meningiomas (4/20 procedures; 20%), followed by adenomas (2/25 procedures; 8%), and craniopharyngiomas (1/25 procedures; 4%); there were no postoperative leaks in patients with Rathke's cleft cysts, chordomas or other pathologies. No postoperative CSF leaks occurred in the last 56 cases. Early in the series, 2 patients underwent uneventful re-operation for overly large fat grafts associated with visual compromise after repair of grade 3 CSF leaks.

Two patients developed delayed epistaxis from the sphenopalatine artery requiring embolization of the internal maxillary arteries.

Illustrative Cases

Giant Invasive Macroadenoma

A 54-year-old man was diagnosed with a bitemporal visual field defect after a routine visual examination. His MRI showed a 60 × 30 × 31 mm solid and cystic suprasellar

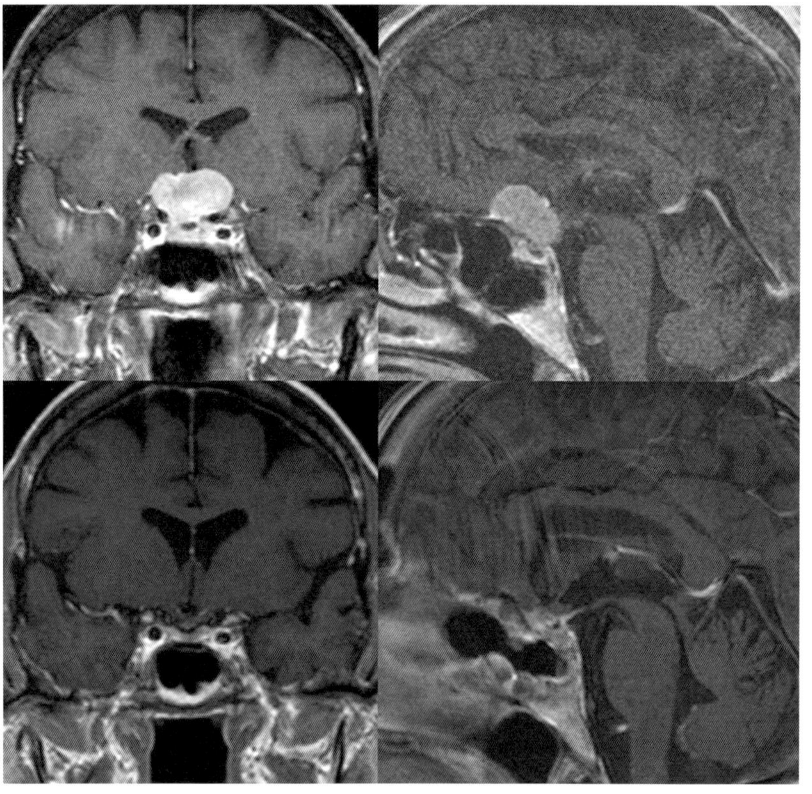

Fig. 7. Preoperative (upper row) and 24-month postoperative (lower row) T_1 post-gadolinium MRI after endonasal removal of a tuberculum sellae meningioma.

mass elevating the chiasm and pushing the pituitary stalk posteriorly. His hormonal tests revealed adrenal insufficiency and a normal prolactin level. He underwent a right endonasal, near total removal with endoscopic assistance. A small residual remained in the left cavernous sinus. His grade 3 CSF leak was repaired uneventfully. His vision returned to normal and his hypopituitarism resolved. At 24 months after surgery, his MRI showed a stable left cavernous sinus residual tumor (fig. 6).

Tuberculum Sellae Meningioma

A 73-year-old woman developed progressive visual loss with bitemporal hemianopsia. Her pituitary MRI showed a 24 × 26 × 13 mm tuberculum sellae meningioma causing severe chiasmal compression with posterior displacement of the pituitary stalk. She underwent right endoscopic-assisted endonasal tumor removal and repair of an intraoperative grade 3 CSF leak repair. She had acute dislodgement of her titanium mesh buttress after vomiting in the recovery room and underwent an uneventful revision of this repair. Twenty-four months after surgery, her MRI shows no residual or recurrent tumor and her vision remains normal (fig. 7).

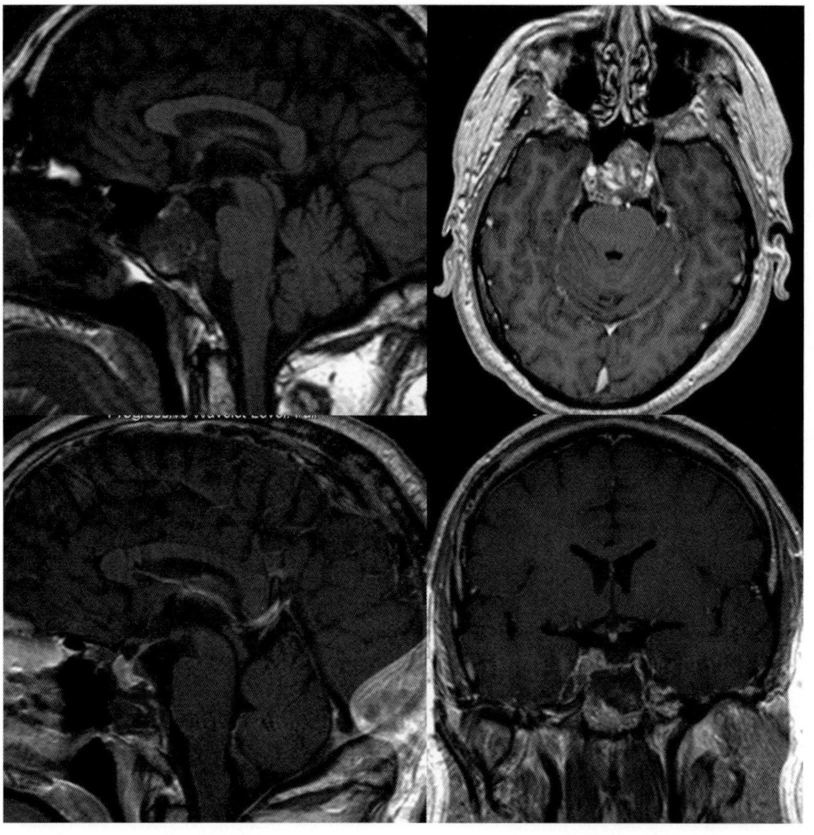

Fig. 8. Preoperative (upper row) and 27-month postoperative (lower row) T_1 post-gadolinium MRI after an extended endonasal removal of a clival chordoma. Note the right cavernous sinus invasion on preoperative scan and the residual postoperative tumor on the postoperative scan.

Chordoma

A 49-year-old man developed diplopia and a cranial nerve VI palsy. His MRI showed a 35 × 30-mm heterogeneously enhancing clival mass with extension to the left and right cavernous sinus. He underwent an uneventful near complete tumor removal via a right endoscopic-assisted endonasal approach using surgical navigation; residual tumor was restricted to the right cavernous sinus as shown on post operative MRI. He underwent stereotactic radiotherapy and has stable disease 27 months after surgery (fig. 8).

Conclusions

The direct endonasal approach with the operating microscope and endoscopic assistance provides an effective minimally invasive route for removal of most parasellar tumors. This skull base approach for removing more challenging tumors, such as tuberculum sellae meningiomas, clival chordomas and craniopharyngiomas, should be attempted only after gaining sufficient experience with simpler sellar lesions such as pituitary adenomas and Rathke's cleft cysts. The success of this approach is also in part dependent upon having the necessary instrumentation including surgical navigation, low profile instrumentation, short endonasal speculums, and high-resolution endoscopy.

References

1 McDonald TJ, Laws ER: Historical aspects of the management of pituitary disorders with emphasis on transsphenoidal surgery; in Laws E, Randall R, Kern E (eds): Management of Pituitary Adenomas and Related Lesions: With Emphasis on Transsphenoidal Microsurgery. New York, Appleton-Century-Crofts, 1982, pp 1–13.

2 Hardy J: Transphenoidal microsurgery of the normal and pathological pituitary. Clin Neurosurg 1969;16:185–217.

3 Ebersold MJ, Quast LM, Laws ER Jr, Scheithauer B, Randall RV: Long-term results in transsphenoidal removal of nonfunctioning pituitary adenomas. J Neurosurg 1986;64:713–719.

4 Fahlbusch R, Buchfelder M, Muller OA: Transsphenoidal surgery for Cushing's disease. J R Soc Med 1986;79:262–269.

5 Kern EB, Pearson BW, McDonald TJ, Laws ER Jr: The transseptal approach to lesions of the pituitary and parasellar regions. Laryngoscope 1979;89:1–34.

6 Wilson CB, Dempsey LC: Transsphenoidal microsurgical removal of 250 pituitary adenomas. J Neurosurg 1978;48:13–22.

7 Laws ER: Transsphenoidal approach to pituitary tumors; in Schmidek H, Sweet W (eds): Operative Neurosurgical Techniques: Indications, Methods, and Results, ed 3. Philadelphia, Saunders, 1995, vol 1, pp 283–292.

8 Liu JK, Das K, Weiss MH, Laws ER Jr, Couldwell WT: The history and evolution of transsphenoidal surgery. J Neurosurg 2001;95:1083–1096.

9 Griffith HB, Veerapen R: A direct transnasal approach to the sphenoid sinus: technical note. J Neurosurg 1987;66:140–142.

10 Cooke RS, Jones RA: Experience with the direct transnasal transsphenoidal approach to the pituitary fossa. Br J Neurosurg 1994;8:193–196.

11 Cappabianca P, Cavallo LM, de Divitiis E: Endoscopic endonasal transsphenoidal surgery. Neurosurgery 2004;55:933–940; discussion 940–931.

12 Kassam A, Snyderman CH, Mintz A, Gardner P, Carrau RL: Expanded endonasal approach: the rostrocaudal axis. I. Crista galli to the sella turcica. Neurosurg Focus 2005;19:E3.

13 Kassam A, Thomas AJ, Snyderman C, Carrau R, Gardner P, Mintz A, Kanaan H, Horowitz M, Pollack IF: Fully endoscopic expanded endonasal approach treating skull base lesions in pediatric patients. J Neurosurg 106:75–86, 2007

14 Kassam A, Gardner P, Snyderman C, Carrau RL, Mintz AH, Prevedello DM: Expanded endonasal approach, a fully endoscopic transnasal approach for the resection of midline suprasellar craniopharyngiomas: a new classification based on the infundibulum. J Neurosurg 2208;108:715–728.

15 Jagannathan J, Prevedello DM, Ayer VS, Dumont AS, Jane JA Jr, Laws ER: Computer-assisted frameless stereotaxy in transsphenoidal surgery at a single institution: review of 176 cases. Neurosurg Focus 2006;20:E9.

16 Prevedello DM, Doglietto F, Jane JA Jr, Jagannathan J, Han J, Laws ER Jr: History of endoscopic skull base surgery: its evolution and current reality. J Neurosurg 2007;107:206–213.

17 Zada G, Kelly DF, Cohan P, Wang C, Swerdloff R: Endonasal transsphenoidal approach for pituitary adenomas and other sellar lesions: an assessment of efficacy, safety, and patient impressions. J Neurosurg. 2003;98:350–358.

18 Catapano D, Sloffer C, Frank G, Pasquini E, D'Angelo V, Lanzino G: Comparision between the microscope and endoscope in the direct endonasal extended transsphenoidal approach: anatomical study. J Neurosurg 2006;104:419–425.

19 Dusick JR, Esposito F, Kelly DF, Cohan P, DeSalles A, Becker DP, Martin NA: The extended direct endonasal transsphenoidal approach for nonadenomatous suprasellar tumors. J Neurosurg 2005;102: 832–841.

20 Esposito F, Becker DP, Villablanca JP, Kelly DF: Endonasal transsphenoidal transclival removal of prepontine epidermoid tumors: technical note. Neurosurgery 2005;56:E443; discussion E443.
21 Esposito F, Kelly DF, Vinters HV, DeSalles AA, Sercarz J, Gorgulhos AA: Primary sphenoid sinus neoplasms: a report of four cases with common clinical presentation treated with transsphenoidal surgery and adjuvant therapies. J Neurooncol 2006; 76:299–306.
22 Fatemi N, Dusick JR, Gorgulho AA, Mattozo CA, Moftakhar P, De Salles AA, Kelly DF: Endonasal microscopic removal of clival chordomas. Surg Neurol 2008;69:331–338.
23 Laws ER: Transsphenoidal approach to pituitary tumors; in Schmidek H, Sweet W (eds): Operative Neurosurgical Techniques: Indications, Methods, and Results, ed 3. Philadelphia, Saunders, 1995, vol 1, pp 283–292.
24 Dusick JR, Esposito F, Malkasian D, Kelly DF: Avoidance of carotid artery injuries in transsphenoidal surgery with the Doppler probe and micro-hook blades. Neurosurgery 2007;60:322–328; discussion 328–329.
25 Fatemi N, Dusick JR, Malkasian D, Emerson J, McArthur DL, Schad W, Kelly DF: Instrumentation assessment: short trapezoidal speculums for suprasellar and infrasellar exposure in endonasal transsphenoidal surgery. Neurosurgery 2008;62(suppl 2): ONS325–329.
26 Fujii K, Chambers SM, Rhoton AL Jr: Neurovascular relationships of the sphenoid sinus: a microsurgical study. J Neurosurg 1979;50:31–39.
27 Renn WH, Rhoton AL Jr: Microsurgical anatomy of the sellar region. J Neurosurg 1975;43:288–298.
28 Yoneoka Y, Watanabe N, Matsuzawa H, Tsumanuma I, Ueki S, Nakada T, Fujii Y: Preoperative depiction of cavernous sinus invasion by pituitary macroadenoma using three-dimensional anisotropy contrast periodically rotated overlapping parallel lines with enhanced reconstruction imaging on a 3-tesla system. J Neurosurg 2008;108:37–41.
29 Esposito F, Dusick JR, Fatemi N, Kelly DF: Graded repair of cranial base defects and cerebrospinal fluid leaks in transsphenoidal surgery. Neurosurgery 2007;60:295–303; discussion 303–294.
30 Dusick JR, Mattozo CA, Esposito F, Kelly DF: BioGlue for prevention of postoperative cerebrospinal fluid leaks in transsphenoidal surgery: a case series. Surg Neurol 2006;66:371–376.

Daniel F. Kelly, MD
Brain Tumor Center
John Wayne Cancer Institute at Saint John's Health Center
2200 Santa Monica Blvd., Santa Monica, CA 90404 (USA)
Tel. +1 310 582 7450, E-Mail kellyd@jwci.org

Kassam AB, Gardner PA (eds): Endoscopic Approaches to the Skull Base.
Prog Neurol Surg. Basel, Karger, 2012, vol 26, pp 222–231

The Learning Curve for Endonasal Surgery of the Cranial Base: A Systematic Approach to Training

Carl H. Snyderman[a] · Harshita Pant[b] · Amin B. Kassam[c] · Ricardo L. Carrau[d] · Daniel M. Prevedello[e] · Paul A. Gardner[f]

Departments of [a]Otolaryngology and [f]Neurosurgery, University of Pittsburgh, Pittsburgh, Pa., USA; [b]Department of Medicine, University of Adelaide, Adelaide, S.A., Australia; [c]Division of Neurosurgery, University of Ottawa, Ottawa, Ont., Canada; Departments of [d]Otolaryngology and [e]Neurological Surgery, Ohio State University, Columbus, Ohio, USA

Abstract

Proper training in endoscopic endonasal surgery of the cranial base is essential to avoid unnecessary morbidity and mortality. An incremental program for the training of skull base surgeons is described that accounts for complex skull base anatomy, technical difficulty, potential risk of neural and vascular injury, extent of intradural dissection, and type of pathology. There are multiple pathways for training in endoscopic skull base surgery. The most important feature of a training program is the building of team surgical skills.

The practice of surgery advances by small steps, reflecting the collective efforts of the medical community. Occasionally, great leaps occur as a result of technological advances, resulting in a rapid change in practice and attitudes: a paradigm shift. Rapid change carries with it unknown risks and unforeseen complications are bound to occur as a new status quo is established. The growing pains of the pioneers and early adopters of new technology can provide useful lessons for those who follow so that mistakes are not repeated and new ones are averted.

One of the biggest advances in surgery over the last two decades has been the introduction of endoscopic techniques as a result of the invention of the Hopkins rod lens. Like a virus, endoscopic techniques have spread from specialty to specialty becoming incorporated into the genome of surgical practice. We have witnessed the introduction of endoscopic surgery in urology, general surgery, and otolaryngology. New applications of endoscopic technology continue to evolve within each of these specialties. One of the last surgical specialties to become 'infected' is neurosurgery, and, secondarily, cranial base surgery [1].

There are a number of challenges in endonasal cranial base surgery that contribute to the long duration of the learning curve [2]. Traditional skull base surgeons are unaccustomed to interpreting skull base anatomy from the endonasal perspective and few sinus surgeons venture into the zone of the skull base. Most skull base surgeons and neurosurgeons have limited experience with the endoscope and consequently lack adequate endoscopic instrumentation and skills. There is a significant risk of neural and vascular injury during endonasal cranial base surgery and surgeons need to develop the necessary skills to be able to deal with hemorrhage effectively. Reconstruction of dural defects also requires different techniques and the risk of a postoperative cerebrospinal fluid leak may be increased initially. Additional challenges include assembling a team of surgeons that can work together consistently and build necessary team skills, having an adequate volume of cases to develop and maintain surgical expertise, and garnering adequate institutional resources and equipment.

Skull Base Modules

Endonasal approaches to the ventral skull base can be categorized into different surgical modules based on their orientation in sagittal and coronal planes relative to the sphenoid sinus [3–5]. The sphenoid sinus is at the crossroads of these approaches and is the starting point for many of the modules due to its central location and relationship to key anatomical structures such as the optic nerve and internal carotid artery (ICA). In the sagittal plane, surgical modules extend from the frontal sinus to the second cervical vertebra. In the coronal plane, surgical modules are divided into anterior, middle, and posterior coronal planes corresponding to the anterior, middle, and posterior cranial fossae. The anterior coronal plane extends laterally across the orbital roof and includes medial transorbital approaches between the medial and inferior rectus muscles. The middle coronal plane extends from the cavernous and paraclival segments of the ICA laterally across the floor of the middle cranial fossa superior to the petrous ICA (suprapetrous). The posterior coronal plane extends from the foramen magnum across the occipital condyle to the jugular foramen and parapharyngeal space. The surgical modules can be combined to tailor the approach to the pathology and each module requires a different level of expertise.

Training Pathways

Surgeons may pursue various pathways to becoming a cranial base surgeon, each with its own merits and shortcomings [6]. Within otolaryngology, cranial base surgery was historically an extension of oncological head and neck surgery and surgeons received additional training through fellowships in cranial base surgery. They were knowledgeable of skull base anatomy, well equipped to repair large dural defects with regional flaps, and shared a philosophy of oncological principles with their head and neck brethren. However, they often lacked endoscopic expertise and did not use the endoscope routinely in other parts of their practice. In contrast, the rhinologist was facile with the endoscope but lacked a thorough understanding of skull base anatomy and did not have the skill set to undertake open approaches to the cranial base and reconstruction if needed. Although most traumatic and spontaneous CSF leaks were being treated endoscopically, there was little experience with the endoscopic reconstruction of large postsurgical dural defects.

The neurosurgeon had multiple potential pathways to cranial base surgery, either through traditional fellowship training in cranial base surgery, pituitary surgery, or vascular surgery. Endoscopic experience, if present, was limited to ventricular surgery and pituitary surgery. Many neurosurgeons have successfully made the transition to endoscopic pituitary surgery. By virtue of surgical volume, pituitary surgery may afford the best opportunity for developing endoscopic skills but pituitary surgeons may be handicapped in performing endonasal surgery beyond the sella. Experience with vascular neurosurgery is essential in dealing with potential vascular complications of endonasal surgery and helps prepare the surgeon for surgical modules that extend laterally around the petrous carotid artery. Finally, experience with open anterior and lateral skull base approaches provides alternative options in case an endonasal approach is inadequate.

Training in only one pathway limits the options for patients and surgeons. Surgeons may be less likely to discuss and offer surgical approaches that they do not perform. Preoperative informed consent should include a discussion of all treatment options, including a range of different surgical approaches, and their respective risks and benefits. Currently, debate still continues over the relative merits of the endonasal approach compared to other approaches but it is becoming a viable option in most medical communities. Of greater concern is the ability to switch between surgical approaches when warranted, to obtain clear resection margins and to deal with complications of hemorrhage or the challenges of reconstruction. Although these can be accomplished by separate teams of surgeons in the same institution, it is preferable if an endonasal surgeon can convert to an open approach in an emergency situation. Finally, training in multiple pathways provides exposure to different surgical philosophies. Importantly, the use of the endoscope should not alter oncological principles and result in less than complete surgery.

Acquisition of Surgical Skills

Surgeons are constantly acquiring new surgical skills throughout their careers. The surgeon who does not pursue additional training quickly becomes obsolete. Following residency training, this is usually accomplished in gradations by taking courses with anatomical models or laboratory skills stations, observing or assisting a surgeon proficient in a new procedure, performing operations under supervision, and ultimately performing the procedures independently. As endonasal procedures become more common, this training will become a routine part of residency and fellowship training. The creation of surgical simulators that teach endonasal anatomy and procedures will facilitate the training of surgeons in all stages of their career.

A review of the introduction of endoscopy in other specialties provides valuable insight. Following the adoption of endoscopic cholecystectomy, there was a sharp increase in the number of bile duct injuries [7]. This gradually declined to a level comparable to open cholecystectomy as surgeons became more proficient. Multiple studies examined the factors that might be predictive of proficiency: proficiency in traditional techniques, endoscopic experience with other procedures, duration of practice, and the number of cases (endoscopic cholecystectomy) [7]. The only significant factor was the number of cases performed doing that specific procedure. There have been attempts to estimate how many operations it took to become proficient. For laparoscopic fundoplication, it is estimated to be approximately 25–30 procedures; for laparoscopic cholecystectomy, 15–20 procedures. An early report on endoscopic hypophysectomy concluded that there was 'no learning curve' as there were no complications in 45 cases [8]. However, this study failed to account for the complexity of cases, the extent of resection, and the experience of the neurosurgeon.

Training Levels

Our own experience with endonasal skull base surgery showed us that there was a long learning curve influenced by multiple factors. We reviewed our experience with our first 700 patients from 1998 to 2006. These were performed for a wide variety of cranial base pathological conditions (fig. 1) and required multiple endoscopic surgical modular approaches (fig. 2). Although most of the operations were transsellar approaches for pituitary adenomas, the majority of the pituitary tumors were extrasellar macroadenomas that required additional surgical modules. Based on our experience, we devised a training program that reflected our own learning (table 1) and incorporates levels of training that is incremental and modular [2]. These levels encompass multiple factors including anatomical knowledge, technical difficulty, potential risk of neural and vascular injury, extent of intradural dissection, and type of pathology. Mastery of each level is recommended before proceeding to the next level. The levels are designed to apply to all endonasal cranial base surgeons, irrespective of their primary specialty.

Level I

Level I procedures are the starting point for all endonasal procedures and reflect a level of expertise that all trainees in otolaryngology should have attained. This includes performing a complete sphenoethmoidectomy and sphenopalatine artery ligation for the management of epistaxis. There is value in neurosurgeons gaining exposure to

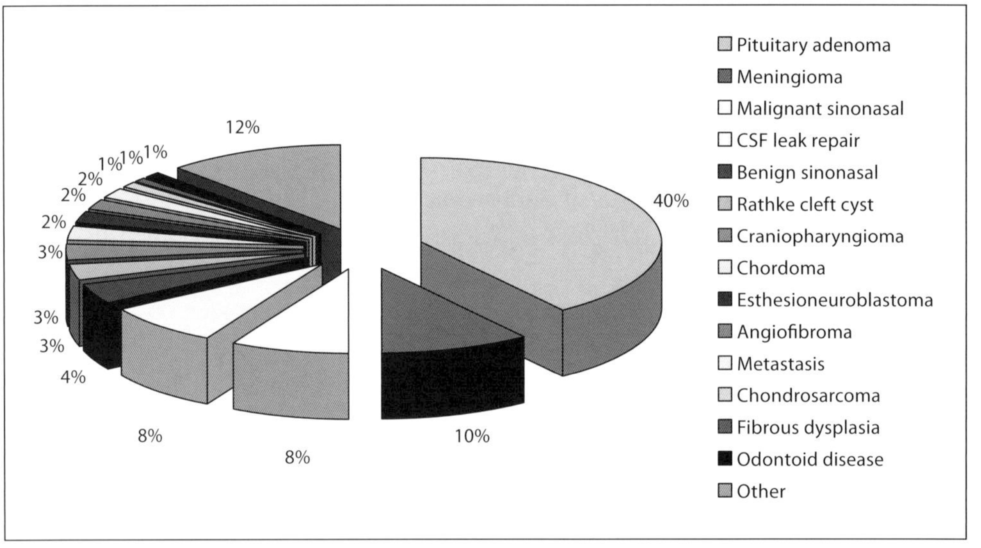

Fig. 1. Pie chart showing the pathology of cranial base lesions in 700 patients that underwent an endoscopic endonasal approach.

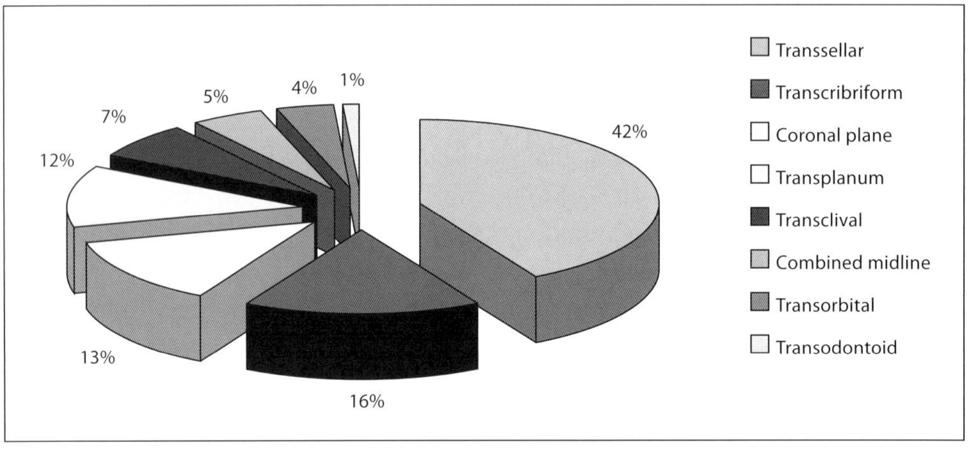

Fig. 2. Pie chart depicting the various endoscopic endonasal approaches performed in 700 patients for removal of cranial base lesions.

basic sinus surgery techniques through beginner courses so that they become familiar with sinus anatomy and instrumentation.

Level II

Level II procedures can be categorized as advanced sinus surgery techniques and includes exposure of the lateral recess of the sphenoid sinus via a transpterygoid

Table 1. Training levels for endonasal skull base surgery

Level I	Sinus surgery
Level II	Advanced sinus surgery Cerebrospinal fluid leak Intrasellar – sella, pituitary
Level III	Extrasellar – sella, pituitary Optic nerve decompression Intraorbital surgery Extradural skull base surgery
Level IV	Intradural skull base surgery A. With cortical cuff Transplanum Transcribriform Type I craniopharyngioma
	Intradural skull base surgery B. Without cortical cuff Type II/III craniopharyngioma Transclival, intradural
Level V	Coronal plane, carotid dissection Vascular surgery

approach, medial decompression of the orbit, and endoscopic frontal sinusotomy (Draf 3 operation, modified Lothrop procedure or frontal drillout). These techniques are a prerequisite for basic skull base modules. Exposure of the lateral recess of the sphenoid sinus is necessary for the repair of spontaneous cerebrospinal fluid leaks associated with meningocoeles of the lateral sphenoid and is a starting point for coronal plane modules that extend along the course of the petrous ICA. Medial decompression of the orbit is necessary for transorbital approaches in the anterior coronal plane, exposure of the anterior and posterior ethmoid arteries for ligation, and optic nerve decompression. Endoscopic frontal sinusotomy is required to obtain an anterior resection margin for tumors that involve the anterior cranial base (olfactory neuroblastoma, olfactory groove meningiomas) and require a 'craniofacial' resection.

Level II also includes endoscopic repair of CSF leaks and endoscopic pituitary surgery for small adenomas with minimal extrasellar extension. Although otolaryngologists can readily repair small CSF leaks independently and neurosurgeons can perform pituitary surgery without assistance, these are valuable opportunities to work together and develop skull base team skills and gain experience with endoscopic visualization and instrumentation. Endoscopic repair of CSF leaks provides necessary experience with the repair of dural defects and endoscopic pituitary surgery provides the opportunity to master hemostatic techniques. It is essential that the surgical team be comfortable performing these procedures together before undertaking more complex skull base procedures.

Level III

Level III procedures can be characterized as extradural skull base surgery. This level includes more advanced pituitary surgery with excision of tumors with extra-sellar extension to the suprasellar area, medial cavernous sinus, and superior clivus. Decompression of the optic nerve in the optic canal may be necessary for the treatment of benign and malignant tumors as well as traumatic fractures. In the sagittal plane, an extradural transclival approach is most frequently performed for chordomas and meningiomas, but may include sinonasal malignancies. A transnasal approach to the upper cervical spine with resection of the odontoid process is most commonly performed for degenerative disease (rheumatoid/osteoarthrisits) affecting the upper cervical spine with pannus formation and basilar invagination. In the coronal plane, transorbital approaches provide access to the orbital roof and intraconal lesions infero-medial to the optic nerve. The petrous apex may be approached medially deep to the paraclival carotid artery for the treatment of expansive petrous apex lesions such as cholesterol granulomas.

For many surgical teams, this is a good place to stop, especially if pituitary surgery is the main focus of the practice. In order to safely perform more complex surgeries with intradural dissection, there should be a sustained commitment to endonasal skull base surgery with regular collaboration between specialties on lower level cases. There should be a sufficient volume of cases so that the surgical team can maintain proficiency. There needs to be a similar commitment on the part of the institution so that adequate resources are available such as equipment, operative time, and support staff. In the absence of training in open cranial base surgery, intradural dissection is not recommended.

Level IV

Level IV procedures are the most complex surgeries that the majority of surgeons will perform. These can be characterized as intradural dissection and limited vascular dissection. They are further divided into levels IVa and IVb based, respectively, on the presence or absence of a cuff of brain tissue between the tumor margin and cerebral vessels. In the sagittal plane, Level IVa includes most transcribriform and transplanum intradural approaches with intradural resection as well as a 'craniofacial' resection for sinonasal malignancies. Type I craniopharyngiomas are in this group [9]. Level IVb includes transclival intradural approaches and type II/III craniopharyngiomas. A transodontoid approach may be used to access intradural tumors at the level of the foramen magnum.

Level V

Level V includes most surgeries in the coronal plane. These include a medial approach to the petrous apex when exposure of the paraclival ICA is necessary. More laterally,

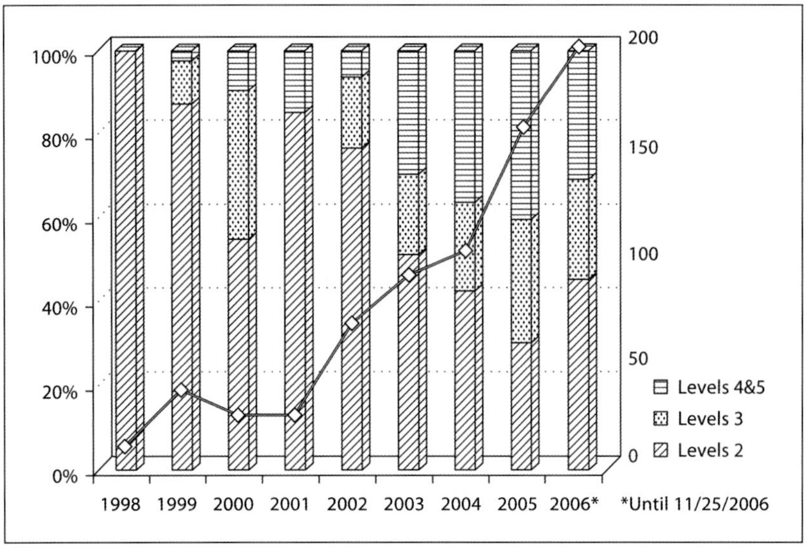

Fig. 3. A bar graph demonstrating the number and complexity (levels 2–5) of endoscopic endonasal approaches for skull base lesions performed between 1998 and 2006.

suprapetrous and infrapetrous approaches to the skull base are included. If exposure of the petrous ICA is necessary, we consider it to be a level V procedure due to the increased difficulty and risks of dissection. Rare level V cases are those with extensive vascularity of the tumor (arteriovenous malformation, large angiofibroma supplied by the ICA) or surgery that is performed for treatment of vascular lesions (aneurysm).

University of Pittsburgh Medical Center (UPMC) Learning Curve

Our own learning curve over the last decade is highlighted in figure 3. It is important to note that the meager volume of cases early in this series reflected a predominantly pituitary practice with level II procedures (intrasellar pituitary adenomas, CSF leaks). Over the first 4–5 years, we gained experience with dural reconstruction and hemostatic techniques, resolved issues with instrumentation, and mastered the complex endonasal anatomy of the skull base [10]. Only then did we start to do more challenging level III and IV procedures. As the complexity of cases increased, the size of dural defects also increased and dural reconstruction became more challenging [11].

Our early experience was plagued by a high incidence of postoperative CSF leaks (40%). In almost all cases, these were resolved with additional endoscopic surgery. Reconstructive techniques evolved over the years to address this problem and included multilayer fascial reconstruction, fat grafts, suturing of dural grafts, intranasal balloon catheter, and finally the vascularized septal mucosal flap [Zanation et al., this vol.], [12]. In addition, lumbar spinal drains were used perioperatively in high risk patients. With the use of septal flaps [13] for reconstruction, the risk of a postoperative CSF leak decreased from approximately 25 to <10%. Currently, the incidence of postoperative CSF leaks in patients reconstructed with a septal mucosal flap is 4% [14].

We looked at the incidence of serious complications such as death, stroke, vascular injury, and intracranial infection in our first 700 endonasal skull base surgeries to determine if serious complications were increased as part of the learning curve. There were no operative mortalities. Four patients died from medical co-morbidities in the perioperative period. The incidence of a major vascular injury was 1% and included two internal carotid artery injuries. Three vascular injuries resulted in a permanent deficit. The incidence of neurological injury was 2.4%; 1.9% were transient and 0.6% were permanent. The incidence of culture-positive meningitis was only 1.2%. These rates of complications compare favorably with open approaches and demonstrate that endonasal skull base surgery can be performed safely. The distribution of serious complications by year demonstrates a steady level of complications over the last decade. A low incidence of early complications is attributed to slow growth of our surgical practice with low complexity cases. Increased experience was offset by increased case complexity in the latter years of the series. Nevertheless, this series demonstrates that serious complications can be avoided during the learning curve by acquisition of anatomical knowledge, a team approach, and adherence to the principles of endoscopic dissection.

Based on our experience, it is difficult to state how many cases are required to achieve surgical proficiency. We propose that at least 30–50 level II surgeries (CSF leaks and pituitary tumors) should be performed before proceeding to level III cases. The introduction of surgical simulators and other teaching aids may help to shorten the learning curve.

Conclusions

A systematic approach to the acquisition of surgical skills for endonasal skull base surgery minimizes the risk of adverse outcomes as surgeons develop expertise. A training program needs to address the complex endoscopic anatomy of the ventral skull base, special instrumentation, visualization with the endoscope, the challenges of hemostasis and dural reconstruction, and working as a team. An incremental training program based on familiarity of the anatomy, technical difficulty, potential risk of neural and vascular injury, extent of intradural dissection, and type of pathology provides a framework for gradual progression and building of team surgical skills. Potential benefits of such a program include standardization of training across centers, institutional oversight and credentialing of surgeons, increased collaboration between specialties, and less patient morbidity and mortality.

References

1 Maroon JC: Skull base surgery: past, present, and future trends. Neurosurg Focus 2005;19:E1.
2 Snyderman C, Kassam A, Carrau R, Mintz A, Gardner P, Prevedello DM: Acquisition of surgical skills for endonasal skull base surgery: a training program. Laryngoscope 2007;117:699–705.
3 Kassam A, Snyderman CH, Mintz A, Gardner P, Carrau RL: Expanded endonasal approach: the rostrocaudal axis. I. Crista galli to the sella turcica. Neurosurg Focus 2005;19:E3.
4 Kassam A, Snyderman CH, Mintz A, Gardner P, Carrau RL: Expanded endonasal approach: the rostrocaudal axis. II. Posterior clinoids to the foramen magnum. Neurosurg Focus 2005;19:E4.
5 Kassam AB, Gardner P, Snyderman C, Mintz A, Carrau R: Expanded endonasal approach: fully endoscopic, completely transnasal approach to the middle third of the clivus, petrous bone, middle cranial fossa, and infratemporal fossa. Neurosurg Focus 2005;19:E6.
6 Snyderman C, Carrau R, Kassam A: Who is the skull base surgeon of the future? Skull Base 2007;17: 353–355.
7 Gibbs VC, Auerbach AD: Learning Curves for New Procedures – the Case of Laparoscopic Cholecystectomy: Making Health Care Safer: A Critical Analysis of Patient Safety Practices. Rockville, Agency for Healthcare Research and Quality, 2001.
8 Sonnenburg RE, White D, Ewend MG, Senior B: The learning curve in minimally invasive pituitary surgery. Am J Rhinol 2004;18:259–263.
9 Kassam AB, Gardner PA, Snyderman CH, Carrau RL, Mintz AH, Prevedello DM: Expanded endonasal approach, a fully endoscopic transnasal approach for the resection of midline suprasellar craniopharyngiomas: a new classification based upon the infundiulum. J Neurosurg 2008;108:715–728.
10 Kassam A, Snyderman CH, Carrau RL, Gardner P, Mintz A: Endoneurosurgical hemostasis techniques: lessons learned from 400 cases. Neurosurg Focus 2005;19:E7.
11 Carrau R, Kassam A, Snyderman C, Duvvuri U, Mintz A, Gardner P: Endoscopic transnasal anterior skull base resection for the treatment of sinonasal malignancies. Operative Techniques in Otolaryngology 2006;17:102–110.
12 Kassam A, Carrau RL, Snyderman CH, Gardner P, Mintz A: Evolution of reconstructive techniques following endoscopic expanded endonasal approaches. Neurosurg Focus 2005;19:E8.
13 Hadad G, Bassagasteguy L, Carrau RL, et al: A novel reconstructive technique after endoscopic expanded endonasal approaches: vascular pedicle nasoseptal flap. Laryngoscope 2006;116:1882–1886.
14 Patel MR, Stadler ME, Snyderman CH, Carrau RL, Kassam AB, Germanwala AV, Gardner P, Zanation AM: How to choose? Endoscopic skull base reconstructive options and limitations. Skull Base 2010;20: 397–404.

Carl H. Snyderman, MD, MBA
Department of Otolaryngology, UPMC
200 Lothrop Street, EEI 500
Pittsburgh, PA 15213 (USA)
Tel. +1 412 647 8186, E-Mail snydermanch@upmc.edu

Author Index

Subject Index